I0044400

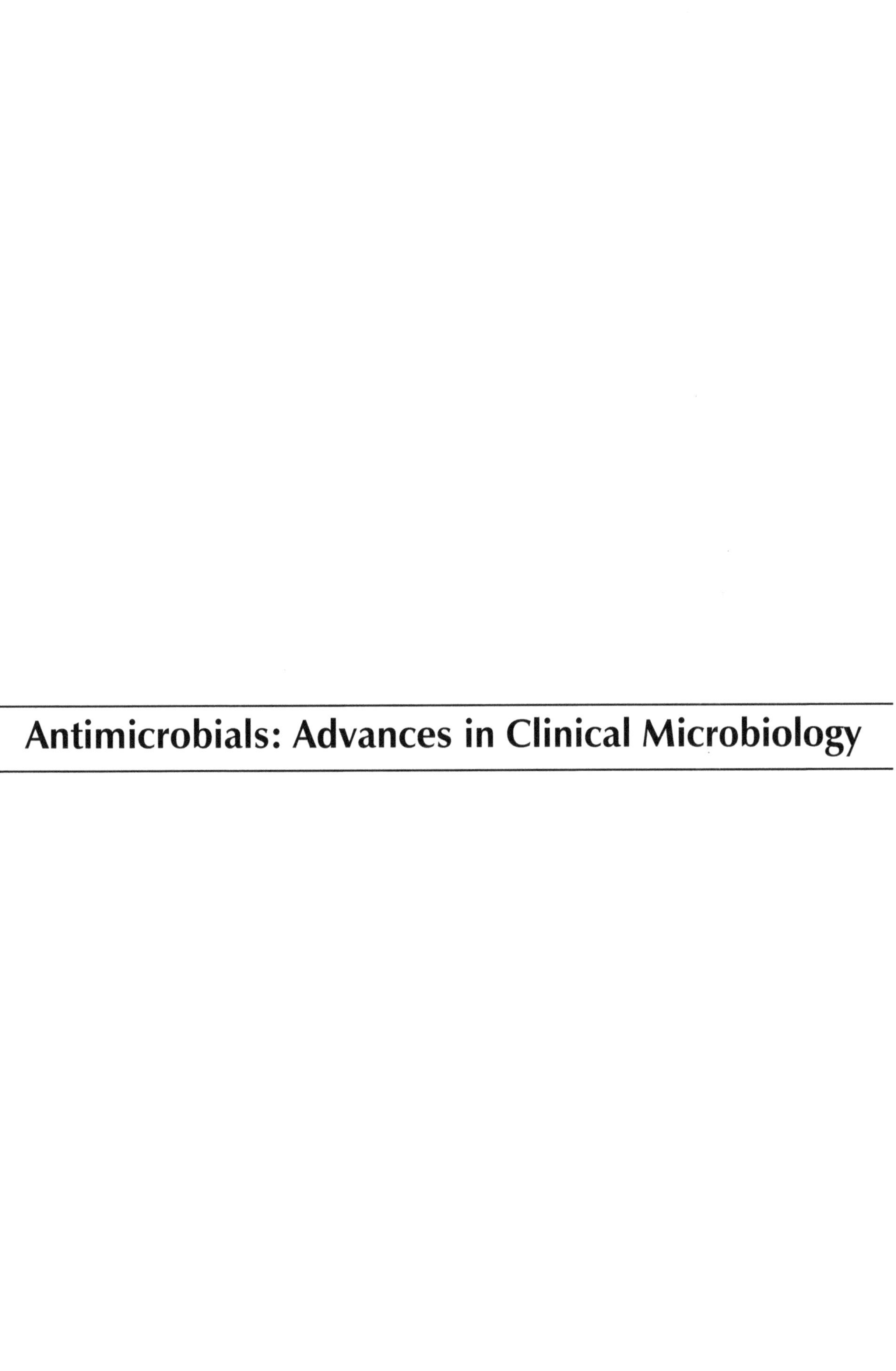

Antimicrobials: Advances in Clinical Microbiology

Antimicrobials: Advances in Clinical Microbiology

Editor: Jessica Hoover

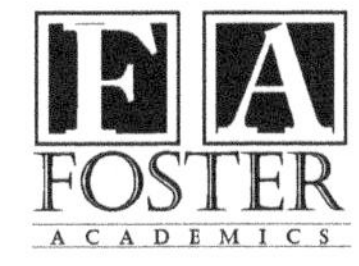

www.fosteracademics.com

www.fosteracademics.com

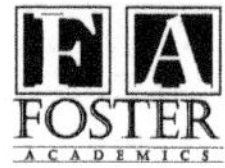

Cataloging-in-Publication Data

Antimicrobials : advances in clinical microbiology / edited by Jessica Hoover.
p. cm.
Includes bibliographical references and index.
ISBN 978-1-63242-702-1
1. Anti-infective agents. 2. Medical microbiology. 3. Diagnostic microbiology.
I. Hoover, Jessica.
RM267 .A58 2019
615.792 2--dc23

Foster Academics,
118-35 Queens Blvd., Suite 400,
Forest Hills, NY 11375, USA

ISBN 978-1-63242-702-1 (Hardback)

Contents

Preface ... IX

Chapter 1 **Efficacy and safety profile of linezolid in the treatment of multidrug-resistant (MDR) and extensively drug-resistant (XDR) tuberculosis** ... 1
Akosua Adom Agyeman and Richard Ofori-Asenso

Chapter 2 **Occurrence of *bla*$_{DHA-1}$ mediated cephalosporin resistance in *Escherichia coli* and their transcriptional response against cephalosporin stress** ... 18
Birson Ingti, Deepjyoti Paul, Anand Prakash Maurya, Debajyoti Bora, Debadatta Dhar Chanda, Atanu Chakravarty and Amitabha Bhattacharjee

Chapter 3 **Emerging azithromycin-resistance among the *Neisseria gonorrhoeae* strains isolated in Hungary** ... 26
Alexandra Brunner, Eva Nemes-Nikodem, Csaba Jeney, Dora Szabo, Marta Marschalko, Sarolta Karpati and Eszter Ostorhazi

Chapter 4 **Antimicrobial resistance in coagulase-negative staphylococci from Nigerian traditional fermented foods** ... 32
P. T. Fowoyo and S. T. Ogunbanwo

Chapter 5 **Stryphnodendron adstringens and purified tannin on *Pythium insidiosum*: in vitro and in vivo studies** ... 39
Rodrigo Trolezi, Juliana Maziero Azanha, Natália Rodrigues Paschoal, Jéssica Luana Chechi, Marcelo José Dias Silva, Viciany Eric Fabris, Wagner Vilegas, Ramon Kaneno, Ary Fernandes Junior and Sandra de Moraes Gimenes Bosco

Chapter 6 **Development of a fast and low-cost qPCR assay for diagnosis of acute gas pharyngitis** ... 46
Mustafa Kolukirik, Mesut Yılmaz, Orhan Ince, Canan Ketre, Ayşe Istanbullu Tosun and Bahar K. Ince

Chapter 7 **Systematic review and meta-analysis of mortality of patients infected with carbapenem-resistant *Klebsiella pneumoniae*** ... 52
Liangfei Xu, Xiaoxi Sun and Xiaoling Ma

Chapter 8 ***Brucella melitensis* VirB12 recombinant protein is a potential marker for serodiagnosis of human brucellosis** ... 64
Shiva Mirkalantari, Amir-Hassan Zarnani, Mahboobeh Nazari, Gholam Reza Irajian and Nour Amirmozafari

Chapter 9 **Activity of AMP2041 against human and animal multidrug resistant *Pseudomonas aeruginosa* clinical isolates** ... 70
Clotilde Silvia Cabassi, Andrea Sala, Davide Santospirito, Giovanni Loris Alborali, Edoardo Carretto, Giovanni Ghibaudo and Simone Taddei

Chapter 10 **Molecular characterization of *Staphylococcus aureus* isolates from various healthcare institutions in Nairobi, Kenya: a cross sectional study** 79
Geoffrey Omuse, Kristien Nel Van Zyl, Kim Hoek, Shima Abdulgader, Samuel Kariuki, Andrew Whitelaw and Gunturu Revathi

Chapter 11 **Performance evaluation of a rapid whole-blood immunoassay for the detection of IgG antibodies against *Helicobacter pylori* in daily clinical practice** 88
Dietmar Enko, Gabriele Halwachs-Baumann, Robert Stolba, Ortrun Rössler and Gernot Kriegshäuser

Chapter 12 **Antibiotic resistance and biofilm production among the strains of *Staphylococcus aureus* isolated from pus/wound swab samples in a tertiary care hospital in Nepal** 93
Ankit Belbase, Narayan Dutt Pant, Krishus Nepal, Bibhusan Neupane, Rikesh Baidhya, Reena Baidya and Binod Lekhak

Chapter 13 **Hematologic manifestations of babesiosis** 98
Tamer Akel and Neville Mobarakai

Chapter 14 **A combination of silver nanoparticles and visible blue light enhances the antibacterial efficacy of ineffective antibiotics against methicillin-resistant *Staphylococcus aureus* (MRSA)** 105
Fatma Elzahraa Akram, Tarek El-Tayeb, Khaled Abou-Aisha and Mohamed El-Azizi

Chapter 15 **Higher atypical enteropathogenic *Escherichia coli* (a-EPEC) bacterial loads in children with diarrhea are associated with PCR detection of the EHEC factor for adherence 1/lymphocyte inhibitory factor A (*efa1/lifa*) gene** 118
Robert Slinger, Kimberley Lau, Michael Slinger, Ioana Moldovan and Francis Chan

Chapter 16 **Smear positive pulmonary tuberculosis and associated factors among homeless individuals in Dessie and Debre Birhan towns, Northeast Ethiopia** 124
Tsedale Semunigus, Belay Tessema, Setegn Eshetie and Feleke Moges

Chapter 17 **Antibiotic consumption in laboratory confirmed vs. non-confirmed bloodstream infections among very low birth weight neonates in Poland** 132
A. Różańska, J. Wójkowska-Mach, P. Adamski, M. Borszewska-Kornacka, E. Gulczyńska, M. Nowiczewski, E. Helwich, A. Kordek, D. Pawlik and M. Bulanda

Chapter 18 **Molecular characterization of clinical IMP-producing *Klebsiella pneumoniae* isolates from a Chinese Tertiary Hospital** 141
Kaisheng Lai, Yanning Ma, Ling Guo, Jingna An, Liyan Ye and Jiyong Yang

Chapter 19 **The efficacy and safety of tigecycline for the treatment of bloodstream infections** 146
Jian Wang, Yaping Pan, Jilu Shen and Yuanhong Xu

Chapter 20 **Dose-dependent artificial prolongation of prothrombin time by interaction between daptomycin and test reagents in patients receiving warfarin: a prospective in vivo clinical study** 156
Makoto Saito, Shuji Hatakeyama, Hideki Hashimoto, Takumitsu Suzuki, Daisuke Jubishi, Makoto Kaneko, Yukio Kume, Takehito Yamamoto, Hiroshi Suzuki and Hiroshi Yotsuyanagi

Chapter 21 **The emergence of a novel sequence type of MDR *Acinetobacter baumannii* from the intensive care unit of an Egyptian tertiary care hospital** 164
Doaa Mohammad Ghaith, Mai Mahmoud Zafer, Mohamed Hamed Al-Agamy, Essam J. Alyamani, Rayan Y. Booq and Omar Almoazzamy

Chapter 22 **Babesiosis in Long Island: review of 62 cases focusing on treatment with azithromycin and atovaquone** 172
Ekaterina A. Kletsova, Eric D. Spitzer, Bettina C. Fries and Luis A. Marcos

Chapter 23 **Prevalence of *Chlamydia trachomatis, Neisseria gonorrhoeae, Mycoplasma genitalium* and *Ureaplasma urealyticum* infections using a novel isothermal simultaneous RNA amplification testing method in infertile males** 179
Ling Qing, Qi-Xiang Song, Jian-Li Feng, Hai-Yan Li, Guiming Liu and Hai-Hong Jiang

Chapter 24 **Factors associated with *Staphylococcus aureus* nasal carriage and molecular characteristics among the general population at a Medical College Campus in Guangzhou, South China** 186
B. J. Chen, X. Y. Xie, L. J. Ni, X. L. Dai, Y. Lu, X. Q. Wu, H. Y. Li, Y. D. Yao and S. Y. Huang

Chapter 25 **Antimicrobial susceptibility among Gram-positive and Gram-negative organisms collected from the Latin American region between 2004 and 2015 as part of the Tigecycline Evaluation and Surveillance Trial** 196
Silvio Vega and Michael J. Dowzicky

Permissions

List of Contributors

Index

Preface

This book has been an outcome of determined endeavour from a group of educationists in the field. The primary objective was to involve a broad spectrum of professionals from diverse cultural background involved in the field for developing new researches. The book not only targets students but also scholars pursuing higher research for further enhancement of the theoretical and practical applications of the subject.

The agents which kill microorganisms or stop their growth are known as antimicrobials. Antimicrobial medicines can be classified according to the microorganisms they act primarily against or according to their function. For instance, antimicrobials used against bacteria are called antibiotics, whereas antimicrobials which kill fungi are called antifungals. Antimicrobial medicines are used in antimicrobial chemotherapy to treat infections. It is further divided into five types, namely, antibacterial chemotherapy, antifungal chemotherapy, anthelminthic chemotherapy, antiprotozoal chemotherapy and antiviral chemotherapy. The topics included in this book on antimicrobials are of utmost significance and bound to provide incredible insights to readers. It aims to shed light on some of the unexplored aspects of clinical microbiology and the recent researches in this field. The book is appropriate for students seeking detailed information in this area.

It was an honour to edit such a profound book and also a challenging task to compile and examine all the relevant data for accuracy and originality. I wish to acknowledge the efforts of the contributors for submitting such brilliant and diverse chapters in the field and for endlessly working for the completion of the book. Last, but not the least; I thank my family for being a constant source of support in all my research endeavours.

Editor

1

Efficacy and safety profile of linezolid in the treatment of multidrug-resistant (MDR) and extensively drug-resistant (XDR) tuberculosis: a systematic review and meta-analysis

Akosua Adom Agyeman* and Richard Ofori-Asenso

Abstract

Background: Treatment options for drug-resistant tuberculosis are still limited. Linezolid has been recommended for treatment of patients with multidrug-resistant (MDR) or extensively-drug-resistant (XDR) tuberculosis, although uncertainties remain regarding its safety and tolerability in these circumstances.

Objective: To systematically evaluate the existing evidence regarding the efficacy and tolerability of linezolid in the treatment of MDR or XDR tuberculosis.

Methods: We conducted a systematic review and meta-analysis in accordance with the PRISMA guidelines. Searches were conducted in PubMed, Web of Science and EMBASE followed by direct search of abstracts in the International Journal of Tuberculosis and Lung Disease to retrieve primary studies published between January 2000 and January 2016 assessing linezolid efficacy and safety in the treatment of drug-resistant TB. We evaluated the occurrence of outcomes including culture conversion, treatment success and incidence of adverse events such as myelosuppression and neuropathy.

Results: Twenty-three (23) studies conducted in fourteen (14) countries and involving 507 patients were retrieved. Only 1 randomized controlled trial was identified and none of the identified studies involved participants from Africa. The pooled proportion for treatment success was 77.36 % (95 % CI = 71.38–82.83 %, $I^2 = 37.6$ %) with culture conversion rate determined as 88.45 % (95 % CI = 83.82–92.38 %, $I^2 = 45.4$ %). There was no strong evidence for both culture conversion ($p = 0.0948$) and treatment success ($p = 0.0695$) between linezolid daily doses ≤ 600 and > 600 mg. Only myelosuppression showed a strong statistical significance ($p < 0.0001$) between dose comparisons. The incidence of neuropathy and other adverse events leading to permanent discontinuation of linezolid also showed no significance upon dose comparisons ($p = 0.3213$, $p = 0.9050$ respectively).

Conclusion: Available evidence presents Linezolid as a viable option in the treatment of MDR/XDR TB although patients ought to be monitored closely for the incidence of major adverse events such as myelosuppression and neuropathy. Additionally, highly powered randomized controlled trials including participants from endemic regions are urgently needed to better inform the magnitude and significance of Linezolid treatment effect in MDR and XDR TB patients.

Keywords: Linezolid, Tuberculosis, Multi-drug resistance, Extensively drug resistant, Meta-analysis, Drug therapy, Infectious diseases

*Correspondence: akosuaadom@gmail.com
Research Unit, Health Policy Consult, Weija, P. O. Box WJ 537, Accra, Ghana

Background

Tuberculosis (TB) is a significant contributor to global morbidity and mortality. About one in three persons representing almost 3 billion individuals worldwide are known to be infected with *Mycobacterium tuberculosis* of which at least 5 % are likely to develop active TB disease during their lifetime [1, 2]. In 2014, more than 9 million new cases of TB were recorded resulting in over 1.5 million deaths [2]. Nearly one in three deaths in HIV-positive individuals are attributable to TB [3]. Disproportionate number of global TB cases are known to occur in areas such as Sub-Saharan Africa and South East Asia [2]. The economic impact of TB is deemed to be enormous as more than 90 % of TB-related deaths occur among adults in the most productive years [4].

Over the last few years, significant progress has been made towards controlling TB and reducing the global burden of the disease. TB incidence has declined in all parts of the world by at least 1.5 % annually since 2000 and is now almost 18 % lower than the rate in 2000 [1, 5]. Additionally, TB mortality has decreased by almost 50 % since 1990, with nearly all of that improvement happening in the era of the millennium development goals (MDGs) [5]. In the context of these TB control successes, it is estimated that over 40 million lives were saved in the period 2000–2014 [1].

However, in spite of the positive developments, the increasing emergence of multidrug-resistant (MDR) and extensively drug-resistant (XDR) TB across the globe has the potential to derail the fight against TB and possibly revert the progress made regarding TB care and control. MDR-TB has been used to represent all forms TB disease in which the causative bacteria is resistant to at least isoniazid and rifampicin, whereas XDR-TB denotes forms of TB in which the bacteria is resistant to rifampicin and isoniazid plus any fluoroquinolone, and at least one of the second line injectable TB drugs (i.e., amikacin, kanamycin, or capreomycin) [6]. By the end of 2013, over 90 countries had documented at least a case of XDR-TB [7]. Almost 5 % of all global TB cases are now estimated to be MDR-TB including over 3 % of newly diagnosed TB cases, and as much as 20 % in previously treated patients [8, 9]. In 2014 alone, more than 400,000 cases of MDR-TB were reported with nearly 10 % of this being XDR-TB [8].

The cost implication of MDR/XDR TB is enormous and one that could impose significant strain on any healthcare system. Diel et al., for instance, estimated the total cost per MDR-TB and XDR-TB case in Germany to be €82,150 and €108,733, respectively [10]. Within the period 2011–2015, as much as USD 1.7 billion was required across the world in tackling MDR-TB [11].

Treatment outcomes for MDR/XDR-TB remain poor even in advanced health systems. In 2007, the World Health Organization (WHO) reported that just around one-third of the over 7000 MDR-TB patients from 13 countries were successfully treated [12]. On the other hand, for nearly four decades no new anti -tubercular drug was registered until the recent introduction of Delamanid and Bedaquiline [13, 14]. Even these new drugs are unable to resolve all the challenges regarding therapy for MDR/XDR-TB [14]. In view of this, diverse treatment approaches have continually been explored including the use of therapies containing linezolid, higher doses of isoniazid and sometimes fluoroquinolones [15].

Linezolid an Oxazolidinone and a relatively newer class of antibiotic has demonstrated potency against drug-resistant *M. tuberculosis* in a number of in vitro studies [16–18]. Since 2006, the WHO has recommended the use of linezolid in the treatment of MDR/XDR-TB with the drug now being included in many TB programmes across the world [19, 20]. Aside its high cost which remains a major barrier to access, there are uncertainties regarding the most effective dose of linezolid with < 600 or ≥ 600 mg daily doses being documented in separate reports [19, 21]. Additionally, serious adverse effects such as neuropathies and hematological adverse reactions have been reported raising huge concerns about the safety of the drug in the treatment of XDR and MDR-TB which usually demands extensive treatment periods [19, 21].

Some reviews have previously sought to assess the efficacy and tolerability/safety of linezolid in the treatment of MDR/XDR-TB [19–23]. The latest of these reviews conducted by Zhang et al. [23], includes primary studies published no later than May 2014. Considering that scientific evidence changes rapidly and according to Whitlock et al. [24], reviews are deemed to be out of date often after few years, there is the need for continuous evaluation of evidence to incorporate new information as they become available. In view of this, we conducted a systematic review and meta-analysis to summarize the existing evidence to date of the safety and efficacy of linezolid in the treatment of DR-TB as an update to previously conducted reviews.

Methods

This systematic review was conducted in accordance with the PRISMA (preferred reporting items for systematic reviews and meta-analyses) guidelines [25].

Search strategy and study selection

We performed searches in PubMed, Web of Science and EMBASE for relevant studies published between January 2000 and January 2016. In addition, we searched the International Journal of Tuberculosis and Lung Disease for original studies published on the subject within the above period. A combination of key words and their synonyms used in all searches were 'multidrug resistant tuberculosis', 'extensively drug resistant tuberculosis', 'linezolid', 'zyvox', 'efficacy' and 'toxicity'. We included 'zyvox' as a keyword as it is the most commonly marketed brand name for linezolid [26]. Search results were limited to human population and English language. References of selected studies and previously published reviews were also screened to identify additional publications. We included only published primary studies involving adult populations of ≥5 patients with sputum culture confirmed (pulmonary or extra pulmonary TB) and available report on efficacy and tolerability (safety). In vitro studies and review articles were excluded as well as case reports with sample size less than 5 patients. Exclusion of studies with relatively small sample size was intended to minimize selection and reporting bias [27].

Study quality assessment

We employed the McMaster critical review for quantitative studies to critically appraise all studies [28, 29]. Further methodological quality assessments of studies were conducted based on the following criteria: linezolid dose stated, DST guided treatment regimen, hospitalization at initiation of linezolid treatment, IRB approval obtained, patients monitored by DOT and outcomes report similar to WHO definitions.

Data extraction

A data extraction form was developed and used to guide the extraction of data from the included studies. First author name, publication year, duration of study, type of study design, control group present, country of study and number of HIV co-infected patients were extracted for epidemiological characteristics. With regards to efficacy and tolerability, data extracted included total number of MDR/XDR TB exposed to linezolid, treatment regimen employed and linezolid dose. Outcome measures on efficacy and tolerability were based on WHO definitions [30]. For efficacy, data were extracted for patients who achieved sputum culture conversion to negative as well as those who were cured. Patients who defaulted, achieved treatment failure, relapsed or died were regarded as unfavorable outcomes. For tolerability, data were extracted for neuropathy, myelosuppression, both temporary and permanent discontinuation of linezolid due to adverse effects and other reported adverse effects associated with linezolid [31]. A summary of the data for outcomes evaluation has been provided as a supplementary material (Additional file 1). All data were extracted by AA and verified by RO. Where there were disagreements, these were resolved by consensus-based discussions.

Statistical analysis

The meta-analysis proportions were conducted using StatsDirect statistical software (Version 3.0.0, StatsDirect Ltd, Cheshire UK) [32]. Individual study proportions were assessed at 95 % confidence interval (CI) as well as the pooled effect. Between-study heterogeneity was assessed by the Quoran (Q) statistic test and the I^2 statistic, which represents the percentage of total variation across studies, attributable to heterogeneity rather than to chance [33]. As we anticipated variations among studies for multiple reasons including study conduct methods, the random effect model (DerSimonian-Laird) was adopted over fixed effect model in the summary of pooled analysis [33]. Publication bias was evaluated by direct observation of funnel plots and the Egger and Begg's tests were applied to measure any asymmetry [34]. For all computations statistical significance was set at $p < 0.05$.

Ethical approval

Ethical approval was not sought for this study as all information used were derived from already published studies available in the public domain.

Results

Studies identification and retrieval

A total of 469 records were retrieved from database search in addition to two records identified through International Journal of Tuberculosis and Lung Disease. Upon removing duplicates and screening by titles and abstracts, 46 articles were found relevant for full-text analysis and reference list screening. Subsequent to this, 23 articles were excluded with reasons (Fig. 1) and 23 studies were identified as eligible for inclusion in the meta-analysis [35–57]. The 23 studies were conducted in 14 countries across the globe. Per regional distribution, more than half (57 %, n = 13), were conducted in Asia. The rest of the studies were conducted in North America (n = 4), South America (n = 1) and Europe (n = 5). None of the selected studies was conducted in Africa. About 57 % (n = 13) of studies were conducted in the last 5 years (2011–2016). Most of the studies were case series (n = 20, 87 %). Only one randomized controlled trial was identified [51]. The two remaining studies consisted of one non-randomized Phase 1 clinical trial [36] and the other a Phase 2a clinical trial [42]. A total of 507 patients received linezolid as part of their treatment regimen and 353 patients were evaluated for definite outcomes (cured, treatment completed, died, failure). About 57 % of patients enrolled tested positive for XDR TB and 3 % had documented HIV positive status (Table 1). Thus the population involved was predominantly HIV negative. In most of the studies, linezolid was included in the

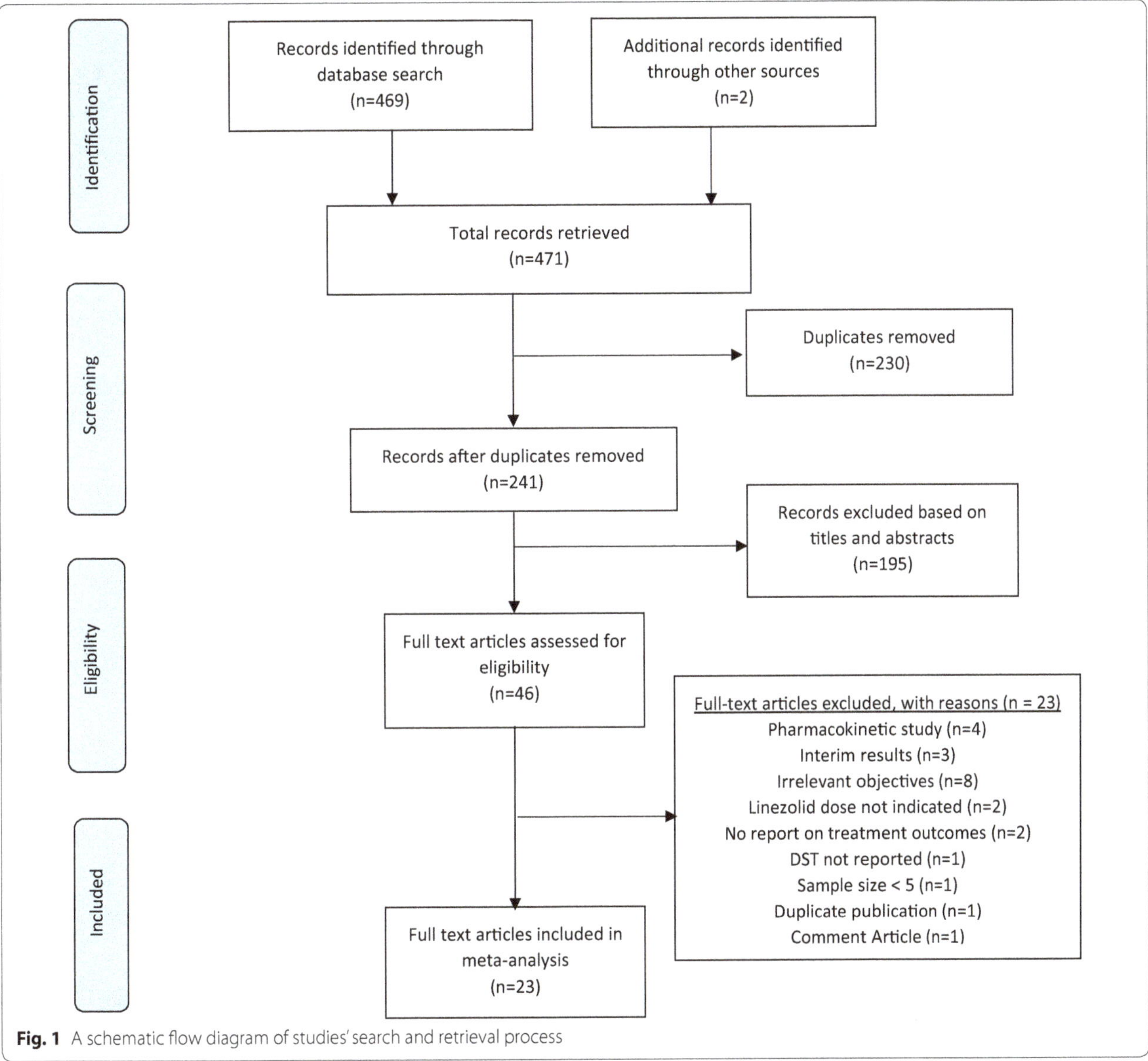

Fig. 1 A schematic flow diagram of studies' search and retrieval process

treatment regimen based on DST following treatment failure to previous treatment regimen. Linezolid was generally administered at a daily minimum dose of 300 mg to a maximum dose of 1200 mg. The duration of treatment ranged from 1 to 36 months. The quality assessment across studies was generally satisfactory. All studies indicated linezolid dose and treatment regimen was individualized based on DST results (Table 2). However, 19 out of 23 studies reported Institutional Review Board (IRB) approval prior to study initiation. The remaining four studies did not report on IRB approval [38, 43, 45, 58]. Hospitalization prior to linezolid treatment was poorly reported; no reporting was done by 15 studies. Nonetheless, 6 studies reported patient hospitalization prior to linezolid treatment and only 2 studies indicated no patient hospitalization. Also, DOT was not reported in 12 out of 13 studies. With respect to treatment success, sixteen (16) studies were similar to WHO definitions whiles four (4) studies did not conform to WHO standards and three (3) studies did not report on their reference guideline.

Efficacy

With the exception of Udwadia et al. [53], all the studies reported on sputum culture conversion with a pooled proportion of 88.45 % (95 % CI = 83.82–92.38 %, $p = 0.0112$) (Fig. 2) and moderate heterogeneity across studies ($I^2 = 45.4$ %; 95 % CI = 0–65.9 %). Eight studies

Table 1 Description of the characteristics of included studies

Study No.	Reference	Year of publication	Country of study	Study design	Control group	Number exposed to Linezolid	Study duration	Number of XDR-TB	LZD dosage	Duration of LZD treatment	Type of anti-TB regimen	HIV infection status
1.	Abbate et al. [35]	2012	Argentina	Retrospective study	No	17	2002–2008	17	600 mg bd	≥12 months after cc	Individualized	All HIV negative
2.	Anger et al. [36]	2010	USA	Retrospective case series	No	16	2000–2006	10	600 mg bd 400 mg bd or 600 mg daily	Mean = 15 Median = 16 Range = 1–29 months	Individualized	3 HIV positive
3.	Condos et al. [37]	2008	USA	Prospective phase 1 clinical trial	No	6[a]	2000–2007	6[a]	600 mg bd 600 mg daily	Range = 9–26 months	Individualized	All HIV negative
4.	De Lorenzo et al. [38]	2012	Italy	Retrospective study	No	12	2009–2010	4	600 mg bd (10 patients) 600 mg daily (1 patient) 450 mg bd (1 patient)	Range = 37–100 days Median = 63.5 days	Individualized	2 HIV negative
5.	Fortún et al. [39]	2005	Spain	Retrospective case series	No	3[b]	1994–2004	0	600 mg bd	Range = 4–24 months Mean = 12 Median = 12	Individualized	1 HIV positive
6.	Koh et al. [40]	2009	South Korea	Retrospective case series	No	24	2007–2008	1	300 mg daily	Median = 12 months	Individualised	All HIV Negative
7.	Koh et al. [41]	2012	South Korea	Retrospective case series	No	51	2007–2009	26	300 mg daily	Median = 413 days IQR = 237–622 days	Individualized	All HIV negative
8.	Lee et al. [42]	2012	South Korea	Phase 2a randomized two-group study	No	38	2008–2011	41	600 mg daily	22 months	Individualized	All HIV negative
9.	Liu et al. [43]	2015	China	Retrospective case series	No	16	2011–2013	16	600 mg daily	Range = 3–21 months Mean = 9.53 months	Individualized	All HIV negative
10.	Migliori et al. [44]	2009	Belarus, Germany, Italy, Switzerland	Retrospective non-randomized unblinded observational study	Yes	85	2001–2007	12	600 mg daily 600 mg bd	Mean = 7 months Median = 3 months	Individualized	3 HIV positive
11.	Nam et al. [45]	2009	South Korea	Retrospective case series	No	11	NR	4	600 mg daily 300 mg bd	Range 3–24 months Mean = 7 months Median 5 months	Individualized	All HIV negative

Table 1 continued

Study No.	Reference	Year of publication	Country of study	Study design	Control group	Number exposed to Linezolid	Study duration	Number of XDR-TB	LZD dosage	Duration of LZD treatment	Type of anti-TB regimen	HIV infection status
12.	Park et al. [46]	2006	South Korea	Prospective non-randomized case series	No	8	2003–2006	5	600 daily 600 bd	Range = 3–18 months Median = 9 months Mean = 11 months	Individualized	All HIV negative
13.	Roongruang-pitayakul et al. [47]	2013	Thailand	Retrospective case series	No	24	2009–2012	7	600 mg daily 300 mg daily	Range = 11.0–21.5 months Mean = 18.7 months	Individualized	All HIV negative
14.	Schecter et al. [48]	2010	USA	Retrospective case series	No	30	2003–2007	3	600 mg daily	Range = 1–36 months Median = 22 months Mean = 19 months	Individualized	17 HIV negative
15.	Singla et al. [49]	2012	India	Prospective case series	No	29	2006–2011	16	600 bd 600 daily	Median = 30 days	Individualized	All HIV negative
16.	Tang et al. [50]	2011	China	Case series	No	14	2009–2010	14	600 mg bd 600 mg daily	Range= 2–11 months Mean: 6.5 months	Individualised	All HIV negative
17.	Tang et al. [51]	2015	China	Prospective multicenter randomized controlled study	Yes	33	2009–2011	65	1200 mg daily 300–600 mg daily	Range = 2–24 months	Individualized	All HIV negative
18.	Tse-Chang et al. [52]	2013	Canada	Retrospective case study	No	13	2000–2011	NR	600 mg daily	Mean = 8.3 months Range = 1.4–22 months	Individualized	1 HIV positive
19.	Udwadia et al. [53]	2010	India	Prospective non-randomized case series	No	18	2000–2007	7	600 mg daily	Mean = 21 months	Individualized	NR
20.	Villar et al. [54]	2011	Portugal	Prospective case series	No	16	2004–2009	12	600 daily 1200 mg daily	Median = 375 days	Individualized	6 HIV positive
21.	Von der Lippe et al. [55]	2006	Norway	Retrospective case series	No	10	1998–2002	0	600 mg bd	Range = 2–10 months Median = 4.25 months	Individualized	1HIV positive
22.	Xu et al. [56]	2012	China	Retrospective case series	No	18	2007–2010	15	600 mg bd 900 mg daily	Range =1.5–10 months Median = 6 months	Individualized	All HIV negative
23.	Zhang et al. [57]	2014	China	Retrospective study	Yes	15	2012–2013	43	600 mg daily	Range = 1–5 months	Individualized	All HIV negative

[a] One paediatric case excluded

[b] Excluded two patients with *M. bovis* infection

Table 2 Summary of the methodological quality assessment of included studies

Study No.	References	IRB approval	LZD dose indicated	Individualised treatment based on DST	Hospital admission prior to LZD treatment	DOT during treatment	Treatment success definition similar to WHO
1.	Abbate et al. [35]	Yes	Yes	Yes	NR	NR	Yes
2.	Anger et al. [36]	Yes	Yes	Yes	NR	Yes	Yes
3.	Condos et al. [37]	Yes	Yes	Yes	NR	NR	Yes
4.	De Lorenzo et al. [38]	NR	Yes	Yes	NR	NR	Yes
5.	Fortún et al. [39]	Yes	Yes	Yes	NR	Yes	Yes
6.	Koh et al. [40]	Yes	Yes	Yes	NR	Yes	Yes
7.	Koh et al. [41]	Yes	Yes	Yes	NR	NR	Yes
8.	Lee et al. [42]	Yes	Yes	Yes	Yes	Yes	No
9.	Liu et al. [43]	NR	Yes	Yes	Yes	NR	NR
10.	Migliori et al. [44]	Yes	Yes	Yes	NR	Yes	Yes
11.	Nam et al. [45]	NR	Yes	Yes	NR	NR	No
12.	Park et al. [46]	Yes	Yes	Yes	NR	NR	Yes
13.	Roongruangpitay-akul et al. [47]	Yes	Yes	Yes	No	Yes	Yes
14.	Schecter et al. [48]	Yes	Yes	Yes	NR	Yes	Yes
15.	Singla et al. [49]	Yes	Yes	Yes	Yes	Yes	No
16.	Tang et al. [50]	Yes	Yes	Yes	NR	NR	NR
17.	Tang et al. [51]	Yes	Yes	Yes	NR	Yes	Yes
18.	Tse-Chang et al. [52]	NR	Yes	Yes	NR	NR	Yes
19.	Udwadia et al. [53]	Yes	Yes	Yes	No	NR	NR
20.	Villar et al. [54]	Yes	Yes	Yes	NR	NR	Yes
21.	Von der Lippe et al. [55]	Yes	Yes	Yes	Yes	Yes	No
22.	Xu et al. [56]	Yes	Yes	Yes	Yes	Yes	Yes
23.	Zhang et al. [57]	Yes	Yes	Yes	Yes	NR	Yes

[35, 36, 39, 46, 48, 50, 54, 55], achieved 100 % sputum culture conversion with a total number of 98 out of 507 patients exposed to linezolid. Among these eight studies, three studies [35, 39, 55] administered linezolid at a dose of 600 mg twice daily with only one study administering at a dose of 600 mg daily. The remaining four studies had mixed dosing regimen in the same cohort of patients. A total of 274 patients achieved treatment success across the 23 studies with a combined proportion of 77.36 % (95 % CI = 71.38–82.83 %, $p = 0.0365$) (Fig. 3) and a low homogeneity test result of 37.6 % (95 % CI = 0–61.3 %). Only two studies [38, 46] had less than 50 % treatment success with linezolid dose regimen between 600 and 1200 mg daily. Three studies [35, 37, 52] reported 100 % treatment success (95 % CI = 78.20–100, 54.07–100 and 66.37–100 %, respectively).

Safety and tolerability

Adverse events related to Linezolid was observes in all the studies. Major adverse events leading to permanent discontinuation of linezolid was observed in 21 studies with pooled proportion of 15.81 % (95 % CI = 9.68–23.11 %, $p < 0.0001$) (Fig. 4). Heterogeneity was observed to be very high at 74 % (95 % CI = 58.0–82.0 %). Two studies did not report whether any permanent discontinuation due to linezolid toxicity had happen or not [53, 54]. On the other hand, in five studies there was no occurrence of permanent discontinuation of linezolid due to adverse events in patients [35, 37, 38, 50, 57]. All 23 studies reported myelosuppression in the form of anemia or neutropenia. The pooled proportion of myelosuppression was observed at 32.93 % (95 % CI = 23.13–43.54 %, $p < 0.0001$) (Fig. 5) and high heterogeneity of 83 %. The Canadian cohort [52] recorded the highest incidence of myelosuppression of 85 % (11 out 13 patients) at a linezolid dose of 600 mg daily. Koh et al. [40] recorded the least occurrence of myelosuppression; 4 % (1 out of 24 patients) with daily 300 mg dose of linezolid. Neuropathy was also recorded in all but one studies with a combined proportion of 29.92 % (95 % CI = 20.53–40.25 %,

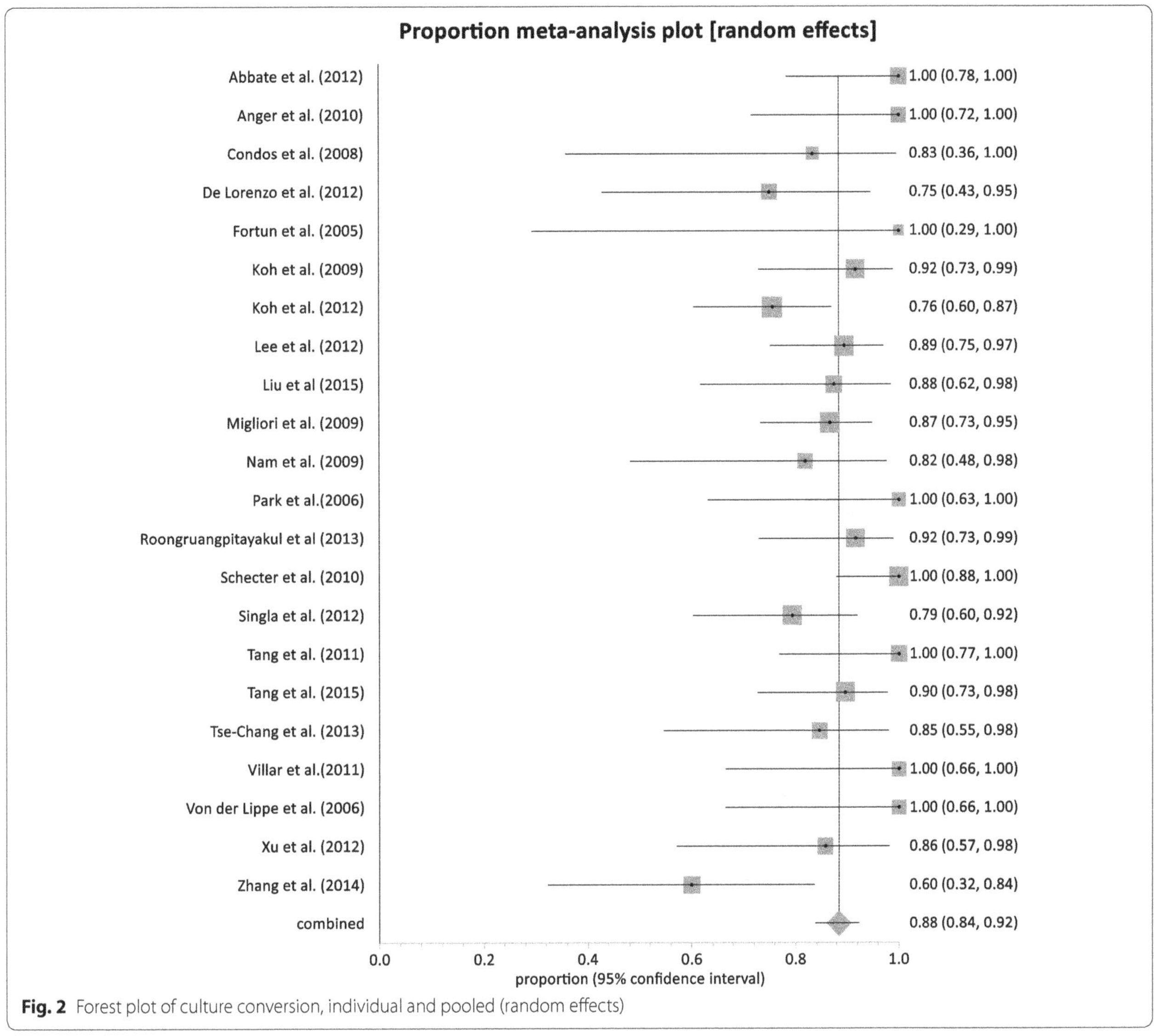

Fig. 2 Forest plot of culture conversion, individual and pooled (random effects)

p < 0.0001) (Fig. 6). None of the patients enrolled in Fortun et al. experienced neuropathy and Linezolid was given at a dose of 600 mg BD [39]. The highest proportion of neuropathy was observed in Nam et al. [45] with a proportion of 81.82 % (95 % CI = 48.22–97.72 %) where linezolid was administered at a maximum dose of 600 mg daily. With the exception of Von der Lippe et al. [55], adverse events other than myelosuppression and neuropathy were reported in the remaining 22 studies. Nausea and vomiting were the most frequently reported. Others included hyperpigmentation of the oral cavity [51] and transient visual impairment [47]. The pooled proportion of reported adverse events other than myelosuppression and neuropathy was 33.60 % (95 % CI = 20.41–48.23 %, p < 0.0001) (Fig. 7).

Outcomes comparison between daily doses ≤ 600 and > 600 mg

Patients receiving linezolid at a dose ≤ 600 mg had lower proportions (85.58 %) of culture conversion compared to those receiving linezolid at doses > 600 mg (95.12 %). There was no strong evidence for both culture conversion (p = 0.0948) and treatment success (p = 0.0695) between linezolid doses ≤ 600 and > 600 mg (Table 3). Nonetheless, higher proportion of patients achieved treatment success in higher doses of linezolid (89.47 %) compared to administering lower doses of linezolid (76.14 %). Linezolid doses > 600 mg observed higher incidence of myelosuppression (50 %) compared with doses ≤ 600 mg (19.58 %). Only myelosuppression showed a strong statistical significance (p < 0.0001) between dose comparisons.

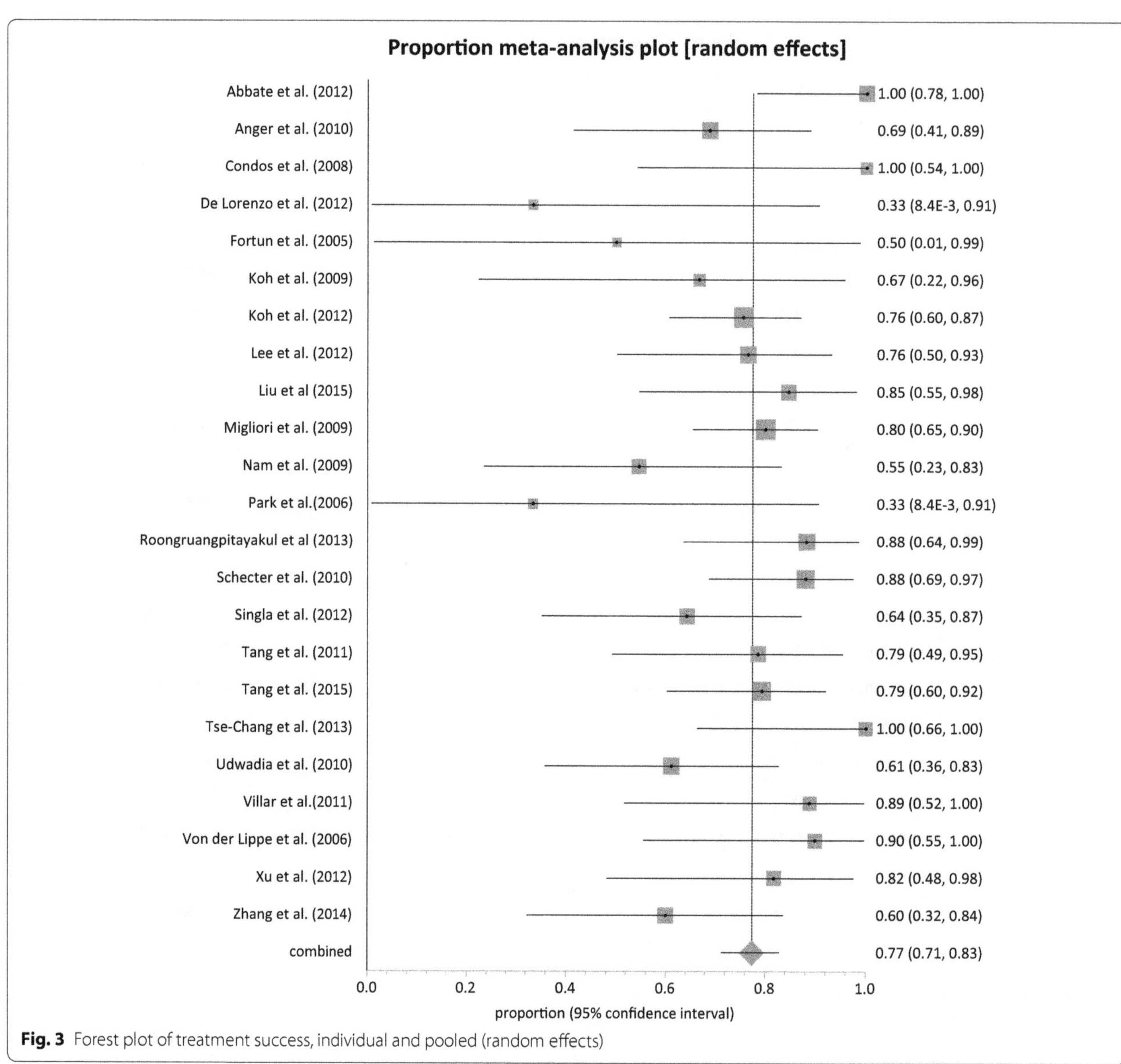

Fig. 3 Forest plot of treatment success, individual and pooled (random effects)

On the contrary, the incidence of neuropathy and adverse events leading to permanent discontinuation of linezolid showed no significance upon dose comparisons ($p = 0.3213$, $p = 0.9050$ respectively).

Publication bias

Begg's and Egger's regression tests were performed to assess publication bias. The shapes of the funnel plots do not show obvious evidence of asymmetry (Fig. 8). However, the *p* value of Egger's test confirmed the existence of publication bias for all the outcomes evaluated [(A) Culture conversion, $p = 0.0144$; (B) treatment success, $p = 0.0006$; (C) myelosuppression, $p = 0.0295$; (D) neuropathy $p = 0.0014$; (E) discontinuation due to linezolid adverse effects, $p = 0.01$ and (F) presence of any other adverse events, $p = 0.0067$].

Discussion

This systematic review and meta-analysis included a larger number of case reports and observational studies than reported in previous reviews which suggests that linezolid is increasingly being used off-label in the management of drug resistant TB. In our systematic review, only one randomized controlled trial (with 'no linezolid intervention' control group) conducted by Tang et al. [51] in China was identified with a total sample size of

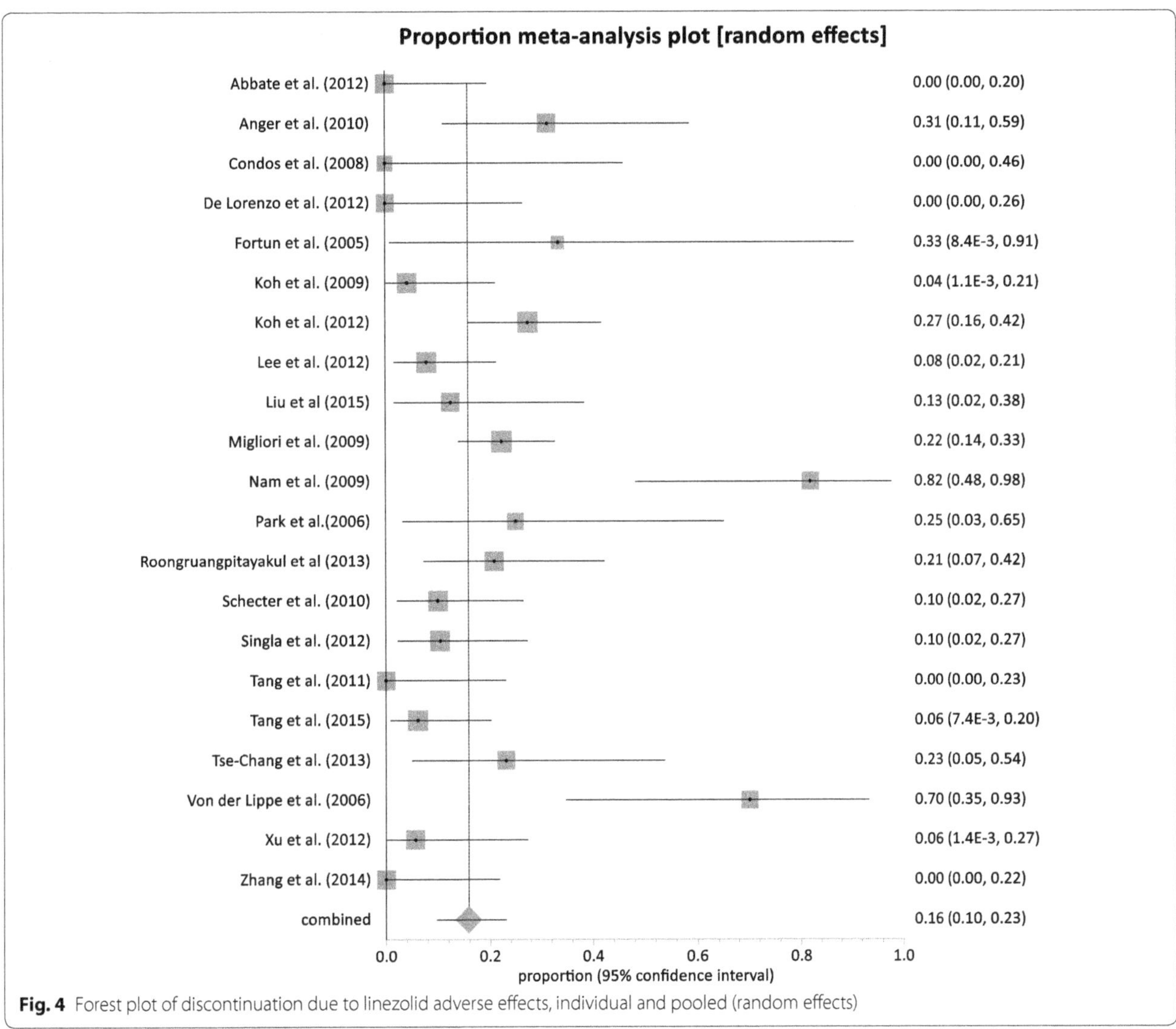

Fig. 4 Forest plot of discontinuation due to linezolid adverse effects, individual and pooled (random effects)

65 patients. This is the first of such kind compared to the randomized trials reported by Lee et al. [42] where both study groups were administered linezolid.

Efficacy

In our review, linezolid was administered in combination with other anti-tubercular drugs to achieve treatment success. Thus treatment success may not be exclusively attributed to linezolid. Nonetheless, since linezolid inclusion mostly followed resistance or treatment failure with other second line drugs, much of the treatment success may be attributed to linezolid. We obtained a pooled culture conversion of 88.45 % (95 % CI 83.82–92.38 %, $p = 0.0112$). Previous reviews by Sotgui et al. [22] and Zhang et al. [23] obtained pooled culture conversion of 93 % ($p = 0.2704$) and 89 % ($p = 0.0217$) respectively. The results from our study shows strong evidence ($p = 0.0112$) of linezolid to achieve culture conversion in MDR/XDRTB patients which is synonymous to that from Zhang et al. ($p = 0.0217$) [23] due to large samples size in these studies compared to Sotgui et al. [22] whose results depicted otherwise.

On the other hand, pooled treatment success was significantly lower [77.36 % (95 % CI 71.38–82.83 %, $p = 0.0365$)] than that obtained for culture conversion. This is also similar to the stated cure rates in the 2015 WHO Global TB report and also results obtained from previous reviews [1, 19, 22, 23]. The 2015 WHO Global report on TB, reports cure rates in 2014 from 43 countries as $\geq$ 75 % with global average cure rate of 50 %. The treatment success proportion obtained in our review in comparison with the culture conversion significantly implies that, most of the MDR/XDR TB patients who achieve sputum culture conversion do not achieve

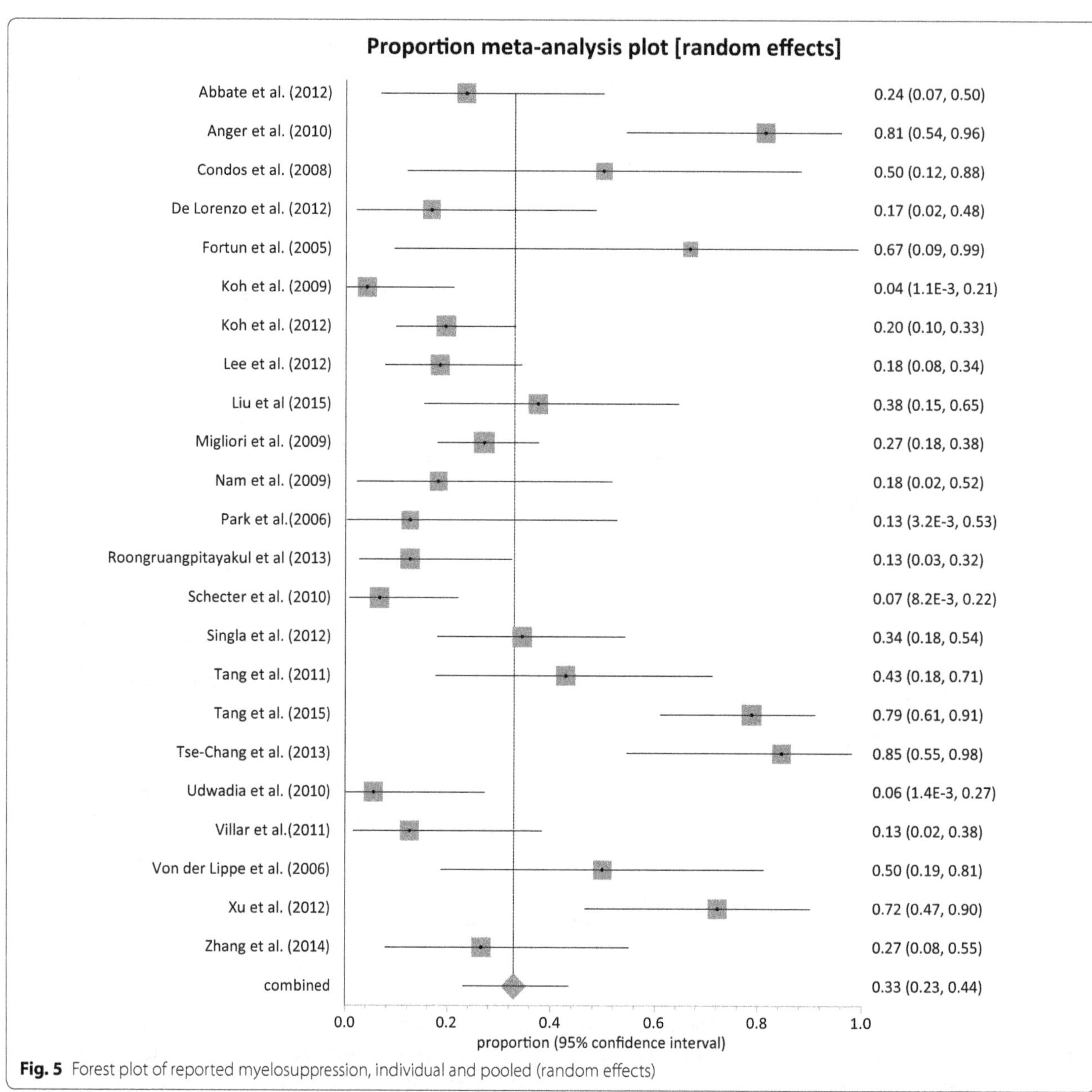

Fig. 5 Forest plot of reported myelosuppression, individual and pooled (random effects)

treatment success. This may be due to default, treatment failure, treatment discontinuation due to adverse effects or relapse. In a study conducted by Xu et al. [56], all patients (n = 18) administered linezolid were culture negative at 7 weeks of treatment during hospital admission. However, at data censor after patient discharge from the hospital, only nine patients (50 %) achieved treatment success whiles three and two patients relapsed and attained treatment failure, respectively. Synonymously, five studies [42, 43, 49, 55, 56] which reported patient admission prior to linezolid administration and discharge after culture conversion also observed higher proportions of culture conversion than treatment success.

Fifteen studies (Table 2) did not report on hospitalization whiles two studies initiated linezolid under outpatient environment [47, 53]. One out of these two studies obtained a lower treatment success (61.10 %) compared to the other [47, 53]. These results contribute to the significance of hospitalization prior to treatment initiation in MDR/XDR TB which enhances therapeutic and adverse events monitoring as well as patient compliance to therapy to achieve high proportions of treatment

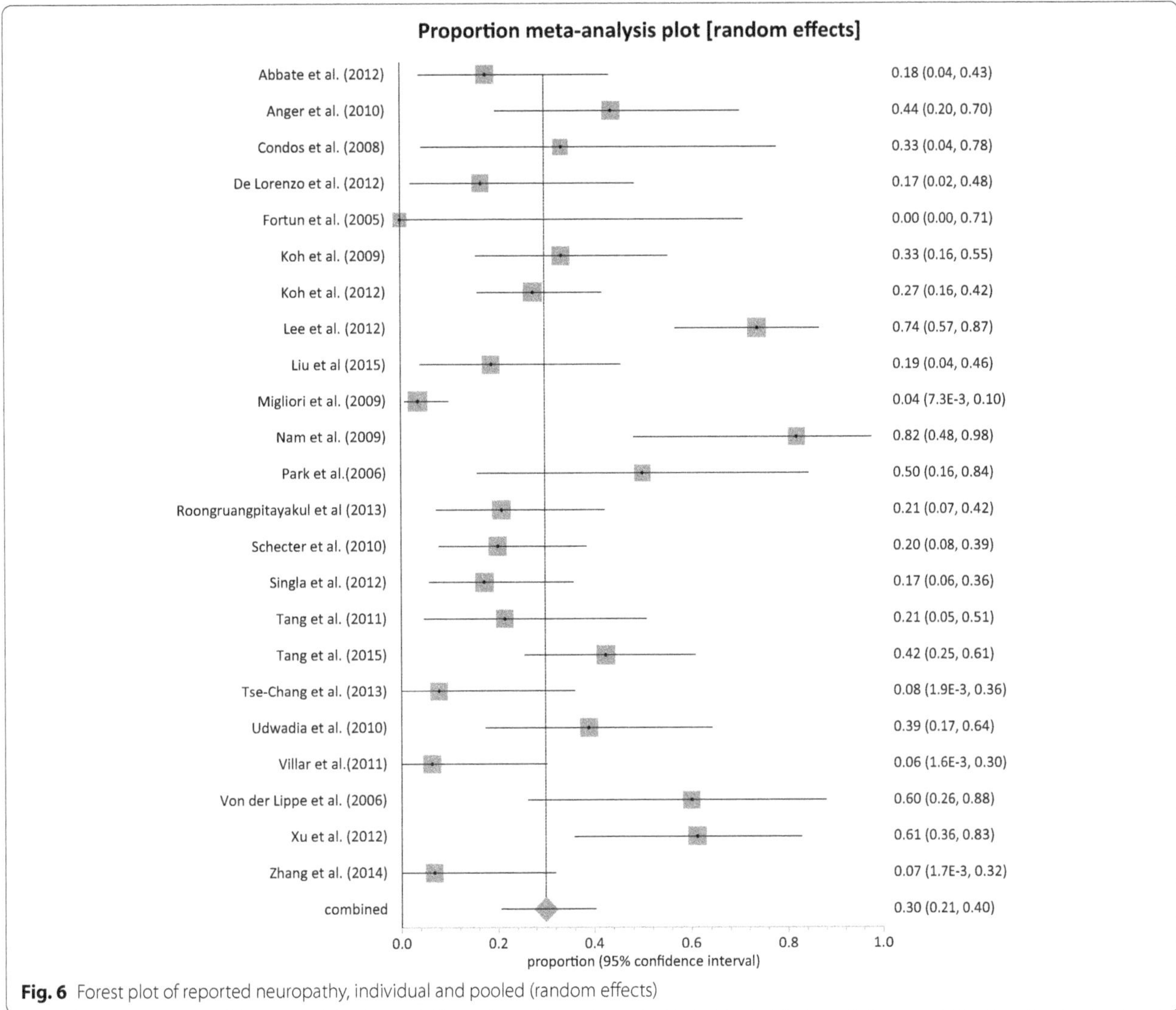

Fig. 6 Forest plot of reported neuropathy, individual and pooled (random effects)

success. Nonetheless, Roongruangpitayakul et al. [47] reports high treatment success proportion (88.2 %) obtained under outpatient conditions. This may imply that with efficient DOT, patients not requiring hospitalization can also be successfully treated with linezolid as long as procedures are in place to monitor incidence of adverse events.

Administering different doses of linezolid did not show any significant difference in culture conversion and treatment success; $p = 0.0948$ and $p = 0.0695$, respectively. A recent systematic review conducted by Zhang et al. also had similar results for culture conversion and favorable outcomes, respectively [23]. Thus, linezolid may be administered at a lower dose to achieve treatment success whiles reducing the incidence of adverse events. However, the dose and duration of linezolid in the treatment of MDR/XDR TB ought to be streamlined based on evidence from randomized controlled trials (RCTs). An RCT conducted by Tang et al. and involving 65 XDR-TB patients reported higher proportions of culture conversion (96 vs. 41 %) and treatment success (79.31 vs. 37.93 %) in the treatment group than the control group [51]. Also in this same RCT, patients were given an initial high dose of linezolid (1200 mg daily) for a period of 4–6 weeks followed by a reduced dose (300–600 mg) in the continuous phase to complete a 24 month treatment regimen. This may propose a successful dosage regimen for MDR/XDR TB involving a maximum tolerable high dose of 1200 mg daily for a short intensive phase, followed by a reduced dose between 300 and 600 mg daily during the continuous phase. Nonetheless, RCTs involving larger patient population need to be conducted to strengthen this evidence. Horsburg et al. proposes a novel method to ascertain optimum duration of antibiotic

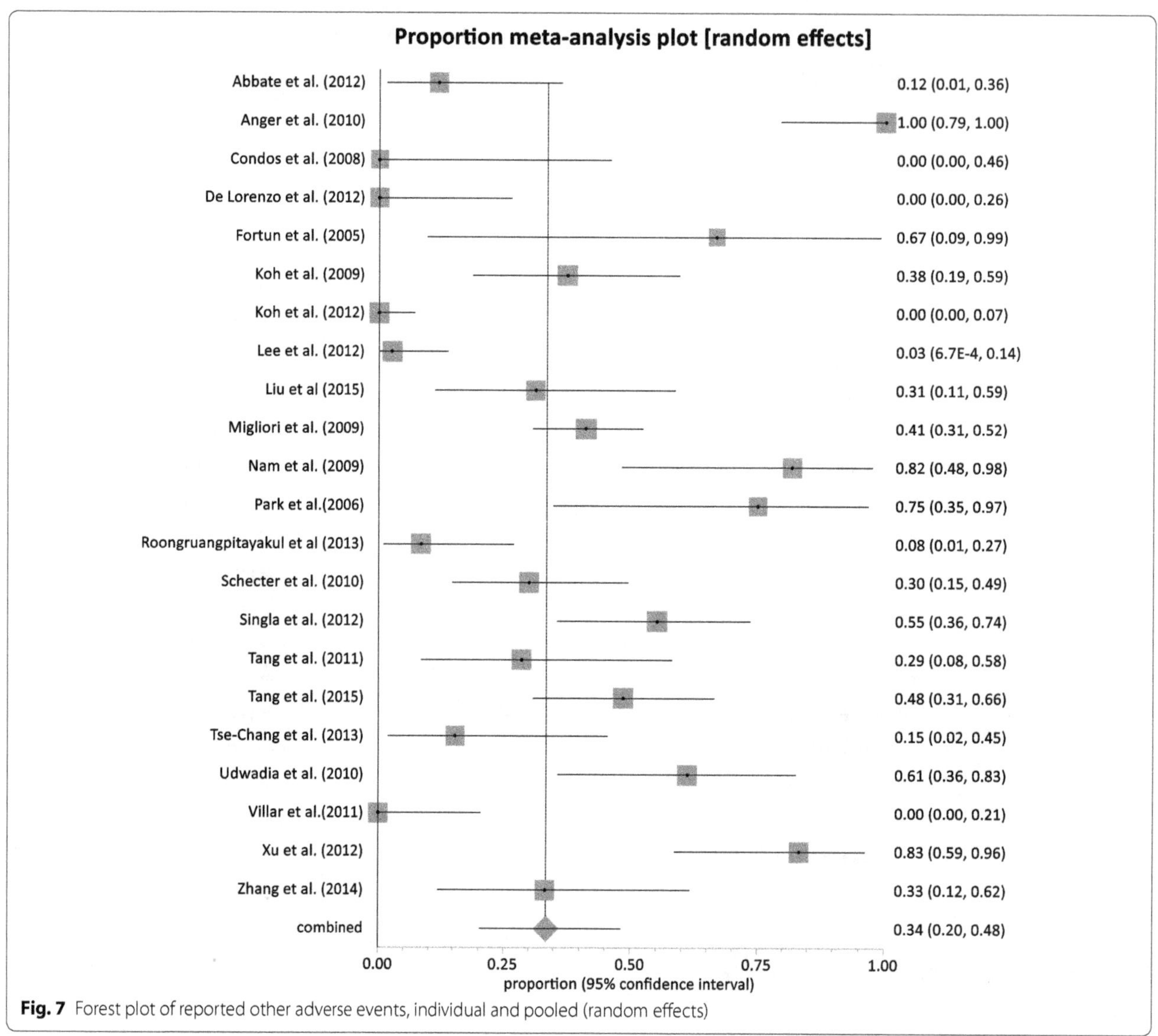

Fig. 7 Forest plot of reported other adverse events, individual and pooled (random effects)

Table 3 Comparison of treatment outcomes of MDR/XDR-TB cases according to daily administered linezolid dose

Outcome	≤600 mg linezolid n (%)	>600 mg linezolid n (%)	Difference (%) (95 % CI)	p value
Culture conversion	184/215 (85.58)	39/41 (95.12)	9.54 (−2.29–16.32 %)	p = 0.0948
Treatment success	134/176 (76.14)	34/38 (89.47)	13.34 (−13.22–23.12 %)	p = 0.0695
Myelosuppression	47/240 (19.58)	24/48 (50.00)	30.42 (15.77–44.94 %)	p < 0.0001
Neuropathy	82/240 (34.17)	20/48 (41.67)	7.5 % (−6.84–22.79 %)	p = 0.3213
Linezolid discontinuation	40/222 (18.02)	9/48 (18.75)	0.73 % (−9.66–14.72 %)	p = 0.9050

treatment regimen [58]. Their proposed model utilizes a logistic regression model in RCT design to ascertain the shortest possible antibiotic treatment duration in relation to corresponding proportions of cured patients. The researchers further highlighted the suitability of this proposed model for anti-tubercular regimen with the aim of minimizing the incidence of resistance, toxicity, costs and pill burden [58].

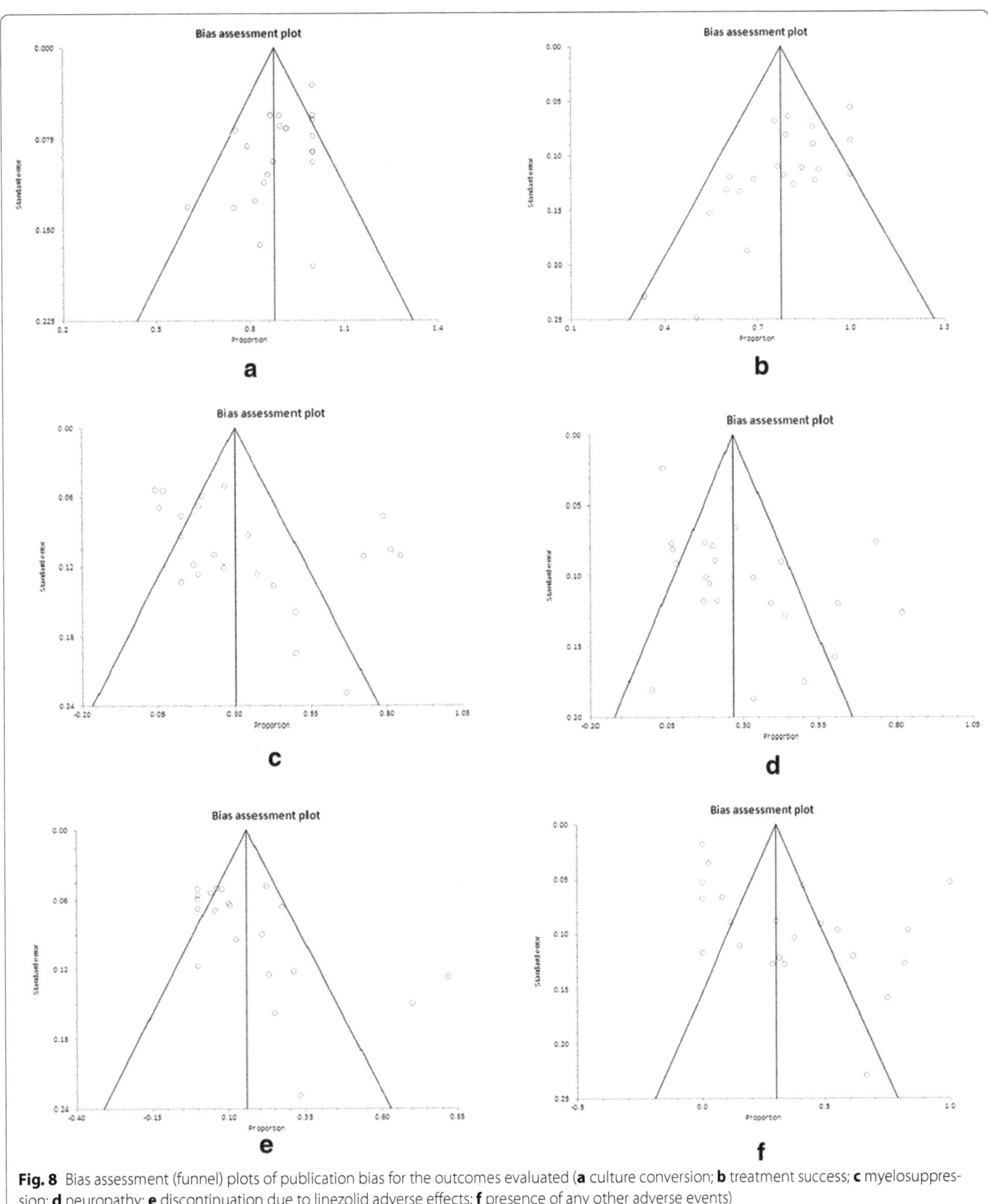

Fig. 8 Bias assessment (funnel) plots of publication bias for the outcomes evaluated (**a** culture conversion; **b** treatment success; **c** myelosuppression; **d** neuropathy; **e** discontinuation due to linezolid adverse effects; **f** presence of any other adverse events)

Safety and tolerability

The major adverse events identified in this review were neuropathy and myelosuppression. Other minor adverse effects which were predominantly gastrointestinal related including nausea and vomiting were reported with a minimum pooled proportion of 33.60 % (95 %

CI = 20.41–48.23 %). Only one case of rhabdomyolysis has been reported by Lee et al. [42] which is an important observation to note in case of an emerging rare adverse effects of linezolid. Myelosuppression occurred at a higher proportion than neuropathy with both adverse events bearing a significant association with linezolid with combined proportions of 32.93 and 29.92 % respectively ($p < 0.0001$). In most studies, myelosuppression and neuropathy effects were managed by temporarily or permanently (15.01 %, $p < 0.0001$) discontinuing linezolid therapy. However, in some patients, incidence of severe anemia was remedied by blood transfusion [37]. Two cases were reported by Von der Lippe et al. for attaining normal full blood count upon withdrawal of linezolid without having to undergo blood transfusion [55]. The incidence of myelosuppression was significantly dose related ($p < 0.0001$) with lower doses associated with lower incidence. The incidence of neuropathy was reported in all studies except one [39]. Roongruangpitayakul et al. observed reversible optic neuropathy and irreversible peripheral neuropathy in patients who suffered these effects following treatment discontinuation and administration of vitamin B supplement [47]. Persistent irreversible neuropathy has also been previously reported by two other studies [53, 55]. From the results obtained ($p = 0.52$), neuropathy was not strongly associated with higher doses of linezolid and as such close monitoring of patients is encouraged irrespective of the dose administered. Therefore, in order to improve tolerability of linezolid regimen in MDR/XDR TB, a combined high dose (1200 mg daily) aimed at a shorter duration and lower dose (300–600 mg) targeted at a longer continuous phase may be employed with effective patient monitoring to inform dose adjustments when required.

Strengths and limitations

The major strength of our study is the large patient population ($n = 507$) which depicts a more significant and stronger evidence compared to previous reviews which included patient population of 218 [19], 121 [22] and 239 [23]. However, there are limitations including the higher proportion of non-randomized case series and retrospective studies ($n = 21$). This increases the likelihood of reporting and selection bias. Additionally, significant heterogeneity among studies are evident including presence of publication bias. Moreover, while this review provides some useful understanding regarding the safety and efficacy of linezolid, only 3 % of the patients involved in the studies' reviewed had documented HIV positive status. This calls for further research targeted at assessing the efficacy and safety of linezolid in HIV patients as they are more likely to develop active TB and TB-related mortality rates among them remains higher than the general population [59]. Also, better data would be needed to evaluate for instance treatment duration that optimally balances favorable clinical outcomes but minimizes occurrence of adverse effects to improve patient safety. Furthermore, while an earlier RCT conducted by Padayatchi et al. [60] was challenged by patient recruitment and retention, this has been overcome by a successfully conducted RCT by Tang et al. [51] while the sample size was relatively small, results from this RCT showed significant treatment success in the treatment group compared to the control group ($p = 0.013$). Nevertheless, there is urgent need for highly powered RCTs with larger sample size across highly endemic regions including participants from Africa to better inform the magnitude and significance of linezolid treatment effect in MDR and XDR TB patients.

Conclusions

Evidence available mainly from observational studies has demonstrated linezolid to be effective in the treatment of MDR/XDR TB. This presents the drug as a viable option towards effective pharmacotherapy for MDR/XDR TB which is increasingly becoming a global health challenge. Nonetheless, patients ought to be monitored closely for the incidence of major adverse events such as myelosuppression and neuropathy. To minimize adverse effects and improve clinical outcomes, a combined high dose (1200 mg daily) for an intensive phase followed by a lower dose (300–600 mg daily) for a continuous phase is proposed along with effective patient monitoring to inform dose adjustments when required. This may however require thorough future research investigation. Specific TB guidelines incorporating the use of linezolid are required and wider commitments from all global health players are needed to address barriers such as the high cost of the drug if successful use and accessibility is to be achieved particularly in low-resourced settings where majority of TB patients live.

Abbreviation

AIDS: acquired immune deficiency syndrome; HIV: human immunodeficiency virus; PRISMA: preferred reporting items for systematic reviews and meta-analyses; WHO: World Health Organization; DOT: directly observed treatment; TB: tuberculosis; MDR: multi-drug resistant; XDR: extensively-drug resistant; DST: drug sensitivity testing; RCT: randomized controlled trial; IRB: Institutional Review Board.

Authors' contribution

AA designed the study and provided guidance from start to finish. Both AA and RO were involved in the studies search, data extraction and analysis. All authors contributed to drafting this manuscript and approve of the content. Both authors read and approved the final manuscript.

Competing interests
The authors declare that they have no competing interests.

Source of funding
None.

References

1. WHO. Global tuberculosis report 2015. http://www.apps.who.int/iris/bitstream/10665/191102/1/9789241565059_eng.pdf?ua=1 Accessed 2 Feb 2016.
2. Maartens G, Wilkinson RJ. Tuberculosis. Lancet. 2007;307(9604):2030–43.
3. WHO. Tuberculosis. http://www.who.int/mediacentre/factsheets/fs104/en/ Accessed 2 Feb 2016.
4. WHO. Tuberculosis: the global burden 2005. http://www.who.int/tb/publications/tb_global_facts_sep05_en.pdf Accessed 2 Feb 2016.
5. Reid A, Grant AD, White RG, Dye C, Vynnycky E, Fielding K, Churchyard G, Pillay Y. Accelerating progress towards tuberculosis elimination: the need for combination treatment and prevention. Int J Tuberc Lung Dis. 2015;19(1):5–9.
6. WHO. Extensively drug-resistant tuberculosis (XDR-TB): recommendations for prevention and control. Wkly Epidemiol Rec. 2006;81(45):425–32.
7. WHO. Multidrug-resistant tuberculosis (MDR-TB). http://www.who.int/tb/challenges/mdr/en/ Accessed 2 Feb 2016.
8. Matteelli A, Roggi A, Carvalho AC. Extensively drug-resistant tuberculosis: epidemiology and management. Clin Epidemiol. 2014;6:111–8.
9. WHO. Multi-drug resistant tuberculosis (MDR-TB): 2015 update http://www.who.int/tb/challenges/mdr/mdr_tb_factsheet.pdf Accessed 3 Feb 2016.
10. Diel R, Nienhaus A, Lampenius N, Rüsch-Gerdes S, Richter E. Cost of multi drug resistance tuberculosis in Germany. Respir Med. 2014;108(11):1677–87.
11. StopTBPartnership. Global plan to stop TB, 2011–2015 http://www.stoptb.org/global/plan/plan1115.asp Accessed 9 Feb 2016.
12. WHO. Towards universal access to diagnosis and treatment of multidrug-resistant and extensively drug resistant tuberculosis by 2015: WHO progress report 2011. Geneva: WHO; 2011 **(WHO/HTM/TB/2011.3)**.
13. Alffenaar JWC, van Altena R, Harmelink IM, Filguera P, Molenaar E, Wessels AMA, et al. Comparison of the pharmacokinetics of two dosage regimens of linezolid in multidrug-resistant and extensively drug-resistant tuberculosis patients. Clin Pharmacokinet. 2010;49(8):559–65.
14. Sotgiu G, Pontali E, Migliori GB. Linezolid to treat MDR-/XDR-tuberculosis: available evidence and future scenarios. Eur Respir J. 2015;45:25–9.
15. Field SK, Fisher D, Jarand JM, et al. New treatment options for multidrug-resistant tuberculosis. Ther Adv Respir Dis. 2012;6:255–68.
16. Alcala L, Ruiz-Serrano JM, Turegano CP, de Viedma GD, Diaz-Infantes M, Marin-Arriaza M, et al. In vitro activities of linezolid against clinical isolates of *Mycobacterium tuberculosis* that are susceptible or resistant to first-line antituberculous drugs. Antimicrob Agents Chemother. 2003;47(1):416–7.
17. Guna R, Munoz C, Dominguez V, Garcia-Garcia A, Galvez J, de Julian-Ortiz J, et al. In vitro activity of linezolid, clarithromycin and moxifloxacin against clinical isolates of Mycobacterium kansasii. J Antimicrob Chemother. 2005;55(6):950–3.
18. Yang C, Hong L, Wang D, Meng X, He J, Tong A, et al. In vitro activity of linezolid against clinical isolates against *Mycobacterium tuberculosis*, including multi-drug resistant and extensively drug-resistant strains from Beijing, China. Jpn J Infect Dis. 2012;65:240–2.
19. Cox H, Ford N. Linezolid for the treatment of complicated drug-resistant tuberculosis: a systematic review and meta-analysis. Int J Tuberc Lung Dis. 2012;16(4):447–54.
20. Jaramillo E, Weyer K, Raviglione M. Linezolid for extensively drug-resistant tuberculosis. N Engl J Med. 2013;368(3):290.
21. Agyeman A, Ofori-Asenso R. Linezolid for the treatment of multi-drug and extensively drug resistant tuberculosis: a systematic review on efficacy and toxicity. Internet J Pharmacol. 2014;13(1).
22. Sotgiu G, Centis R, D'Ambrosio L, Alffenaar JW, Anger HA, Caminero JA, Castiglia P, De Lorenzo S, Ferrara G, Koh WJ, Schecter GF, Shim TS, Singla R, Skrahina A, Spanevello A, Udwadia ZF, Villar M, Zampogna E, Zellweger JP, Zumla A, Migliori GB. Efficacy, safety and tolerability of linezolid containing regimens in treating MDR-TB and XDR-TB: systematic review and meta-analysis. Eur Respir J. 2012;40(6):1430–42.
23. Zhang X, Falagas ME, Vardakas KZ, Wang R, Qin R, Wang J, Liu Y. Systematic review and meta-analysis of the efficacy and safety of therapy with linezolid containing regimens in the treatment of multidrug-resistant and extensively drug-resistant tuberculosis. J Thorac Dis. 2015;7(4):603–15.
24. Whitlock EP, Lin JS, Chou R, Shekelle P, Robinson KA. Using existing systematic reviews in complex systematic reviews. Ann Intern Med. 2008;148(10):776–82.
25. Moher D, Liberati A, Tetzlaff J, Altman DG. Preferred reporting items for systematic reviews and meta-analyses: the PRISMA statement. Ann Intern Med. 2009;151(4):264–9.
26. Wikipedia. Linezolid. https://www.en.wikipedia.org/wiki/Linezolid Accessed 2 Feb 2016.
27. Chan K, Bhandari M. Three-minute critical appraisal of a case series article. Indian J Orthop. 2011;45(2):103–4.
28. Law M, Stewart D, Pollock N, Letts L, Bosh J, Westmorland M. Critical review form-quantitative studies. McMaster University 1998 (28th July, 1998). http://www.srs-mcmaster.ca/wp-content/uploads/2015/04/Critical-Review-Form-Quantitative-Studies-English.doc. Accessed 1 Jan 2016.
29. Deenadayalan Y, Perraton L, Machotka Z, Kumar S. Day therapy programs for adolescents with mental health problems: a systematic review. Internet J Allied Health Sci Pract. 2010;8(1):1–14.
30. WHO. Treatment of tuberculosis: guidelines 2010 http://www.whqlibdoc.who.int/publications/2010/9789241547833_eng.pdf. Accessed 2 Feb 2016.
31. TBOnline. Linezolid. http://www.tbonline.info/posts/2011/8/24/linezolid/ Accessed 2 Feb 2016.
32. StatsDirect. Proportion meta-analysis http://www.statsdirect.com/help/default.htm#meta_analysis/proportion.htm. Accessed 4 February 2016.
33. Higgins JPT, Thompson SG, Deeks JJ, Altman DG. Measuring inconsistency in Meta-analyses. Br Med J. 2003;327(7414):557–60.
34. Song F, Khan KS, Dinnes J, Sutton AJ. Asymmetric funnel plots and publication bias in meta-analyses of diagnostic accuracy. Int J Epidemiol. 2002;31(1):88–95.
35. Abbate E, Vescovo M, Natiello M, Cufre M, Garcia A, Gonzalez Montaner P, et al. Successful alternative treatment of extensively drug-resistant tuberculosis in Argentina with a combination of linezolid, moxifloxacin and thioridazine. J Antimicrob Chemother. 2012;67(2):473–7.
36. Anger HA, Dworkin F, Sharma S, Munsiff SS, Nilsen DM, Ahuja SD. Linezolid use for treatment of multidrug-resistant and extensively drug-resistant tuberculosis, New York City, 2000–2006. J Antimicrob Chemother. 2010;65(4):775–83.
37. Condos R, Hadgiangelis N, Leibert E, Jacquette G, Harkin T, Rom WN. Case series report of a linezolid-containing regimen for extensively drug-resistant tuberculosis. Chest. 2008;134(1):187–92.
38. De Lorenzo S, Centis R, D'Ambrosio L, Sotgiu G, Migliori GB. On linezolid efficacy and tolerability. Eur Respir J. 2012;39(3):770–2.
39. Fortún J, Martín-Dávila P, Navas E, Pérez-Elías MJ, Cobo J, Tato M, De la Pedrosa EG, Gómez-Mampaso E, Moreno S. Linezolid for the treatment of multidrug-resistant tuberculosis. J Antimicrob Chemother. 2005;56(1):180–5.
40. Koh WJ, Kwon OJ, Gwak H, Chung JW, Cho SN, Kim WS, et al. Daily 300 mg dose of linezolid for the treatment of intractable multidrug-resistant and extensively drug-resistant tuberculosis. J Antimicrob Chemother. 2009;64(2):388–91.
41. Koh WJ, Kang YR, Jeon K, Jung Kwon O, Lyu J, Kim WS, et al. Daily 300 mg dose of linezolid for multidrug-resistant and extensively drug-resistant tuberculosis: updated analysis of 51 patients. J Antimicrob Chemother. 2012;67(6):1503–7.
42. Lee M, Lee J, Carroll MW, Choi H, Min S, Song T, et al. Linezolid for treatment of chronic extensively drug-resistant tuberculosis. N Engl J Med. 2012;367(16):1508–18.
43. Liu Y, Bao P, Wang D, Li Y, Tang L, Zhou Y, Zhao W. Clinical outcomes of linezolid treatment for extensively drug-resistant tuberculosis in

Beijing, China: a hospital-based retrospective study. Jpn J Infect Dis. 2015;68(3):244–7.

44. Migliori GB, Eker B, Richardson MD, Sotgiu G, Zellweger JP, Skrahina A, Ortmann J, Girardi E, Hoffmann H, Besozzi G, Bevilacqua N, Kirsten D, Centis R, Lange C, TBNET Study Group. A retrospective TBNET assessment of linezolid safety, tolerability and efficacy in multidrug-resistant tuberculosis. Eur Respir J. 2009;34(2):387–93.
45. Nam HS, Koh WJ, Kwon OJ, Cho SN, Shim TS. Daily half-dose linezolid for the treatment of intractable multidrug-resistant tuberculosis. Int J Antimicrob Agents. 2009;33(1):92–3.
46. Park IN, Hong SB, Oh YM, Kim MN, Lim CM, Lee SD, et al. Efficacy and tolerability of daily-half dose linezolid in patients with intractable multidrug-resistant tuberculosis. J Antimicrob Chemother. 2006;58(3):701–4.
47. Roongruangpitayakul C, Chuchottaworn C. Outcomes of MDR/XDR-TB patients treated with linezolid: experience in Thailand. J Med Assoc Thai. 2013;96(10):1273–82.
48. Schecter GF, Scott C, True L, Raftery A, Flood J, Mase S. Linezolid in the treatment of multidrug-resistant tuberculosis. Clin Infect Dis. 2010;50(1):49–55.
49. Singla R, Caminero JA, Jaiswal A, Singla N, Gupta S, Bali RK, et al. Linezolid: an effective, safe and cheap drug for patients failing multidrug-resistant tuberculosis treatment in India. Eur Respir J. 2012;39(4):956–62.
50. Tang SJ, Zhang Q, Zeng LH, Sun H, Gu J, Hao XH, et al. Efficacy and safety of linezolid in the treatment of extensively drug-resistant tuberculosis. Jpn J Infect Dis. 2011;64(6):509–12.
51. Tang S, Yao L, Hao X, Zhang X, Liu G, Liu X, Wu M, Zen L, Sun H, Liu Y, Gu J, Lin F, Wang X, Zhang Z. Efficacy, safety and tolerability of linezolid for the treatment of XDR-TB: a study in China. Eur Respir J. 2015;45(1):161–70.
52. Tse-Chang A, Kunimoto D, Der E, Ahmed R. Assessment of linezolid efficacy, safety and tolerability in the treatment of tuberculosis: a retrospective case review. Can J Infect Dis Med Microbiol. 2013;24(3):e50–2.
53. Udwadia ZF, Sen T, Moharil G. Assessment of linezolid efficacy and safety in MDR- and XDR-TB: an Indian perspective. Eur Respir J. 2010;35:936–8.
54. Villar M, Sotgiu G, D'Ambrosio L, Raymundo E, Fernandes L, Barbedo J, et al. Linezolid safety, tolerability and efficacy to treat multidrug- and extensively drug-resistant tuberculosis. Eur Respir J. 2011;38(3):730–3.
55. Von Der Lippe B, Sandven P, Brubakk O. Efficacy and safety of linezolid in multidrug resistant tuberculosis (MDR-TB)—a report of ten cases. J Infect. 2006;52(2):92–6.
56. Xu HB, Jiang RH, Li L, Xiao HP. Linezolid in the treatment of MDR-TB: a retrospective clinical study. Int J Tuberc Lung Dis. 2012;16(3):358–63.
57. Zhang L, Pang Y, Yu X, Wang Y, Gao M, Huang H, Zhao Y. Linezolid in the treatment of extensively drug-resistant tuberculosis. Infection. 2014;42(4):705–11.
58. Horsburgh CR, Shea KM, Phillips P, Lavalley M. Randomized clinical trials to identify optimal antibiotic treatment duration. Trials. 2013;28(14):88.
59. CDC. Drug-resistant TB. http://www.cdc.gov/tb/topic/drtb/ Accessed May 5 2016.
60. Padayatchi N, Mac Kenzie WR, Hirsch-Moverman Y, Feng PJ, Villarino E, Saukkonen J, Heilig CM, Weiner M, El-Sadr WM. Lessons from a randomized clinical trial for multidrug-resistant tuberculosis. Int J Tuberc Lung Dis. 2012;16(12):1582–7.

2

Occurrence of bla_{DHA-1} mediated cephalosporin resistance in *Escherichia coli* and their transcriptional response against cephalosporin stress: a report from India

Birson Ingti[1], Deepjyoti Paul[1], Anand Prakash Maurya[1], Debajyoti Bora[3], Debadatta Dhar Chanda[2], Atanu Chakravarty[2] and Amitabha Bhattacharjee[1*]

Abstract

Background: Treatment alternatives for DHA-1 harboring strains are challenging as it confers resistance to broad spectrum cephalosporins and may further limit treatment option when expressed at higher levels. Therefore, this study was designed to know the prevalence of DHA genes and analyse the transcription level of DHA-1 against different β-lactam stress.

Methods: Screening of AmpC β-lactamase phenotypically by modified three dimensional extract method followed by Antimicrobial Susceptibility and MIC determination. Genotyping screening of β-lactamase genes was performed by PCR assay followed by their sequencing. The bla_{DHA-1} transcriptional response was evaluated under different cephalosporin stress by RT PCR. Transferability of bla_{DHA} gene was performed by transformation and conjugation and plasmid incompatibility typing, DNA fingerprinting by enterobacterial repetitive intergenic consensus sequences PCR.

Results: 16 DHA-1 genes were screened positive from 176 *Escherichia coli* isolates and primer extension analysis showed a significant increase in DHA-1 mRNA transcription in response to cefotaxime at 8 μg/ml (6.99×10^2 fold), ceftriaxone at 2 μg/ml (2.63×10^3 fold), ceftazidime at 8 μg/ml (7.06×10^3 fold) and cefoxitin at 4 μg/ml (3.60×10^4 fold) when compared with untreated strain. These transcription data were found significant when analyzed statistically using one way ANOVA. Four different ESBL genes were detected in 10 isolates which include CTX-M (n = 6), SHV (n = 4), TEM (n = 3) and OXA-10 (n = 1), whereas, carbapenemase gene (NDM) was detected only in one isolate. Other plasmid mediated AmpC β-lactamases CIT (n = 9), EBC (n = 2) were detected in nine isolates. All DHA-1 genes detected were encoded in plasmid and incompatibility typing from the transformants indicated that the plasmid encoding bla_{DHA-1} was carried mostly by the FIA and L/M Inc group.

Conclusion: This study demonstrates the prevalence of DHA-1 gene in this region and highlights high transcription of DHA-1 when induced with different β-lactam antibiotics. Therefore, cephalosporin treatment must be restricted for the patients infected with pathogen expressing this resistance determinant.

Background

Escherichia coli (E. coli) possess a chromosomal cephalosporinase gene, which is regulated by a weak promoter and a transcriptional attenuator. The gene confers resistance only to narrow-spectrum cephalosporins [1, 2]. However, spontaneous mutations in the promoter, as well as transcriptional attenuator region of the AmpC gene may induce constitutive overproduction of the cephalosporinase resulting in resistance to penicillins and broad-spectrum cephalosporins (e.g. cefotaxime, ceftazidime, ceftriaxone, aztreonam etc.) [3, 4]. Besides hyper-production of the chromosomally encoded enzyme, the presence of one or more plasmid-mediated AmpC β-lactamases along with other intrinsic mechanisms in *E. coli* leads to resistance

*Correspondence: ab0404@gmail.com
[1] Department of Microbiology, Assam University, Silchar 788011, India
Full list of author information is available at the end of the article

against multiple antimicrobial agents, compromising the efficacy of treatment [5–7]. Six families of plasmid-encoded AmpC β-lactamases were described based on their sequence similarities as CIT, FOX, MOX, DHA, EBC, and ACC [8]. The most commonly recognized plasmid-mediated AmpC among the strains of *E. coli* includes the CMY-2 type which belongs to the CIT family [9, 10].

DHA-1, another plasmid-mediated AmpC β-lactamase, belonging to DHA family was found increasingly among Enterobacteriaceae in many parts of the world and was a growing concerned in the medical world as it leads to treatment failure [7]. It was first characterized in a *Salmonella enteritidis* which has the ability to hydrolyze penicillins, cephamycin, including broad spectrum cephalosporin leaving physicians with limited antibiotic choices. It was also the first plasmid-encoded β-lactamase found to be inducible and can be expressed in high levels [11, 12]. So far a total of 24 gene types of DHA family have been reported (http://www.ncbi.nlm.nih.gov/projects/pathogens/submit_beta_lactamase). The regulation of this β-lactamase expression is closely linked to cell wall recycling and involves at least three genes: *ampR* (codes for a transcriptional regulator of the LysR family), *ampG* (codes for a transmembrane permease) and *ampD* (codes for a cytosolic *N*-acetyl-anhydromuramyl- L-alanine amidase) [13].

Though it was well established that β-lactam antibiotics are potent inducers of class C in most of the members of the family Enterobacteriaceae [7], there is no relevant information on the level of AmpC expression taking place when the strains with incomplete regulatory elements were under antibiotic stress. Therefore, this study was undertaken to investigate the transcriptional response of DHA-1 under various cephalosporin's stresses.

Methods

Bacterial strains

A total of 176 consecutive, non-duplicate *Escherichia* isolates were collected from different clinical specimens (mostly from urine followed by pus) obtained from different Wards/OPD of Silchar Medical College and Hospital, India from October 2012 to March 2013. The isolates were identified by cultural characteristics, biochemical reactions and further confirmed by 16S rDNA sequencing using primers, a forward primer 5′-AGAGTTTGATCMTGGCTCAG-3′ and a reverse primer 5′-TACGGYTACCTTGTTACGACTT-3′.

Screening of AmpC β-lactamase by cefoxitin disc test and modified three dimensional extract method

Preliminary screening of AmpC β-lactamase was carried out on Mueller–Hinton Agar plates containing cefoxitin (30 μg) (Hi Media, Mumbai). Isolates with inhibition zones of less than 18 mm, were considered as screen positives [14]. The suspected AmpC β-lactamase producers were further confirmed by modified three dimensional extract test (M3DET) [15]. *Escherichia coli* ATCC 25922 and *Enterobacter cloacae* P99 were used as negative and positive control respectively.

Antimicrobial susceptibility and minimum inhibitory concentrations (MIC's) determination

Antimicrobial susceptibility was determined by Kirby Bauer disc diffusion method on Mueller–Hinton Agar plates. Following antibiotics were used: amikacin (30 μg), gentamicin (10 μg), ciprofloxacin (30 μg), trimethoprim/sulphamethoxazole (1.25/23.75 μg), tigecycline (15 μg) (Hi Media, Mumbai). MIC's of various antibiotics were also determined on Mueller–Hinton Agar plates by agar dilution method according to CLSI and EUCAST guidelines [16, 17]. Following antibiotics were used: cefotaxime, ceftazidime, ceftriaxone, cefepime, imipenem, meropenem, ertapenem and aztreonam (Hi-Media, Mumbai, India).

Detection of DHA gene by polymerase chain reaction

Polymerase chain reaction (PCR) was performed targeting all the DHA genes by using a pair of primers as listed in Table 1. Isolates positive for DHA genes were further investigated for the presence of other AmpC gene families, namely: CIT, ACC, FOX and EBC [18]. PCR amplification was performed using 30 μl of total reaction volume. Reactions were run under the following conditions: initial denaturation at 95 °C for 2 min, 34 cycles of 95 °C for 15 s, 51 °C for 1 min, 72 °C for 1 min and final extension at 72 °C for 7 min.

PCR products were purified by QIAquick Gel Extraction Kit (QIAGEN, Germany) and sequenced. Sequence results were analysed using a BLAST suite program of NCBI (http://blast.ncbi.nlm.nih.gov/Blast.cgi).

Molecular characterization of ESBL and carbapenemase genes by multiplex PCR

For amplification and characterization of ESBL genes, a set of five primers were used, namely: TEM, CTX-M, SHV, OXA-2, and PER [19]. Reactions were run under the following conditions: initial denaturation at 94 °C for 5 min, 33 cycles of 94 °C for 35 s., 51 °C for 1 min, 72 °C for 1 min and a final extension at 72 °C for 7 min.

For amplification and characterization of carbapenemase genes, a set of seven primers were used, namely: KPC, IMI, NMC, SME, VIM, IMP, and NDM (Table 1). Reactions were run as described previously.

Transcriptional expression analysis of $bla_{DHA\text{-}1}$ by quantitative realtime PCR

Expression of the $bla_{DHA\text{-}1}$ gene was studied in response to cefoxitin, cefotaxime, ceftriaxone and ceftazidime

Table 1 List of oligonucleotide primers for amplification of β-lactamase genes

Serial no.	Targets	Primers pairs	Sequence (5′→3′)	Product size (bp)	Reference
1	DHA-1 and DHA-2	DHA F DHA R	TGATGGCACAGCAGGATATTC GCTTTGACTCTTTCGGTATTCG	997	[18]
2	KPC	KPC F KPC R	5′-CATTCAAGGGCTTTCTTGCTGC-3′ 5′-ACGACGGCATAGTCATTTGC-3′	538	[20]
3	IMI/NMC	IMI/NMC F IMI/NMC R	5′-CCATTCACCCATCACAAC-3′ 5′-CTACCGCATAATCATTTGC-3′	440	[21]
4	SME	SME F SME R	5′-AACGGCTTCATTTTTGTTTAG-3′ 5′-GCTTCCGCAATAGTTTTATCA-3′	831	[22]
5	VIM	VIM F VIMR	5′-GATGGTGTTTGGTCGCATA-3′ 5′-CGAATGCGCAGCACCAG-3′	390	[23]
6	IMP	IMP F IMP R	5′-TTGACACTCCATTTACDG-3′ 5′-GATYGAGAATTAAGCCACYCT-3′	139	[23]
7	NDM	NDM F NDM R	5′-GGGCAGTCGCTTCCAACGGT-3′ 5′-GTAGTGCTCAGTGTCGGCAT-3′	476	[24]
8	DHA-1	DHA-RT F DHA-RT R	5′-TGATGGCACAGCAGGATATTC-3′ 5′-TACTTACAGATCCGAGCTCAA-3′	144	This study

stress at different concentrations (2, 4, 8 μg/ml) and was determined by inoculating the organisms harboring $bla_{\text{DHA-1}}$ in Luria–Bertani broth (Hi-media, Mumbai, India). Isolate without any antibiotic pressure was used as a control. A total RNA was isolated using Qiagen RNase Mini Kit (Qiagen, Germany), immediately reverse transcribed into cDNA by using QuantiTect® reverse transcription kit (Qiagen, Germany). The cDNA was quantified by Picodrop (Pico 200, Cambridge, UK) and quantitative real time PCR was performed using Power Sybr Green Master Mix (Applied Biosystem, Warrington, UK) in step one plus real time detection system (Applied Biosystem, USA). The house keeping gene *rpsel* of *E. coli* was used as an internal standard [25]. DHA-1 positive isolates showing resistance to broad spectrum cephalosporins and also devoid of other β-lactamases was selected for this study. The primer used for amplification of DHA-1 is listed in Table 1. PCR reactions were performed in triplicates for the isolate. The reaction was run under the following conditions: 95 °C for 2 min, 32 cycles of 95 °C for 20 s, 48 °C for 40 s and 72 °C for 1 min. The relative expression of $bla_{\text{DHA-1}}$ at a different antibiotics pressure was determined by the $\Delta\Delta C_t$ method. Relative quantification was compared with strain grown for 16 h without any antibiotic pressure.

Statistical analysis

The changes in DHA-1 mRNA expression in response to different β-lactam antibiotic stresses at different concentration were analyzed using one-way ANOVA followed by Tukey–Kramer (Tukey's W) multiple comparison test using SPSS version 17.0. Differences were considered statistically significant at both 5 and 1% level when $p < 0.05$. Data are presented as mean fold change + standard error of the mean.

Plasmid preparation

The bacterial isolates were cultured in Luria–Bertani broth (LB broth) containing 0.25 μg/ml of cefotaxime. Cultures were incubated on shaker incubator overnight at 37 °C, 160 rpm. Plasmids were purified by QIA prep Spin Miniprep Kit (QIAGEN, Germany).

Transferability of bla_{DHA} gene by transformation and conjugation

The transformation experiments were carried out by heat shock method [26] using *E. coli* DH5α as the recipient. Transformants were selected on cefotaxime (0.5 μg/ml) containing LB Agar plates.

Conjugation experiments were carried out between clinical isolates as donors and a streptomycin resistant *E. coli* strain B (Genei, Bangalore) as the recipient. An overnight culture of the bacteria was diluted in Luria–Bertani broth (Hi-Media, Mumbai, India) and was grown at 37 °C till the O.D. of the recipient and donor culture reached 0.8–0.9 at A_{600}. Donor and recipient cells were mixed at 1:5 donor-to-recipient ratios and transconjugants were selected L.B Agar plates supplemented with cefotaxime (0.5 μg/ml) and streptomycin (600 μg/ml).

Plasmid incompatibiltiy typing

For detection of incompatibility group type of plasmid carrying bla_{DHA}, PCR based replicon typing was carried out, targeting 18 different replicon types, to perform five multiplex and three simplex PCRs to amplify the FIA,

FIB, FIC, HI1, HI2, I1-Ig, L/M, N, P, W, T, A/C, K, B/O, X, Y, F and FIIA replicons [27].

DNA fingerprinting by enterobacterial repetitive intergenic consensus sequences PCR

Typing of all bla_{DHA-1} producing *E. coli* isolates was done by enterobacterial repetitive intergenic consensus (ERIC) PCR as described previously [28]. Isolates were put into cluster based on banding pattern and dendogram was prepared by NTSYS software.

Results

During the study period, a total of 176 *E. coli* isolates were obtained from different clinical samples. Among these, 110 (62.5%) were resistant to cefoxitin and 63 (35.8%) isolates were found to show AmpC activity by M3DET. By performing PCR, 16 isolates were detected for DHA genes and showed a sequence identical to that of DHA-1 (Table 1). These isolates harboring DHA-1 gene were selected for further study. Among DHA-1 positive isolates four different ESBL genes were detected in 10 isolates which include CTX-M (n = 6), SHV (n = 4), TEM (n = 3) and OXA-10 (n = 1). Carbapenemase gene (NDM-1) was detected only in one isolate. Other plasmid mediated AmpC β-lactamase CIT (n = 9), EBC (n = 2) were detected in nine isolates that carried either CTX-M (n = 3),SHV (n = 1), TEM (n = 1), NDM (n = 1) alone or CTX-M plus SHV(n = 2), CTX-M plus TEM (n = 1) and OXA-10 plus SHV (n = 1) (Table 2). These isolates harboring AmpC β-lactamase were mostly obtained from Surgery and medicine ward. To demonstrate whether DHA-1 expression would take place in the presence of different cephalosporins at a different concentration, an *E.coli* strain BM-567 (Table 2) harboring only DHA-1 β-lactamase and showing resistance to broad spectrum cephalosporins was selected. The fold increase in mRNA production was measured using primer extension analysis. It was observed that there was a significant increase in the expression of DHA-1 gene in response to cefotaxime, ceftriaxone, ceftazidime but not as high as those for cefoxitin when compared with the basal level without antibiotic pressure (Fig. 1). Though increased in transcription was observed in response to these β-lactam antibiotics, high transcript level were achieved when induced by cefotaxime at 8 μg/ml (6.99×10^2 fold), ceftriaxone at 2 μg/ml (2.63×10^3 fold), ceftazidime at 8 μg/ml (7.06×10^3 fold) and cefoxitin at 4 μg/ml (3.60×10^4 fold) (Fig. 1). The ANOVA and Tukey–Kramer (Tukey's W) multiple comparison test for checking the differences in the expression of DHA-1 was found to be significant (p value is less than 0.05; Table 3).

Typing by ERIC-PCR confirmed 16 different haplotypes (Fig. 2) indicating the diversity of the isolates. The susceptibility pattern of these bla_{DHA-1} harboring isolates showed resistance towards β-lactam including broad spectrum cephalosporin but most of them were susceptible against a carbapenem group of drugs. They also show susceptibility to tigecycline and moderate to high resistance against amikacin, gentamycin, co-trimoxazole, ciprofloxacin. The MICs of selected β-lactam antibiotics for all the parental strains harboring DHA-1 were found to be above breakpoint level (Table 2). The transformation experiment could establish that DHA-1 was encoded in plasmid however, conjugation experiment revealed that only 4 isolates could conjugatively transfer DHA-1 gene in *E. coli* strain B which was confirmed by PCR analysis. On performing incompatibility typing it was established that most of the transformants with DHA-1 were associated with K, FIA, L/M, FIB, HI1, B/O & I1 *Inc* group (Table 2).

Discussion

The first plasmid mediated AmpC β-lactamase, to be reported was CMY-1, in 1989 [29]. Since then, several plasmid-encoded AmpC β-lactamases (ACC, FOX, MOX, CMY, ACT, etc.) have been reported in several genera of bacteria, including *Salmonella* spp., *Pseudomonas* spp., *Proteus mirabilis* and *Klebsiella pneumoniae* [7]. Among them plasmid encoded DHA-1; a clinically important AmpC β-lactamase was the first β-lactamase found to be inducible and can be expressed at higher levels in strains having AmpR regulatory gene [11, 30]. This plasmid- mediated β-lactamase is now being increasingly detected in a strain of *E. coli* worldwide [31–33] and early detection of this β-lactamase (DHA-1) is mandatory for better antibiotic therapy and also to prevent further spread. The present study reports the prevalence of DHA-1 (9%) among *E. coli* strains in this region which is quite high compared to other studies [30, 32, 33] and typing of these DHA-1 harboring isolates by ERIC PCR revealed diverse haplotypes, indicating the spread of the DHA-1 gene through horizontal transfer. Based on the present susceptibility data (Table 2) and previous studies [11, 12], carbapenem and other non-β-lactam antibiotics such as tigecycline could be better drugs of choice for the treatment of infections caused by *E. coli* producing DHA-1.

From the earlier study, it appears that *E. coli* lack one of the regulatory component (AmpR gene), which leads to the lower level, non-inducible expression of AmpC [34]. However, inducible cephalosporinase (bla_{CMY-13}) found associated with an AmpR gene was detected recently in a strain of *E. coli* [35]. Several broad spectrum cephalosporins were believed to increase the expression of AmpC β-lactamase [36], although the concentration which leads to increase in the expression of AmpC β-lactamase was not established.

Table 2 Clinical history, their molecular details and resistance profile of DHA-1 gene-positive *E. coli* isolates

Sl. No.	Sample ID	Age (years)	Sex	Ward/clinics	Type of clinical specimen	[a]ESBL genes detected	Carbapen-emase genes detected	Other plas-mid AmpC genes	(Inc type)	Resistance profile	MIC of β-lactam (mg/l)							
											CTX	CAZ	CRO	FEP	ATM	IMP	MEM	ETP
1	BM12	35	Male	Surgery	Pus	–	–	–	K	AMK, GEN, SXT	>512	>512	256	>512	64	16	8	8
2	BM26	107	Female	Pediatrics	Urine	TEM	–	–	FIA,	CIP, AMK, GEN, SXT	64	128	64	8	64	<2	<2	<2
3	BM59	55	Female	Medicine	Urine	–	–	–	FIA	CIP, AMK, GEN, SXT	128	64	64	16	128	<2	<2	<2
4	BM63	60	Female	Surgery	Pus	CTX-M	–	CIT	–	CIP, AMK, GEN, SXT	128	128	256	16	64	<2	<2	<2
5	BM130	27	Female	Surgery	Pus	TEM	–	CIT, EBC	HI1, L/M	CIP, AMK, GEN, SXT	>512	512	>512	64	256	16	4	4
6	BM138	45	Male	Surgery	Pus	CTX-M	–	–	–	CIP, GEN, SXT	64	128	128	32	128	<2	<2	<2
7	BM197	30	Female	Surgery	Pus	–	–	CIT	L/M	CIP, AMK, GEN, SXT	512	>512	256	64	512	2	<2	<2
8	BM230	43	Female	Surgery	Pus	CTX-M, SHV	–	CIT	L/M	CIP, AMK, GEN, SXT	64	128	256	32	256	16	8	16
9	BM252	7	Female	Paediatrics	Urine	SHV	–	CIT, EBC	F1B, FIA	CIP, AMK, GEN, SXT	>512	>512	>512	128	256	8	<2	<2
10	BM355	10	Male	Paediatrics	Urine	–	NDM	CIT	FIA	CIP, AMK, SXT	>512	512	>512	8	256	<2	<2	<2
11	BM409	61	Male	Medicine	Urine	CTX-M	–	CIT	K	CIP, AMK, GEN, SXT	64	64	32	16	128	<2	<2	<2
12	BM441	40	Male	Medicine	Stool	CTX-M, SHV	–	–	FIA	CIP, AMK, GEN, SXT	32	64	128	32	256	<2	<2	<2
13	BM508	48	Male	Surgery	Pus	–	–	CIT	I1	CIP, AMK, GEN	32	32	32	16	256	<2	<2	<2
14	BM520	55	Female	Surgery	Pus	OXA-10, SHV	–	–	–	CIP, GEN, SXT	16	128	128	32	32	<2	<2	<2
15	BM567	30	Male	Medicine	Urine	–	–	–	–	CIP, AMK, GEN, SXT	128	256	256	32	256	<2	<2	<2
16	BM576	40	Female	Medicine	Urine	CTX-M, TEM	–	CIT	K, B/O	AMK, GEN, SXT	>512	>512	>512	128	>512	16	16	32

AMK amikacin; *GEN* gentamycin; *CIP* ciprofloxacin; *SXT* cottrimoxazole; *CTX* cefotaxime; *CAZ* ceftazidime; *CRO* ceftriaxone; *FEP* cefepime; *ATM* aztreonam; *IMP* imipenem; *MEM* meropenem; *ETP* ertapenem

[a] Extended spectrum β-lactamase

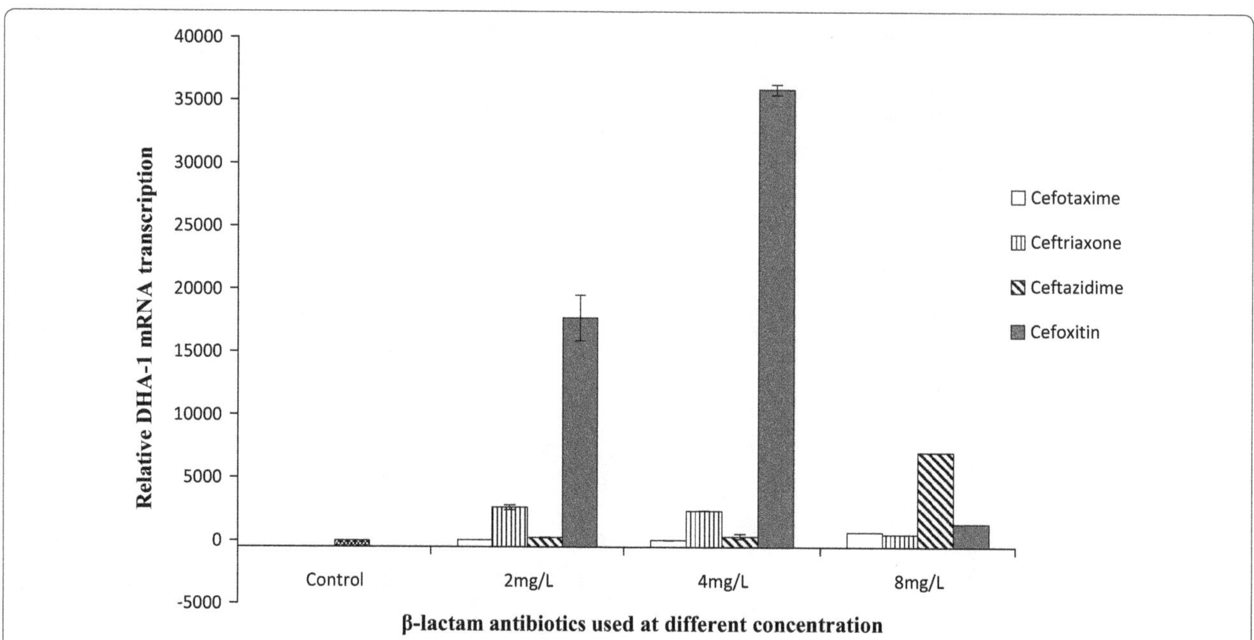

Fig. 1 Transcriptional analysis of DHA-1 espression by RT-PCR. Total bacterial RNA was isolated from mid-log- phase cultures of *E. coli*. The *error bars* represent the standard deviations of the means of triplicate samples

Table 3 Statistical analysis of changes in DHA-1 mRNA expression in response to different-lactam antibiotic stress at different concentration using one way ANOVA

Sl no.	β-lactam antibiotics	Value (Mean ± SEM)				p value
		NA	2 mg/l	4 mg/l	8 mg/l	
1	Cefotaxime	1.00 ± 0	56.66 ± 1.18	58.10 ± 0.58	699.25 ± 5.27	0.001*
2	Ceftriaxone	1.00 ± 0	2634.69 ± 16.58	2383.97 ± 20.73	510.70 ± 6.04	
3	Ceftazidime	1.00 ± 0	249.50 ± 11.63	356.27 ± 14.20	7059.48 ± 60.91	
4	Cefoxitin	1.00 ± 0	17721.31 ± 608.47	35855.21 ± 1050.38	1363.69 ± 237.37	

NA no antibiotic; *SEM* standard error of the mean

* Significant ($p < 0.05$)

This study demonstrates higher transcription of DHA-1 when induced with different cephalosporins. These differences in the relative amounts of RNA transcription of DHA-1 gene, when induced with different cephalosporins at a concentration below MIC level suggest that the transcription varies depending on the level of antibiotics stress. Higher AmpC production was supported by another finding, where *bla*MIR-1, a plasmid-encoded *AmpC* gene exhibited a 95-fold increase in expression relative to WT *AmpC* [37]. Concentration dependent expression of AmpC cephalosporinase was also observed in a strain of *Pseudomonas aeruginosa*, when the strain was induced with cefoxitin or clavulanic acid at 8, 16 and 50 μg/ml [38]. So far, the factors behind the quantitative differences of AmpC expression in *E.coli* strain when exposed to different β-lactam concentration is unknown. A transformation experiment could establish that all the DHA-1 gene were encoded in a plasmid which is in agreement with the previous study [12, 30–33] and Incompatibility typing from the transformants indicated that the plasmid encoding bla_{DHA-1} was carried mostly by FIA and L/M Inc group as found in another study [39]. Although detection of other Inc group, namely HI1, FIB, I1, K in the present study was mostly associated with CMY-2 and ACC harboring strains [39]. Plasmids carrying genes for AmpC β-lactamases often carry ESBL genes such as CTX-M [40, 41] as found in the present study, where most of these DHA-1 harboring isolates co-harbour ESBL genes (Table 2). Co-existence of New Delhi metallo-β-lactamase (NDM) gene was also observed in one isolate as the high prevalence of the *E. coli* harboring a metallo-β-lactamase known as the NDM has been increasingly observed in the Indian subcontinent [42].

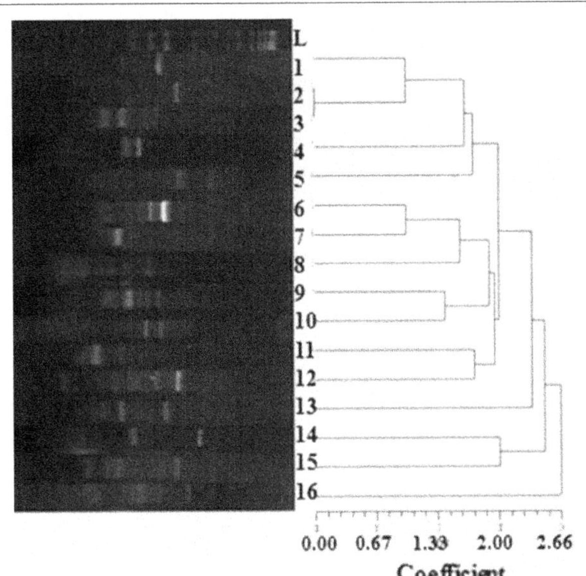

Fig. 2 ERIC PCR analysis of *E. coli* producing DHA-1 β-lactamase. *Lane* L: molecular weight marker; *lanes* 1–16: isolates harboring DHA-1 β-lactamase

Conclusion

Strains harboring plasmid mediated AmpC (DHA-1) genes are often resistant to multiple antimicrobial agents and the overexpression of this resistant determinant when induced with different cephalosporins stress will further limit treatment option. The present study demonstrates that higher expression of DHA-1 takes place when induced with specific concentrations of β-lactam antibiotics, although further research is required to understand the factors behind the upregulation of DHA-1 gene in the future. Therefore, revision in cephalosporin usage policy is required for effective treatment of patients infected with pathogen harboring this mechanism.

Authors' contributions

BI performed the experimental work, data collection and analysis and prepared the manuscript. AB supervised the research work and participated in designing the study and drafting the manuscript. DP and APM participated in sample collection and part of experiments. DB participated in statistical analysis. DD and AC Participated in experiment designing and manuscript correction. All authors read and approved the final manuscript.

Author details

[1] Department of Microbiology, Assam University, Silchar 788011, India. [2] Department of Microbiology, Silchar Medical College and Hospital, Silchar 788014, India. [3] Department of Statistics, Dibrugarh University, Dibrugarh, India.

Acknowledgements

The authors would like to acknowledge the help of HOD, Microbiology, Assam University for providing infrastructure. The authors sincerely acknowledge the financial support provided by University Grants Commissions (UGC-MRP) Government of India. Authors also acknowledge the help from Assam University Biotech Hub for providing laboratory facility to complete this work.

Competing interests

The authors declared that they have no competing interests.

Consent for publication

All the authors read and approved the final version of the manuscript.

Ethical approval

The work was approved by Institutional Ethical committee of Assam University, Silchar vide Reference Number: IEC/AUS/C/2014-003. The authors confirm that participants provided their written informed consent to participate in this study.

Funding

University grants commission (UGC-MRP) and (UGC-RGNF) to Birson Ingti Vide letter no. F1-17.1/2013-14/RGNF-2013-14-ST-ASS-38069/(SAIII/Website).

References

1. Jaurin B, Grundstrom T. AmpC cephalosporinase of *Escherichia coli* K-12 has a different evolutionary origin from that of β-lactamases of the penicillinase type. Proc Natl Acad Sci USA. 1981;78:4897–901.
2. Bergstrom S, Normark S. β-Lactam resistance in clinical isolates of *Escherichia coli* caused by elevated production of the *ampC* mediated chromosomal β-lactamase. Antimicrob Agents Chemother. 1979;16:427–33.
3. Caroff N, Espaze E, Gautreau D, Richet H, Reynaud A. Analysis of the effects of −42 and −32 ampC promoter mutations in clinical isolates of *Escherichia coli* hyperproducing ampC. J Antimicrob Chemother. 2000;45:783–8.
4. Jaurin B, Grundstrom T, Edlund T, Normark S. The *E. coli* β-lactamase attenuator mediates growth rate-dependent regulation. Nature. 1981;290:221–5.
5. Deshpande LM, Jones RN, Fritsche TR, Sader HS. Occurrence of plasmidic AmpC type β-lactamase-mediated resistance in *Escherichia coli*: report from the SENTRY Antimicrobial Surveillance Program (North America, 2004). Int J Antimicrob Agents. 2006;28:578–81.
6. Mammeri H, Nordmann P, Berkani A, Eb F. Contribution of extended-spectrum AmpC (ESAC) β-lactamases to carbapenem resistance in *Escherichia coli*. FEMS Microbiol Lett. 2008;282:238–40.
7. Jacoby GA. *AmpC* β-lactamases. Clin Microbiol Rev. 2009;22:161–82.
8. Pérez-Pérez FJ, Hanson ND. Detection of plasmid-mediated AmpC β-lactamase genes in clinical isolates by using multiplex PCR. J Clin Microbiol. 2002;40:2153–62.
9. Naseer U, Haldorsen B, Simonsen GS, Sundsfjord A. Sporadic occurrence of CMY-2-producing multidrug-resistant *Escherichia coli* of ST-complexes 38 and 448, and ST131 in Norway. Clin Microbiol Infect. 2010;16:171–8.
10. Pavez M, Neves P, Dropa M, et al. Emergence of carbapenem resistant *Escherichia coli* producing CMY-2-type AmpC β-lactamase in Brazil. J Med Microbiol. 2008;57:1590–2.
11. Gaillot O, Clement C, Simonet M, Philippon A. Novel transferable β-lactam resistance with cephalosporinase characteristics in *Salmonella enteritidis*. J Antimicrob Chemother. 1997;39:85–7.
12. Barnaud G, Arlet G, Verdet C, Gaillot O, Lagrange PH, Philippon A. *Salmonella enteritidis*: AmpC plasmid-mediated inducible β-lactamase (DHA-1) with an *ampR* gene from *Morganella morganii*. Antimicrob Agents Chemother. 1998;42:2352–8.
13. Hanson ND, Sanders CC. Regulation of inducible AmpC β-lactamase expression among Enterobacteriaceae. Curr Pharm Des. 1999;5:881–94.
14. Lorian V. Antibiotics in laboratory medicine. 5th ed. Philadelphia: Lippincott Williams and Wilkins; 2005.
15. Coudron PE, Moland ES, Thomson KS. Occurrence and detection of AmpC β-lactamases among *Escherichia coli*, *Klebsiella pneumoniae*, and *Proteus mirabilis* isolates at a Veterans Medical Center. J Clin Microbiol. 2000;38:1791–6.

16. Clinical and Laboratory Standards Institute. Performance standards for antimicrobial susceptibility testing; twenty-third informational supplement. M100-S23. Wayne: CLSI; 2013.
17. European committee on antimicrobial susceptibility testing. Breakpoint tables for interpretation of MICs and zone diameters, version 6.0; 2016.
18. Caroline D, Anaelle DC, Dominique D, Christine F, Guillaume A. Development of a set of multiplex PCR assays for the detection of genes encoding important β-lactamases in Enterobacteriaceae. J Antimicrob Chemother. 2010;65:490–5.
19. Lee S, Park YJ, Kim M, Lee HK, Han K, Kang CS. Prevalence of Ambler class A and D β-lactamases among clinical isolates of *Pseudomonas aeruginosa* in Korea. J Antimicrob Chemother. 2005;56:122–7.
20. Nass T, Cuzon G, Villegas MV, Lartigue MF, Quinn JP, Nordmann P. Genetic structures at the origin of acquisition of the β-lactamase blaKPC gene. Antimicrob Agents Chemother. 2008;52:1257–63.
21. Rasmussen BA, Bush K, Keeney D, Yang Y, Hare R, Gara CO, et al. Characterization of IMI-1 betalactamase, a class A carbapenem-hydrolyzing enzyme from Enterobacter cloaceae. Antimicrob Agents Chemother. 1996;40:2080–6.
22. Nass T, Vandel L, Sougakoff W, Livermore DM, Nordmann P. Cloning and sequence analysis of the gene for a carbapenem hydrolyzing class A β-lactamase, SME-1, from Serratia marcescens S6. Antimicrob Agents Chemother. 1994;38:1262–70.
23. Jh Y, Yi K, Lee H, Yong D, Lee K, Kim JM, et al. Molecular characterization of metallo-β-lacatamaseproducing Acinetobacter baumannii and Acinetbacter genomospecies 3 from Korea: identification of two new integrons carrying the blaVIM-2 gene cassettes. J Antimicrob Chemother. 2002;49:837–40.
24. Yong D, Toleman MA, Giske CG, Cho HS, Sundman K, Lee K, et al. Characterization of a New Metallo-β-Lactamase Gene, blaNDM-1, and a Novel Erythromycin Esterase Gene Carried on a Unique Genetic Structure in Klebsiella pneumoniae Sequence Type 14 from India. Antimicrob Agents Chemother. 2009;53:5046–54.
25. Swick MC, Morgan-Linnell SK, Carlson KM, et al. Expression of multidrug efflux pump genes *acrAB-tolC*, *mdfA* and *norE* in *Escherichia coli* clinical isolates as a function of fluroquinolone and multidrug resistance. Antimicrob Agents Chemother. 2011;55:921–4.
26. Sambrook J, Fritsch EF, Maniatis T. Molecular cloning: a laboratory manual. 2nd ed. New York: Cold Spring Harbor Laboratory Press; 1989.
27. Carattoli A, Bertini A, Villa L, Falbo V, et al. Identification of plasmids by PCR-based replicon typing. J Microbiol Methods. 2005;63:219–28.
28. Versalovic J, Koeuth T, Lupski JR. Distribution of repetitive DNA sequences in eubacteria and application to fingerprinting of bacterial genomes. Nucleic Acids Res. 1995;19:6823–31.
29. Bauernfeind A, Chong Y, Schweighart S. Extended broad spectrum β-lactamase in *Klebsiella pneumoniae* including resistance to cephamycins. Infection. 1989;17:316–21.
30. Yong D, Limc Y, Song W, et al. Plasmid-mediated, inducible AmpC β-lactamase (DHA-1)-producing Enterobacteriaceae at a Korean hospital: wide dissemination in *Klebsiella pneumoniae* and *Klebsiella oxytoca* and emergence in *Proteus mirabilis*. Diagn Microbiol Infect Dis. 2005;53:65–70.
31. Pham JN, Chambers I, Poirel L, Nordmann P, Bell SM. Detection of a plasmid-mediated inducible cephalosporinase DHA-1 from *Escherichia coli*. Pathology. 2010;42(2):196–7.
32. Giakkoupi P, Tambic-Andrasevic A, Vourli S, et al. Transferable DHA-1 cephalosporinase in *Escherichia coli*. Int J Antimicrob Agents. 2006;27:77–80.
33. Song W, Kim JS, Kim HS, et al. Emergence of *Escherichia coli* isolates producing conjugative plasmid-mediated DHA-1 β-lactamase in a Korean University Hospital. J. Hospital Infection. 2006;63:459–64.
34. Honore N, Nicolas MH, Cole ST. Inducible cephalosporinase production in clinical isolates of *Enterobacter cloacae* is controlled by a regulatory gene that has been deleted from *Escherichia coli*. EMBO J. 1986;5(13):3709–14.
35. Miriagou V, Tzouvelekis LS, Villa L, Lebessi E, Vatopoulos AC, Carattoli A, et al. CMY-13, a novel inducible cephalosporinase encoded by an *Escherichia coli* plasmid. Antimicrob Agents Chemother. 2004;48:3172–4.
36. Livermore DM. Clinical significance of β-lactamase induction and stable derepression in gram-negative rods. Eur. J. Clin. Microbiol. 1987;6:439–45.
37. Reisbig MD, Ashfaque H, Nancy DH. Factors influencing gene expression and resistance for gram-negative organisms expressing plasmid-encoded *ampC* genes of *Enterobacter* origin. J Antimicrob Chemother. 2003;2003(51):1141–51.
38. Lister PD, Gardner VM, Sanders CC. Clavulanate induces expression of the *Pseudomonas aeruginosa* AmpC cephalosporinase at physiologically relevant concentrations and antagonizes the antibacterial activity of ticarcillin. Antimicrob Agents Chemother. 1999;43:882–9.
39. Mata C, Miro E, Alvarado A, et al. Plasmid typing and genetic context of AmpC β-lactamases in Enterobacteriaceae lacking inducible chromosomal ampC genes: findings from a Spanish hospital 1999–2007. J Antimicrob Chemother. 2012;67:115–22.
40. Migma DT, Hyang NM, Geum CJ, Su RK, Myung HC, Suk CJ, et al. Molecular characterization of extended-spectrum-β-lactamase- producing and plasmid-mediated AmpC β-lactamase-producing *Escherichia coli* isolated from stray dogs in South Korea. Antimicrob Agents Chemother. 2012;56:2705–12.
41. Lee CH, Liu JW, Li CC, Chien CC, Tang YF, Su LH. Spread of IS*CR1* elements containing bla_{DHA-1} and multiple antimicrobial resistance genes leading to increase of flomoxef resistance in extended-spectrum-β-lactamase producing *Klebsiella pneumoniae*. Antimicrob Agents Chemother. 2011;55:4058–63.
42. Kumarasamy KK, Toleman MA, Walsh TR, Bagaria J, Butt F, Balakrishnan R, et al. Emergence of a new antibiotic resistance mechanism in India, Pakistan, and the UK: a molecular, biological, and epidemiological study. Lancet Infect. Dis. 2012;10:597–602.

3

Emerging azithromycin-resistance among the *Neisseria gonorrhoeae* strains isolated in Hungary

Alexandra Brunner[1], Eva Nemes-Nikodem[2], Csaba Jeney[3], Dora Szabo[3], Marta Marschalko[1], Sarolta Karpati[1] and Eszter Ostorhazi[3*]

Abstract

Background: In the 1990s, azithromycin became the drug of choice for many infectious diseases but emerging resistance to the drug has only been reported in the last decade. In the last 5 years, the National *Neisseria gonorrhoeae* Reference Laboratory of Hungary (NNGRLH) has also observed an increased number of *N. gonorrhoeae* strains resistant to azithromycin. The aim of this study was to determine the most frequent sequence types (ST) of *N. gonorrhoeae* related to elevated levels of azithromycin MIC (minimal inhibitory concentration). Previously and currently isolated azithromycin-resistant strains have been investigated for the existence of molecular relationship.

Methods: Maldi-Tof technic was applied for the identification of the strains isolated from outpatients attending the reference laboratory. Testing antibiotic susceptibility of azithromycin, cefixime, ceftriaxone, tetracycline, spectinomycin and ciprofloxacin was carried out for all the identified strains, using MIC strip test Liofilchem®. *N. gonorrhoeae* multiantigen sequence typing (NG-MAST) was performed exclusively on azithromycin-resistant isolates. A phylogenetic tree was drawn using MEGA6 (Molecular Evolutionary Genetics Analysis Version 6.0) Neighbour-Joining method.

Results: Out of 192 *N. gonorrhoeae* isolates, 30.0 % (58/192) proved resistant to azithromycin (MIC > 0.5 mg/L). Of the azithromycin-resistant isolates, ST1407, ST4995 and ST11064 were the most prevalent. Based on the phylogenetic analysis, the latter two STs are closely related.

Conclusions: In contrast to West-European countries, in our region, resistance to azithromycin has increased up to 30 % in the last 5 years, so the recommendation of the European Guideline −500 mg of ceftriaxone combined with 2 g of azithromycin as first choice therapy against *N. gonorrhoeae*- should be seriously considered in case of Hungary.

Keywords: Azithromycin-resistance, *Neisseria gonorrhoeae*, Sequence types, Phylogenetic tree

Background

The treatment of gonorrhoea infection poses a continuous problem as *Neisseria gonorrhoeae* has developed resistance to each antimicrobials used in the past 70 years [1]. Therefore, it is necessary to enhance the surveillance of gonococcal antimicrobial resistance, especially for the drugs of first choice: ceftriaxone and azithromycin [2]. In Hungary, resistance to ceftriaxone has not yet been reported. In contrast, the appearance and spread of azithromycin-resistance have been observed in the last 4 years [3].

Since the 1990s, azithromycin has become the drug of choice for many infections, such as sexually transmitted diseases (STDs), community-acquired pneumonia, acute bacterial sinusitis, otitis media, tonsillitis, pharyngitis, skin infections or acute bacterial exacerbations of chronic obstructive pulmonary disease [4]. Of STDs, azithromycin is used to treat uncomplicated gonorrhoea in patients with cephalosporin allergy, *Chlamydia trachomatis* co-infection, *Heamophilus ducreyii, Ureaplasma urealyticum, Mycoplasma genitalium* infections. This antibiotic

*Correspondence: ostorhazi.eszter@med.semmelweis-univ.hu
[3] Institute of Medical Microbiology, Semmelweis University, 4 Nagyvárad Square, Budapest, Hungary
Full list of author information is available at the end of the article

revolutionised the therapy as it shortened treatment time from 7–14 days to 1–5 days and improved patient compliance due to high tissue levels and long half-life. New administration formulations such as sustained-release microspheres allowed higher doses to be administered and reduced gastrointestinal side-effects, so azithromycin seemed to be capable of approaching the concept of an ideal antibiotic [5]. However, recently decreased antimicrobial susceptibility to azithromycin may disprove this assumption.

According to the data of the European Surveillance of Antimicrobial Consumption (ESAC), in Hungary the outpatient consumption of antimicrobials was 16.0 defined daily doses (DDD) per 1000 inhabitants per day. This number can be subdivided into major antibiotic classes such as penicillins topping the list by DDD of 7.19, macrolides taking the second place with DDD of 2.94 and, finally, cephalosporins with DDD of 2.13 [6].

Nevertheless, at the National *Neisseria gonorrhoeae* Reference Laboratory of Hungary (NNGRLH), we observed the appearance and rapid spread of azithromycin-resistance in Hungary between 2010 and 2013. We aimed to survey the antimicrobial susceptibility in 2014 and compare it with the data of the last 4 years and characterise the azithromycin-resistant strains by NG-MAST.

Molecular evolutionary analysis was conducted and genetic relationships were estimated between the STs spreading in Hungary in 2014.

Methods

Bacterial strains and medical records

The NNGRLH at the STD Centre in the Department of Dermatology, Venerology and Dermatooncology of Semmelweis University, Budapest, Hungary collected samples from consecutive symptomatic gonorrhoea patients and from their asymptomatic contacts in 2014. The samples were cultured, characterised and stored on Cryobank breads (Mast Diagnostic, Germany) at −80 °C. Clinical data such as sex, age, sexual orientation, anatomic site of infection were recorded. *C. trachomatis* co-infection was also screened. Patients' data were analysed according to law 1997/CLIV 26§ taking into account maximum privacy rights and anonymity of patients [7].

Antibiotic susceptibility

Clinical samples -cervical, anal, urethral and pharyngeal swabs- were obtained and grown on preheated VCA3 agar (Biomérieux, Budapest, Hungary) and on non-selective PVX chocolate agar (Biomérieux, Budapest, Hungary) at 37 °C in an atmosphere of 5 % of carbon dioxide for 24–48 h. Minimum inhibitory concentrations (MIC; mg/L) were determined for azithromycin, cefixime, ceftriaxone, tetracycline, spectinomycin and ciprofloxacin on PVX chocolate agar (Biomérieux, Budapest, Hungary) using MIC strip tests (Liofilchem® s.r.l., Roseto degli Abruzzi, Italy) according to the manufacturer's instructions, using a direct colony suspension equivalent to McFarland standard of 0.5. Testing conditions also included incubation at 36.5 °C and 5 % of carbon dioxide for 24 h. All results were interpreted by using breakpoints for susceptibility and resistance according to the European Committee on Antimicrobial Susceptibility Testing (EUCAST) [8]. Concerning the MIC breakpoints of azithromycin, strains with MICs over 0.25 mg/L but below 0.5 mg/L were considered to be of intermediate resistance. Isolates with MICs higher than 0.5 mg/L were considered resistant. *N. gonorrhoeae* ATCC 49226, with an azithromycin MIC of 0.12 mg/L, was used as a control strain to ensure the quality of the susceptibility tests.

Molecular methods

Out of the 58 resistant and 42 intermediately resistant strains 29 and 21 were selected for *N. gonorrhoeae* multiantigen sequence typing (NG-MAST) according to a previously described method [9]. The sequences of *porB* and *tbpB* PCR products were determined after their preliminary purification by the Exosap IT purification kit (Affymetrix, USA). BigDye® Terminator v3.1 Cycle Sequencing Kit (Life Technologies, USA) was used and the same forward and reverse primers were applied as for *porB* and *tbpB* PCR methods. Last purification was carried out by NucleoSEQ Column PCR Purification Kit (Macherey–Nagel, Germany). Nucleotide sequences were determined by capillary electrophoresis, with a capillary length of 50 cm and POP-7 polymer on ABI 3130xl Genetic Analyzer (Applied Biosystems, Foster City, CA, USA).

NG-MAST STs including the new alleles and STs were assigned on the NG-MAST website (www.ng-mast.net).

Phylogenetic tree was constructed by MEGA6 (Molecular Evolutionary Genetics Analysis Version 6.0) Neighbour-Joining algorithm, using maximum composite likelihood model [10]. The degree of similarity was determined using the highly similar sequence (Megablast) BLASTN Program of the National Library of Medicine of the National Center for Biotechnology Information [11].

Results

In 2014, 192 *N. gonorrhoeae* strains were isolated at the STD Centre of the Department of Dermatology, Venerology and Dermatooncology of Semmelweis University, Budapest, Hungary. The number of patients attending our STD centre makes up about 10 % of the total number of notified gonorrhoea infections in Hungary year by year. However, the ratio of *N. gonorrhoeae* positive patients to total patients examined increased from 7.8 %

in 2013 to 10.85 % by the end of 2014. Of the 192 *N. gonorrhoeae*, 85 % were isolated from male patients (median age 32 years); the remaining strains were collected from females (median age 26 years).

Urethritis was found in 77.3 % of male patients, while in females the dominant anatomical site of infection was the urethra (68.9 %) and cervix (65.5 %). Symptomatic infections or asymptomatic carrier states were detected in the anus (20.2 %/44.8 %) and in the pharynx (17.9 %/24.1 %) in male/female patients, respectively.

All the 192 isolates were susceptible to ceftriaxone and spectinomycin. The prevalence of ciprofloxacin and tetracycline resistance −39.8 and 70 %, respectively-remained as high as in previous years in Hungary. However, the MIC averages of ceftriaxone and cefixime have increased in the last few years. Cefixime MIC exceeded the resistant breakpoints in 1.57 % of the strains.

Of the 192 strains, 92 (48 %) were susceptible to azithromycin and 100 (52 %) exhibited reduced susceptibility. Fifty-eight of these 100 strains −30.0 % of all the strains- were resistant to azithromycin, according to the breakpoints of EUCAST. The percentage of azithromycin resistance showed a significant increase from 15.9 % in 2013 to 30.0 % in 2014 ($\chi^2 = 11.4437$, P value is 0.000717, $P < 0.001$). Concerning the strains with reduced susceptibility to azithromycin, we can say that the ratio of female/male patients was 1–7.3. MICs of ≥ 1 mg/L for azithromycin were observed in 7.0 % (13/192) of the isolated *N. gonorrhoeae* strains out of which three had an MIC of 1.5 mg/L (Additional file 1: Figure S1).

The prevalence of *C. trachomatis* infection detected by multiplex RT-PCR was only 6.7 % in 2014 at the NNGRLH, but *N. gonorrhoeae* positivity was found in 12.2 % of cases. Only 14.7 % of the gonorrhoea-positive samples were co-infected with *C. trachomatis*.

The 50 *N. gonorrhoeae* resistant or intermediate-resistant isolates to azithromycin were divided into 34 NG-MAST sequence types, and a unique NG-MAST sequence type was found for 10 isolates. The three dominant strains were ST1407, ST4995 and ST11064, each represented by 5 isolates (10–10 %). Regarding frequency, these were followed by ST 4417 represented by 3 isolates, then by ST 995 and ST 8517, each represented by 2 isolates. The 29 other STs were represented by only one isolate. Ten new STs, which had not been previously described in the world, were assigned as ST 11699 to ST 11708 on NG-MAST website. Four of them, ST 11703, 11706-11708, due to new allele combinations of known *porB* and *tbpB* alleles, were assigned on the website. The other 6 new STs had new *porB* or *tbpB* alleles (Table 1).

According to the phylogenic tree in Fig. 1, the azithromycin-resistant and intermediately resistant strains isolated in NNGLRH in 2014 were divided into three major groups based on closer relationship. From the most prevalent STs, the first group contained ST225; ST1407 belonged to the second group, whereas the third group contained ST4995 and ST11064. A similarity of at least 96 % can be shown for all members of the third group. The biggest similarity-99 %- was detected between ST21, ST11064 and ST11703. A 98 % similarity between

Table 1 Incidence of sequence types, *porB* and *tbpB* allels among azithromycin-resistant or intermediate-resistant *N. gonorrhoeae* strains isolated in Hungary in 2014

ST	*porB* allele	*tbpB* allele	Number of strains	Azithromycin susceptibility category, number of strains	
				I	R
10081	5921	29	1	1	–
10083	3031	29	1	1	–
995	28	29	2	–	2
4417	2707	894	3	1	2
10087	35	29	1	–	1
5333	3229	137	1	–	1
225	4	4	1	–	1
10088	2700	4	1	1	–
11706	1183	1388	1	–	1
7232	1489	1388	1	–	1
11702	6870	1582	1	1	–
8706	35	1582	1	1	–
11704	6871	2003	1	–	1
11708	1183	18	1	–	1
8465	4864	18	1	–	1
2400	1489	563	1	–	1
8115	3942	563	1	–	1
11707	4864	563	1	–	1
10101	4160	110	1	1	–
8517	1142	1531	2	1	1
3378	2043	110	1	1	–
8826	5213	110	1	–	1
1407	908	110	5	2	3
11699	6867	138	1	1	–
21	14	33	1	–	1
11064	14	1131	5	2	3
11703	1582	1131	1	1	–
10593	581	1131	1	1	–
11700	6868	1131	1	1	–
4995	3031	33	5	3	2
5343	6195	1131	1	–	1
11337	6630	1131	1	–	1
11705	6872	2004	1	1	–
11701	6869	1131	1	–	1
$\Sigma=$			50	21	29

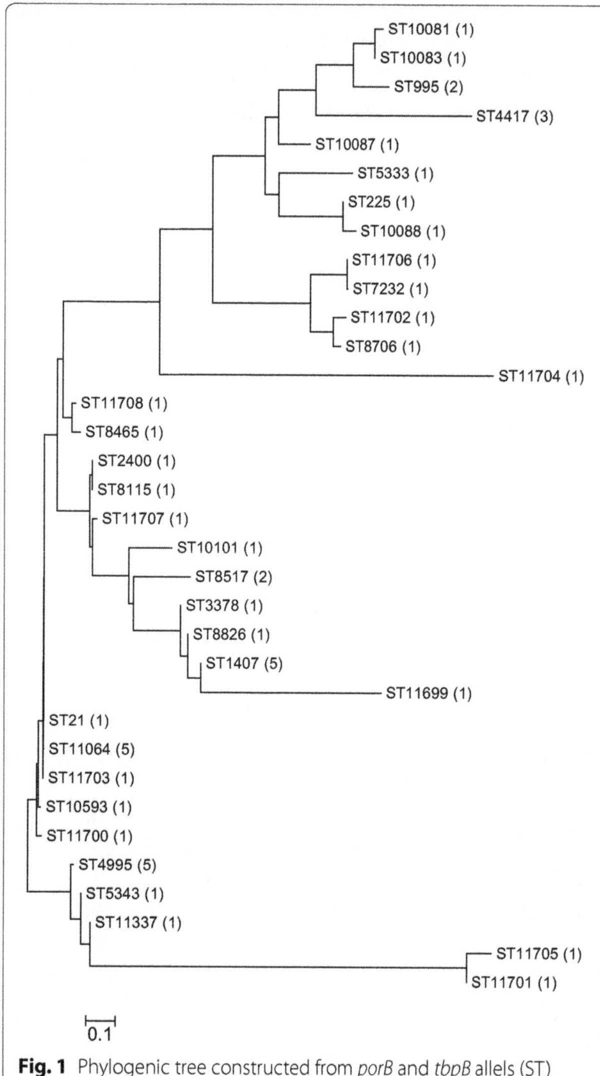

Fig. 1 Phylogenic tree constructed from *porB* and *tbpB* alleles (ST) from 50 azithromycin-resistant or intermediate-resistant strains isolated in 2014 in Hungary. Number of isolates according to the appropriate STs is indicated in parenthesis

ST11703 and ST10593, or between ST10593 and ST11700 was detected, but ST11700 and ST11703 demonstrated only a 97 % similarity. With the latter two STs, ST4995 showed a similarity of 96 %. Between ST 4995 and ST5343 or ST11337 a similarity of 97 % was detected.

Discussion

For the treatment of gonorrhoea, the European Guideline, published in 2012, recommends 500 mg of ceftriaxone combined with 2 g of azithromycin as first choice therapy [2]. This dual therapy is supported by European epidemiological surveys, mostly based on western European data. These European epidemiological surveys demonstrate that *C. trachomatis* co-infection is so common in young heterosexual patients under 30 and in MSM with gonorrhoea that 1 g of azithromycin administered orally as a single dose or 100 mg of doxycycline administered orally twice daily for 7 days should be given unless co-infection has been excluded by NAAT testing.

Since resistance to azithromycin increased from 0 to 30 % in Hungary in the last 5 years, and WHO recommended [1] that an antimicrobial should not be used when >5 % of the strains are resistant, we aimed to conduct an active surveillance to detect recent emergence in Hungary. Our theory for the increasing azithromycin resistance is that, according to ESAC, azithromycin has become the second most commonly used antimicrobial in Hungary. Hence, patients might have been treated previously with azithromycin for an infection, microbiome in the pharynx or anus, could have been exposed to this antibiotic several times, could have acquired resistance and acted as reservoirs of genes [12]. Azithromycin-resistant samples were frequently isolated from the pharynx (21 %) or the anus (32.5 %), which may refer to the fact that the asymptomatic carrier state provides an opportunity for commensal microbiome and *N. gonorrhoeae* to exchange their resistance genes, resulting in a hyperexpression of the efflux pump MtrCDE or mutation in the 23S rRNA [13, 14]. The high percentage of infections in the pharynx and anus do not only involve the risk of acquiring resistance, but also the risk of developing a disseminated infection and the spread of asymptomatic gonorrhoea.

Previously, the most frequent isolated STs were ST2992, ST1407, ST4995 and ST225 in Hungary [15]. In our recent study, three groups of STs based on closer relationship, were observed among azithromycin-resistant or intermediate-resistant *N. gonorrhoeae* strains isolated in Hungary in 2014. The first group contains the previously described ST225; ST1407 belongs to the second group, while ST4995 and ST11064 are included in the third group (Fig. 1). The latter two STs represent the 20 % of the azithromycin-resistant strains but, according to the data of Table 1 and Fig. 1, it can be presumed that more than 30 % of the azithromycin-resistant isolates are closely related in the third group of STs (similarity is at least 96 %). The previously described uniquely high prevalence of ST4995 in Hungary confirms the theory that the isolates of the third neighbourhood group are successful strains in this country, and may cause therapeutic failure in our region in the future. Nevertheless, based on the exact definition of genogroup—one identical allele is shared and the other allele shows a similarity of ≥99 % [16]—only ST21, ST11064 and ST11703 make up a genogroup. This genogroup is named G11064, since ST11064 is the predominant ST within the group.

The other prevalently isolated strains in the second group of neighbourhood are associated with ST1407, i.e.

the ST previously described as resistant to ciprofloxacin, tetracycline and strongly associated with decreased susceptibility to cephalosporins [16, 17]. Poorly controlled use of antibiotics may promote the selection and spread of multidrug-resistant strains from this group [18].

The rapid selection of azithromycin-resistant strains in Hungary shows that azithromycin might not be optimised for the treatment of gonorrhoea, neither in monotherapy nor in dual therapy. On the one hand, the question is whether the combination of cephalosporins with azithromycin decreases the MICs of cephalosporins or not. There are some studies which report in vitro synergy between third-generation cephalosporins and azithromycin [19], but others do not [20]. The clinical efficacy of the dual therapy with ceftriaxone and azithromycin could be lower than ceftriaxone monotherapy since the combination was less bactericidal as ceftriaxone alone in a time-kill experiment [21].

On the other hand, we have to investigate the prevalence of *C. trachomatis* co-infection. In Europe, according to ECDC's data, *Chlamydia* is the most frequently reported STD. In 2011, 346911 cases were notified in 25 European countries, and 39179 cases of gonorrhoea were registered. By contrast, in our laboratory twice as many gonorrhoea infections were identified as *Chlamydia* infections; 6.7 % of the samples of the STD centre were *Chlamydia*-positive and 12.2 % were gonorrhoea-positive. These data correlate with those of the National Epidemiological Laboratory, where 1077 cases of *Chlamydia* and 1525 cases of gonorrhoea were recorded in 2013. While the surveys of IUSTI refer to the common prevalence of co-infection, in our laboratory only 14.7 % of the gonorrhoea-positive samples were co-infected with *C. trachomatis*. This also raises the question whether combination therapy is the appropriate treatment in Hungary for gonorrhoea infection. Furthermore, as the increasing azithromycin-resistance and also the emerging cefixime and ceftriaxone MICs threaten the currently recommended therapies for gonorrhoea, it would be essential to replace these antimicrobials with novel ones which have not been used before for gonorrhoea infection in our country. The use of solithromycin, gentamicin, gemifloxacin might be a short term solution, but developing novel antimicrobials is essential [22, 23].

Conclusions

In Hungary, the treatment of gonorrhoea infections relies on the combination therapy of ceftriaxone and azithromycin, recommended by the international guidelines. However, the data of this study should not only draw attention to caution in the use of azithromycin as the sole treatment for gonorrhoea but also to that in the use of combination therapy in Hungary. This study indicates that the rate of azithromycin-resistant strains is growing in our country year by year. We observed a unique emergence of azithromycin-resistant *N. gonorrhoeae* strains the amount of which has doubled in a period of 1e year. Besides, the strains being the most common in Hungary in 2013, also appeared in 2014 and were associated with azithromycin-resistance. This experience restricts the usefulness of this antibiotic recommended as first-line treatment for gonorrhoea worldwide and argues for regular surveillance to determine azithromycin-susceptibility.

Abbreviations

ECDC: European Centre for Disease Prevention and Control; ESAC: European Surveillance of Antimicrobial Consumption; EUCAST: European Committee on Antimicrobial Susceptibility Testing; DDD: defined daily doses; IUSTI: International Union against Sexually Transmitted Infections; NG-MAST: *N. gonorrhoeae* multiantigen sequence typing; MEGA6: Molecular Evolutionary Genetics Analysis Version 6.0; MIC: minimal inhibitory concentration; MSM: men who have sex with men; NNGRL: National *Neisseria gonorrhoeae* Reference Laboratory of Hungary; ST: sequence type; STD: sexually transmitted diseases.

Authors' contributions

BA, OE wrote the manuscript. BA, NNE conducted the review of the literature relevant to the paper. MM and SK examined and treated the patients. NNE and OE performed identification and susceptibility testing of the strains. BA, JCS and SZD made the molecular examinations of the strains and prepared the phylogenetic tree. Each author contributed suggestions to the manuscript. All authors read and approved the final manuscript.

Author details

[1] Department of Dermatology, Venerology and Dermatooncology, Semmelweis University, 41 Mária Street, Budapest, Hungary. [2] Department of Laboratory Medicine, Semmelweis University, 41 Mária Street, Budapest, Hungary. [3] Institute of Medical Microbiology, Semmelweis University, 4 Nagyvárad Square, Budapest, Hungary.

Competing interests

The authors declare that they have no competing interests and no specific funding was provided for this study.

References

1. Tapsall JW. Antibiotic resistance in *Neisseria gonorrhoeae*. Clin Infect Dis. 2005;41:263–8.
2. Bignell C, Unemo M, European STI Guidelines Editorial Board. European guideline on the diagnosis and treatment of Gonorrhoea in adults. Int J STD AIDS. 2013;24:85–92.
3. Brunner A, Nemes-Nikodem E, Mihalik N, Marschalko M, Karpati S, Ostorhazi E. Incidence and antimicrobial susceptibility of *Neisseria gonorrhoeae* isolates from patients attending the national *N. gonorrhoeae* reference laboratory of Hungary. BMC Infect Dis. 2014;14:433.

4. Steingrimsson O, Olafsson JH, Thorarinsson H, Ryan RW, Johnson RB, Tilton RC. Azithromycin in the treatment of sexually transmitted disease. J Antimicrob Chemother. 1990;25:109–14.
5. Amrol D. Single-dose azithromycin microsphere formulation: a novel delivery system for antibiotics. Int J Nanomed. 2007;2:9–12.
6. European Centre for Disease Prevention and Control (ECDC). Antimicrobial consumption interactive database (ESAC-Net). 2015. http://www.ecdc.europa.eu/en/healthtopics/antimicrobial_resistance/esac-net-database/Pages/database.aspx.
7. Országos Epidemiológiai Központ (OEK)/National Epidemiological Centre. Szexuális úton terjedő betegségek Magyarországon/Sexually transmitted diseases in Hungary 2013. IV. Epinfo. 2014;5:45–50.
8. The European Committee on Antimicrobial Susceptibility Testing. Breakpoint tables for interpretation of MICs and zone diameters. Version 4.0. 2014. http://www.eucast.org.
9. Martin IM, Ison CA, Aanensen DM, Fenton KA, Spratt BG. Rapid sequence-based identification of gonococcal transmission clusters in a large metropolitan area. J Infect Dis. 2004;189:1497–505.
10. Tamura K, Stecher G, Peterson D, Filipski A, Kumar S. MEGA6: molecular evolutionary genetics analysis Version 6.0. Mol Biol Evol. 2013;30:2725–9.
11. http://blast.ncbi.nlm.nih.gov/Blast.cgi?PAGE_TYPE=BlastSearch&PROG_DEF=blastn&BLAST_PROG_DEF=megaBlast&BLAST_SPEC=blast2seq.
12. Kenyon C, Osbak K. Certain attributes of the sexual ecosystem of high-risk MSM have resulted in an altered microbiome with an enhanced propensity to generate and transmit antibiotic resistance. Med Hypotheses. 2014;83:196–202.
13. Starnino S, Stefanelli P. *Neisseria gonorrhoeae* Italian Study Group. Azithromycin-resistant *N. gonorrhoeae* strains recently isolated in Italy. J Antimicrob Chemother. 2009;63:1200–4.
14. Ng LK, Martin I, Liu G, Bryden L. Mutation in 23S rRNA associated with macrolide resistance in *Neisseria gonorrhoeae*. Antimicrob Agents Chemother. 2002;46:3020–5.
15. Nemes-Nikodém É, Brunner A, Pintér D, Mihalik N, et al. Antimicrobial susceptibility and genotyping analysis of Hungarian *Neisseria gonorrhoeae* strains in 2013. Acta Microbiol Immunol Hung. 2014;61:435–45.
16. Chisholm SA, Unemo M, Quaye N, et al. Molecular epidemiological typing within the European gonococcal antimicrobial resistance surveillance programme reveals predominance of a multidrug-resistant clone. Euro Surveill. 2013;18:20358.
17. Palmer HM, Young H, Graham C, Dave J. Prediction of antibiotic resistance using *Neisseria gonorrhoeae* multi-antigen sequence typing. Sex Transm Infect. 2008;84:280–4.
18. Chisholm SA, Wilson J, Alexander S, Tripodo F, Al-Shahib A, Schaefer U, Lythgow K, Fifer H. An outbreak of high-level azithromycin resistant *Neisseria gonorrhoeae* in England. Sex Transm Infect. 2015;92:365–7. doi:10.1136/sextrans-2015-052312.
19. Furuya R, Nakayama H, Kanayama A, et al. *In vitro* synergistic effects of double combinations of beta-lactams and azithromycin against clinical isolates of *Neisseria gonorrhoeae*. J Infect Chemother. 2006;12:172–6.
20. Barbee LA, Soge OO, Holmes KK, Golden MR. In vitro synergy testing of novel antimicrobial combination therapies against *Neisseria gonorrhoeae*. J Antimicrob Chemother. 2014;69:1572–8.
21. Hauser C, Hirzberger L, Unemo M, Furrer H, Endimiani A. *In vitro* activity of fosfomycin alone and in combination with ceftriaxone or azithromycin against clinical *Neisseria gonorrhoeae* isolates. Antimicrob Agents Chemother. 2015;59:1605–11.
22. Ross JDC, Lewis DA. Cephalosporin resistant *Neisseria gonorrhoeae*: time to consider gentamicin? Sex Transm Infect. 2012;88:6–8.
23. Lewis DA. Global resistance of *Neisseria gonorrhoeae*: when theory becomes reality. Curr Opin Infect Dis. 2014;27:62–7.

4

Antimicrobial resistance in coagulase-negative staphylococci from Nigerian traditional fermented foods

P. T. Fowoyo[1*] and S. T. Ogunbanwo[2]

Abstract

Background: Coagulase-negative staphylococci have become increasingly recognized as the etiological agent of some infections. A significant characteristic of coagulase-negative staphylococci especially strains isolated from animals and clinical samples is their resistance to routinely used antibiotics although, resistant strains isolated from fermented foods have not been fully reported.

Methods: A total of two hundred and fifty-five CoNS isolates were subjected to antimicrobial susceptibility test using the disc diffusion technique. The minimum inhibitory concentration of the isolates to the tested antibiotics was determined using the microbroth dilution method. Methicillin resistant strains were confirmed by detection of methicillin resistant genes (*mecA*) and also employing cefoxitin screening test.

Results: The isolates were confirmed to be methicillin resistant by the detection of *mecA* genes and the cefoxitin screening test. The isolates demonstrated appreciable resistance to ampicillin (86.7%), sulfomethoxazole–trimethoprim (74.9%), amoxicillin–clavulanic acid (52.5%) and oxacillin (35.7%). Methicillin resistance was exhibited by 13 out of the 255 isolates although no *mecA* gene was detected. It was also observed that the methicillin resistant isolates were prevalent in these traditional foods; *iru*, *kindirmo*, *nono* and *wara*.

Conclusion: This study has ameliorated the incidence of multiple antibiotic resistant coagulase-negative staphylococci in Nigerian fermented foods and if not tackled adequately might lead to horizontal transfer of antibiotic resistance from food to man.

Keywords: Antibiotic resistance, Coagulase-negative staphylococci, Fermented foods, Methicillin resistance, *mecA* gene

Background

Coagulase-negative staphylococci were previously dismissed as contaminants and were found to occur mostly in hospitalized patients, individuals suffering from nosocomial infections and infections arising from the use of catheter or other intra-uterine devices however, it has been shown that CoNS from fermented foods also exhibit virulent traits [1]. The major challenge of CoNS-related infections has been the difficulty in therapy due to antimicrobial resistance. Antimicrobial agents used in therapy and as feed supplements to promote growth in food animals may increase the spread of drug-resistant bacteria. Such bacteria may contaminate milk or meat and are subsequently found in fermented food made of such raw material [2]. The levels of antibiotic resistant infections in the developing world have increased steadily in the last few decades as a result of combination of microbial characteristics and the selective pressure of antimicrobial use [3]. Microbial mechanisms of overcoming the activities of antimicrobial agents include the production of structure-altering or inactivating enzymes (e.g. beta-lactamase or amino glycoside-modifying enzymes), alteration of penicillin-binding proteins or other cell-wall target sites, altered DNA gyrase targets, permeability mutations,

*Correspondence: seunpt@yahoo.com
[1] Biosciences Department, Salem University, P.M.B. 1060 Lokoja, Kogi State, Nigeria
Full list of author information is available at the end of the article

active efflux and ribosomal modification [4–6]. Multidrug-resistant bacteria in both the hospital and community environment are important concern to the clinician, as it is the major cause of failure in the treatment of infectious diseases, increased morbidity, and mortality and the evolution of new pathogens [7, 8].

Penicillin was initially the drug of choice for treatment of infections caused by *Staphylococcus* however, penicillin resistance in CoNS became very high since 1968 [9]. Nowadays, resistance is around 91% in clinical strains [10]. Two mechanisms confer penicillin resistance in staphylococci; the first and the most important is the production of β-lactamase which inactivates penicillin by the hydrolysis of its β-lactam ring. The second is primarily associated with human isolates and confers resistance due to a penicillin-binding protein, PBP2a, encoded by *mecA* [2]. The *blaZ* has also been identified as the cause of penicillin resistance among coagulase-negative staphylococci (CoNS) suggesting that *blaZ* is one of the main mechanism of penicillin resistance in staphylococci [2]. Methicillin resistance in *Staphylococcus* is caused by the expression of PBP2a encoded by the *mecA* gene [11]. Resistance of staphylococci to methicillin and all β-lactam antibiotics is associated with the low affinity of a penicillin-binding protein, PBP2a, which is not present in susceptible staphylococci [12–17]. This protein is encoded by the *mecA* gene, which is located in the mec region in which the DNA is of foreign origin [18]. There is evidence of horizontal transfer of SCC cassette between staphylococcal species [19] which implies that CoNS could serve as a reservoir for the spread of resistance genes. Transfer of resistance genes between CoNS and *S. aureus* has been reported thus indicating that CoNS may act as a resistance gene reservoir for *S. aureus*. It is thus possible that the different species of staphylococci that are present in the same microenvironment, for example on the skin of dairy cows can exchange *mecA* and *blaZ*, if the appropriate bacterial factors are met [2].

In this study, the incidence of antibiotic resistance against 9 antibiotics among 255 strains of coagulase-negative staphylococci of fermented food associated CoNS were investigated using disc diffusion technique according to the CLSI guidelines. The antibiotic resistant phenotypes were confirmed molecularly by the detection of *mecA* genes and cefoxitin screening test.

Methods

CoNS strains used in this study

In total, 255 CoNS strains were used in this study. The strains were isolated from six different Nigerian fermented foods, including *kindirmo* (66), *nono* (44) *iru* (58), *wara* (32), *ogi* (28) and *kunu* (27). The isolates were identified using both conventional and molecular methods employing 16S rRNA sequencing [20].

Antibiotic susceptibility testing

In vitro susceptibility of the test isolates to the antibiotics was determined using Kirby-Bauer disc diffusion [21]. A sterile wire loop was used to pick a discrete colony of the 18 h old culture of each of the test isolate cultured on mannitol salt agar (MSA) and used to inoculate sterile brain heart infusion broth inside a test tube and incubated at 37 °C for 4 h. The inoculum was standardized using the 0.5 McFarland turbidity standard which corresponds to 1.5×10^8 cfu/ml of cells. A sterile cotton swab was dipped into the adjusted suspension and excess inoculum was removed by pressing the swab firmly on the inside wall of the tube. The dried surface of a Mueller–Hinton agar plate was inoculated by streaking the swab over the entire surface. This procedure was repeated by streaking two more times, rotating the plate approximately 60° each time to ensure an even distribution of inoculum. The antimicrobial discs were placed firmly on the surface of the inoculated agar plate using sterile forceps. The plates were left for 1 h after which they were incubated at 35 °C for 18 h. After 16–18 h of incubation, the plates were examined and the diameters of the zones of inhibition were measured. The discs used were ampicillin (30 μg), amoxicillin-clavulanic acid (30 μg), cefotaxime (30 μg), oxacillin (1 μg), ciprofloxacin (5 μg), trimethoprim–sulphomethaxazole (5 μg), erythromycin (25 μg), gentamycin (10 μg) and ofloxacin (5 μg). All the antibiotic discs were procured from Oxoid, Germany. The results were classified as susceptible, intermediate, or resistant according to the approved guidelines of the Clinical and Laboratory Standards Institute [22].

Determination of minimum inhibitory concentration (MIC) using the broth micro-dilution method

The method by [21] was employed. A 96-well microtitre plate was used. Twofold serial dilutions of the different antibiotics were prepared and dispensed into the microtitre plates. The antimicrobial solutions were prepared at twice the desired final concentration and the wells filled with 0.05 ml of the antibiotic instead of 0.1 ml. Each tray labeled had a growth control well and a sterility (uninoculated) well.

The inoculum used for the broth micro-dilution was prepared using the direct colony suspension method. An 18 h old culture of CoNS was grown on blood agar. Distinct colonies were picked and each inoculated into 5 ml of Mueller–Hinton broth in a test tube. The broth culture was incubated at 35 °C for 4 h. The turbidity of the actively growing broth culture was adjusted with sterile broth using 0.5 McFarland standard. The resulting suspension contained approximately $1–2 \times 10^8$ cfu/ml. 2 ml of the suspension was dispensed into 38 ml of water (1:20 dilution). The prong of the inoculator was used to transfer 0.01 ml (1:10 dilution) into each well. The MIC panel was inoculated carefully to avoid splashing from one well to another. The microdilution trays were incubated inside a plastic bag at 35 ± 2 °C for 16–20 h in an ambient air incubator within 15 min of adding the inoculum. The amount of growth in the wells containing the antimicrobial agent was compared with the amount of growth in the growth control wells (no antimicrobial agent) used in each set of tests when determining the growth end points. A test was considered valid when acceptable growth was ≥2 mm turbidity at the bottom of the well or when a definite turbidity was observed.

Detection of methicillin resistance genes (*mecA*)

The methicillin resistant genes present in the coagulase-negative staphylococci strains were detected by polymerase chain reaction according to the method of [23]. DNA was extracted using the QIA Amp mini kit (QIAgen). Polymerase chain reaction for detection of the gene *mecA* (513 bp) was carried out using the following primers: A22f (5′ AAA ATC GAT GGT AAA GGT TGG C 3′) and A22r (AGT TCT GCA GTA CCG GAT TTG C) as described by [11]. Amplification cycles for *mecA* was carried out according to the method of [23] Considering 40 cycles of 94 °C for 30 s, 55 °C for 30 s, 72 °C for 1 min with a final extension of 72 °C for 5 min. *Staphylococcus aureus* ATCC43300 *mecA* + was used as positive control [21]. The amplicons were evaluated by agarose gel electrophoresis followed by staining in ethidium bromide (0.5 mg/ml), visualized on UV transilluminator (UVP, Inc USA) and documented by the program QuantiOne (BioRad) using molecular weight markers of 100 bp (Fermentas ®).

Results

A total of 221 (86.7%) of the isolates were resistant to ampicillin, however majority of the resistant CoNS occurred in *wara* (93.8%), *nono* (88.6%), *kindirmo* (92.4%) and *iru* (86.2%). 74.9% of the CoNS isolates were resistant to trimethoprim-sulfamethoxazole with high incidence in *iru* (84.5%), *wara* (84.4%) and *kindirmo* (72.7%). The highest resistance of amoxicillin-clavulanic acid was noted in CoNS isolated from *ogi* (60.7%), *iru* (60.3%), *nono* and *wara* (59.4%). The highest oxacillin resistance isolates were from *ogi* (42.9%), *nono* (40.9%) and *wara* (43.8%). The resistance to the other antibiotics cefotaxime, ciprofloxacin, erythromycin, gentamycin and ofloxacin were not as high as the other antibiotics as shown in Table 1.

Table 2 shows the resistance phenotype of the CoNS species. Thirty-four (13%) of the isolates were not resistant to any of the antibiotic tested. CoNS species having resistance phenotype to only ampicillin and trimethoprim-sulfamethoxazole were only 57 in number. *Staphylococcus epidermidis* (92%) demonstrated the highest resistance to ampicillin while *S. caprae* (69%) had the

Table 2 Phenotypic antimicrobial resistance patterns of CoNS species from fermented food samples

Profile	Resistance phenotypes	Number of strains	Number of antibiotic classes
1	None	34	0
2	AMP	30	1
3	AMP, SXT	57	2
4	AMP, SXT, AMC	43	2
5	AMP, SXT, AMC, OX	30	2
6	AMP, SXT, AMC, OX, CIP	21	3
7	AMP, SXT, AMC, OX, CIP, E	11	4
8	AMP, SXT, AMC, OX, CIP, E, CN	10	5
9	AMP, SXT, AMC, OX, CIP, E, CN, OFX	10	5
10	AMP, SXT, AMC, OX, CIP, E, CN, OFX, CTX	9	5

AMP ampicillin, *SXT* sulphomethoxazole–trimethoprim, *AMC* Amoxicillin–clavulanic acid, *OX* oxacillin, *CIP* ciprofloxacin, *E* erythromycin, *CN* gentamicin, *OFX* ofloxacin, *CTX* cefotaxime

Table 1 Distribution and Percentage Antimicrobial Resistance of Coagulase-Negative Staphylococci from Fermented Food Samples

Antibiotics	% Resistance of CoNS from foods						
	Total	*Iru*	*Ogi*	*Nono*	*Kindirmo*	*Kunu zaki*	*Wara*
	(255)	n = 58	n = 28	n = 44	n = 66	n = 27	n = 32
Ampicillin	221 (86.7%)	50 (86.2%)	21 (75%)	39 (88.6%)	61 (92.4%)	20 (74.1%)	30 (93.8%)
Trimethoprim–sulfamethoxazole	191 (74.9%)	49 (84.5%)	18 (64.3%)	31 (70.5%)	48 (72.7%)	18 (66.7%)	27 (84.4%)
Amoxicillin–clavulanic acid	134 (52.5%)	35 (60.3%)	17 (60.7%)	26 (59.1%)	29 (43.9%)	8 (29.6%)	19 (59.4%)
Cefotaxime	9 (3.5%)	2 (3.4%)	0 (0%)	3 (6.8%)	2 (3.0%)	1 (3.7%)	1 (3.1%)
Oxacillin	91 (35.7%)	17 (29.3%)	12 (42.9%)	18 (40.9%)	21 (31.8%)	9 (33.3%)	14 (43.8%)
Ciprofloxacin	61 (23.9%)	12 (20.7%)	3 (10.7%)	10 (22.7%)	18 (27.3%)	5 (18.5%)	13 (40.6%)
Erythromycin	40 (15.7%)	8 (13.8%)	2 (7.1%)	10 (22.7%)	11 (16.7%)	0 (0%)	9 (28.1%)
Gentamicin	29 (11.4%)	4 (6.9%)	2 (7.1%)	9 (20.5%)	7 (16.7%)	0 (0%)	7 (21.9%)
Ofloxacin	18 (7.1%)	2 (3.4%)	1 (3.6%)	4 (9.1%)	4 (6.1%)	1 (3.7%)	6 (18.8%)

least percentage of resistance to ampicillin. For trimethoprim-sulfamethoxazole, the highest resistance of 81% was recorded in *S. xylosus* with *S. caprae* having the least resistance (53%) to the antibiotic. *Staphylococcus simulans* (68%) recorded the highest resistance to amoxicillin-clavulanic acid while the least resistance was shown in *S. epidermidis* (41%). Oxacillin resistance in *S. xylosus* was 32% which was the highest and the least was in *S. kloosii* (14%). *Staphylococcus caprae* exhibited the highest resistance to ciprofloxacin, ofloxacin, gentamycin, erythromycin and cefotaxime as shown in Fig. 1.

Table 3 shows the minimum inhibitory concentration (MIC) distribution of the CoNS species. Based on the Clinical and Laboratory Standards Institute (CLSI) guidelines for MIC reading, the percentage of CoNS species resistant to the ampicillin, trimethoprim-sulfomethoxazole, amoxicillin-clavulanic acid and oxacillin were 85.5, 67.8, 49.8 and 25.9% respectively.

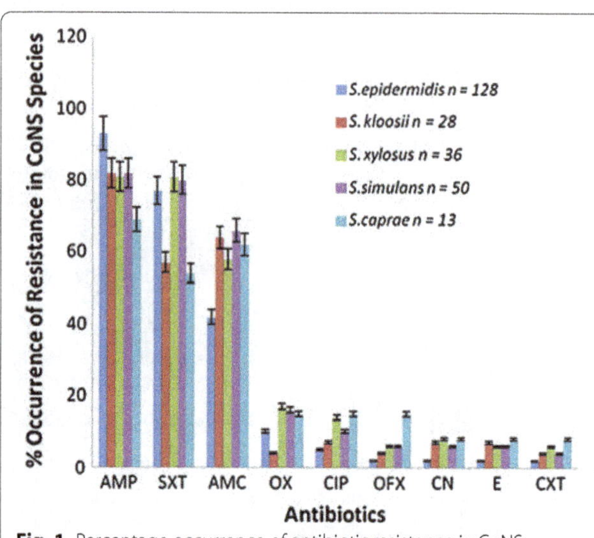

Fig. 1 Percentage occurrence of antibiotic resistance in CoNS Species. *Error bars* represent standard deviation of mean of replicate determinations

Cefoxitin screening test was carried out on the isolates so as to establish their status as methicillin resistant strains. Thirteen (5.1%) of the tested isolates were positive to cefoxitin screening test and most of them were multidrug resistant with the highest occurrence of the methicillin resistant species in *nono*. The species were *S. kloosii* (KIL 4), *S. xylosus* (WAIL 3, KIL 2 and WAJ 5),

Table 4 Coagulase negative Staphylococci isolates showing methicillin resistance using cefoxitin screening

ID	Source	C–S	Resistance phenotype
S. xylosus KIL 2	*Kindirmo*	+	AMP, OX, SXT, AMC, CIP, E, CXT, CN. OFX
S. xylosus WAIL 3	*Wara*	+	AMP, OX, SXT, CIP, E, CXT, CN. OFX
S. kloosii KIL 4	*Kindirmo*	+	AMP, OX, SXT, AMC, CIP, E, CN OFX
S. epidermidis OGIL 3	*Ogi*	+	AMP, OX, AMC, CIP, E, OFX
S. epidermidis IRIL 7	*Iru*	+	AMP, OX, SXT, AMC, CIP, CN OFX
S. epidermidis NOMA 10	*Nono*	+	AMP, OX, SXT, AMC, CIP, E, CXT, CN OFX
S. simulans NOJ 6	*Nono*	+	AMP, OX, CIP, E, CXT, OFX
S. simulans KIM 5	*Kindirmo*	+	AMP, OX, SXT, AMC, CIP, E,
S. xylosus WAJ 5	*Wara*	+	AMP, OX, SXT, AMC, E, CXT
S. caprae NOMA 5	*Nono*	+	AMP, OX, SXT, AMC, CIP, E, CXT, OFX
S. caprae NOMA 6	*Nono*	+	AMP, OX, SXT, CIP, E, CN OFX
S. epidermidis NOL 3	*Nono*	+	AMP, OX, SXT, AMC, E, CXT CN OFX
S. epidermidis IRIL 5	*Iru*	+	AMP, OX, SXT, CIP, E, CN OFX

Table 3 Minimum inhibitory concentration (MIC) of antibiotics against CoNS isolated from fermented food samples

Antimicrobial agents	Numbers of CoNS with MIC[a]											Resistant isolates (%)
	≤0.12	0.25	0.5	1	2	4	8	16	32	64	128	
Ampicillin	24	13	*11*	*62*	*55*	*27*	*0*	*0*	*43*	*18*	*2*	218 (85.5%)
Trimethoprim–sulfomethoxazole	11	37	19	15	0	*0*	*0*	*0*	*0*	*70*	*103*	173 (67.8%)
Amoxicillin–clavulanic acid	101	0	27	0	0	0	*0*	*0*	*0*	*40*	*87*	127 (49.8%)
Oxacillin	53	136	0	*0*	*0*	*47*	*0*	*0*	*19*	*0*	*0*	66 (25.9%)
Ciprofloxacin	84	43	14	0	**52**	*0*	*7*	*24*	*9*	*9*	*13*	62 (24.3%)
Ofloxacin	21	12	22	69	**121**	*0*	*0*	*0*	*0*	*0*	*10*	10 (3.9%)
Gentamicin	15	151	16	**26**	**10**	**0**	*21*	*7*	*0*	*0*	*0*	37 (14.5%)
Erythromycin	98	91	15	0	0	0	*0*	*6*	*0*	*40*	*0*	46 (18.0%)
Cefotaxime[b]	0	181	20	0	0	49	0	0	0	3	2	–

[a] Based on the CLSI breakpoints. MICs indicative for susceptible isolates are displayed on a white background, those for intermediate on a bold and those for resistant on a italics

[b] Susceptility of staphylococci to cefotaxime may be detected from testing only penicillin and either cefoxitin or oxacillin

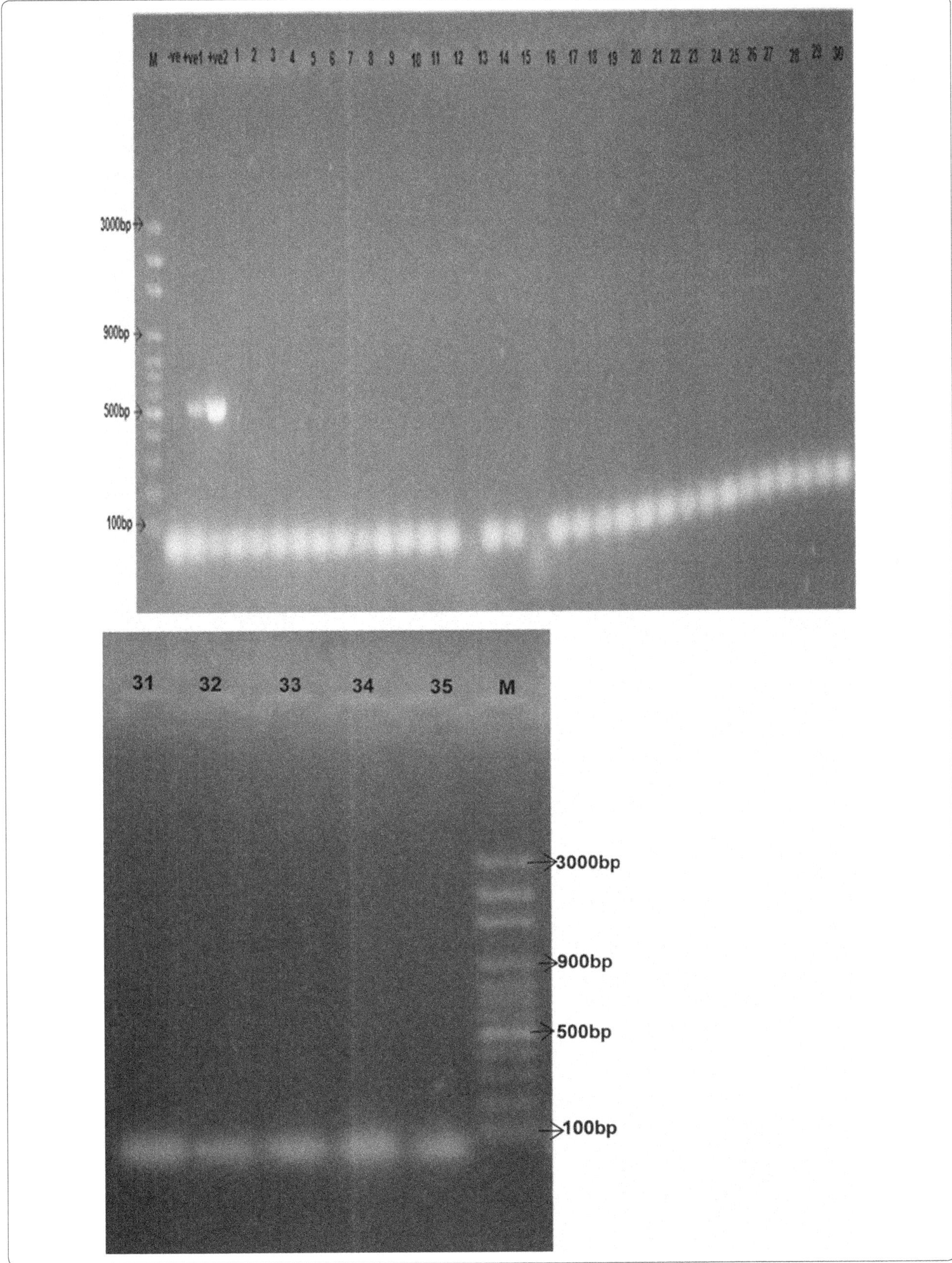
M -ve +ve1 +ve2 1 2 3 4 5 6 7 8 9 10 11 12 13 14 15 16 17 18 19 20 21 22 23 24 25 26 27 28 29 30
3000bp
900bp
500bp
100bp
31 32 33 34 35 M
3000bp
900bp
500bp
100bp

(See figure on previous page.)
Fig. 2 Gel electrophoresis micrograph of PCR product screen for *mecA* from extracted DNA (1–35) *Left* to *right*: M = O'GeneRuler 100 bp plus molecular weight marker (Thermo Scientific Fermentas™), Well 2 = Negative control for *mecA* gene, well 3 = Positive control 2, well 4 = Positive control 2 for *mecA* gene, wells 5–30 = Isolates 1–30. Weight of *mecA* gene = 513 bp. Positive isolates- none

S. epidermidis (OGIL 3, IRIL 7, NOMA 10, NOL 3 and IRIL 5), *S. simulans* (NOJ 6 and KIM 5) and *S. caprae* (NOMA 5 and NOMA 6) as indicated in Table 4. The molecular expression for *mecA* genes revealed that none of the isolates possessed the resistant genes (Fig. 2).

Discussion

Majority of the CoNS strains exhibited resistance to ampicillin, amoxicillin-clavulanic acid, sulphomethoxazole–trimethoprim, and oxacillin. A large percentage of the strains were susceptible to the antibiotics ciprofloxacin, erythromycin, gentamicin, cefotaxime and ofloxacin. *Staphylococcus epidermidis* demonstrated the highest resistance to ampicillin while *S. xylosus* exhibited the highest resistance to sulfomethoxazole–trimethoprim. The highest percentage resistance to amoxicillin-clavulanic acid was demonstrated by *S. simulans*. Oxacillin resistance was highly demonstrated by *S. xylosus*. The resistance exhibited by a large percentage of CoNS to these routinely used antibiotics in treatment of staphylococcal infections necessitates the search for newer and more effective antibiotics against this group of organisms.

There was discrepancy between the detection of methicillin resistance phenotypically using cefoxitin screening and the absence of *mecA* gene in the CoNS strains. This may be attributed to methicillin resistance being caused by other mechanisms other than expression of *mecA* gene [24]. Also the sensitivity of PCR in the detection of *mecA* may have been compromised by the presence of PCR inhibitors or other physical factors [25, 26]. The work by [27] showed that out of 15 isolates showing oxacillin resistant phenotype, only one possessed the *mecA* gene, it was noted that there were unusual methicillin resistant CoNS that have a resistance mechanism other than the production of PBP2a and they have been reported as borderline methicillin resistant strains [28]. The borderline methicillin resistant strains are resistant to oxacillin due to their plasmid borne determinants including hyper-produced penicillinases, genes conferring resistance to cadmium or other gene products [29, 30]. It is also possible that the *mecA* negative oxacillin resistant CoNS may possess *mecA* alleles which could not be detected by the primers used in this study. Many CoNS strains also show diversity in *mecA* sequences and have different impact on β-lactam resistance.

Conclusions

The high percentage of antimicrobial resistance demonstrated by the strains shows that food may serve as reservoirs for antibiotic resistance and allow for horizontal gene transfer from farm animals or their products to humans. Indigenous fermented food products may represent a critical risk for transfer of antimicrobial resistance to humans. As a consequence, transfer of antimicrobial resistance genes between bacteria after ingestion by humans may occur. Antimicrobial resistant CoNS present in food constitute a direct risk to public health as they increase the gene pool from which pathogenic bacteria can pick up resistance traits. The resistance of the organisms to routinely used antimicrobials also calls for the search for new antimicrobials and more effective management of diseases caused by CoNS in the event of an outbreak.

Abbreviations

CoNS: coagulase-negative staphylococci; *mecA*: methicillin resistant gene; PBP2a: penicillin binding protein; DNA: deoxyribonucleic acid; CLSI: Clinical and Laboratory Standards Institute; MIC: minimum inhibitory concentration.

Authors' contributions

FP carried out the laboratory analysis, OS was a major contributor in writing the manuscript. Both authors read and approved the final manuscript.

Author details

[1] Biosciences Department, Salem University, P.M.B. 1060 Lokoja, Kogi State, Nigeria. [2] Microbiology Department, University of Ibadan, Ibadan, Oyo State, Nigeria.

Acknowledgements

Not applicable.

Competing interests

The authors declare that they have no competing interests.

Funding

This research was self funded.

References

1. Fowoyo PT, Ogunbanwo ST. Occurrence and characterisation of coagulase-negative staphylococci from Nigerian traditional fermented foods. Food Sci Qual Manag. 2016;50:49–55.

2. Normanno G, Salandra GL, Dambrosio A, Quaglia NC, Corrente M, Parisi A, Olsen JE, Christensen H, Aarestrup F. Diversity and evolution of *blaZ* from *Staphylococcus aureus* and coagulase-negative staphylococci. J Antimicrob Chemother. 2006;57(3):450–60. doi:10.1093/jac/dki492.
3. Blondeau JM, Tillotson GS. Antimicrobial susceptibility patterns of respiratory pathogens-a global perspective. Semin Respir Infect. 2000;15:195–207.
4. Gold HS, Moellering RC. Antimicrobial-drug resistance. N Engl J Med. 1996;335(19):1445–53.
5. Aaterson DL. Extended-spectrum betalactamases: the European experience. Curr Opin Infect Dis. 2001;14:697–701.
6. Levy SB. Factors impacting on the problem of antibiotic resistance. J Antimicrob Chemother. 2002;49(1):25–30. doi:10.1093/jac/49.1.25.
7. Hacker J, Blum-Oehler G, Muhldorfer I, Tschape H. Pathogenicity islands of virulent bacteria: structure, function and impact on microbial evolution. Mol Microbiol. 1997;23:1089–97.
8. Jones RN, Phaller MA. Bacterial resistance; a worldwide problem. Diagn Microbiol Infect Dis. 1998;31:379–88.
9. Corse J, Williams REO. Antibiotic resistance of coagulase-negative staphylococci and micrococci. J Clin Pathol. 1968;21:722.
10. Koksal F, Yasar H, Samasti M. Antibiotic resistance patterns of coagulase negative *Staphylococcus* strains isolated from blood cultures of septicemic patients in Turkey. Microbiol Res. 2007;164(4):404–10.
11. Kumurya AS. Loss of the meca gene during storage of methicillin resistant *Staphylococcus aureus* isolates in Northwestern Nigeria. J Public Health Epidemiol. 2013;5(10):410–5. doi:10.5897/JPHE12.105.
12. Hartman BJ, Tomasz A. Low-affinity penicillin-binding protein associated with beta-lactam resistance in *Staphylococcus* aureus. J Bacteriol. 1984;158(2):513–6.
13. Pierre J, Williamson R, Bornet M, Gutmann L. Presence of an additional penicillin-binding protein in methicillin-resistant *Staphylococcus epidermidis, Staphylococcus haemolyticus, Staphylococcus hominis, and Staphylococcus simulans* with a low affinity for methicillin, cephalothin, and cefamandole. Antimicrob Agents Chemother. 1990;34:1691–4.
14. Chambers HF. Coagulase-negative staphylococci resistant to beta-lactam antibiotics in vivo produce penicillin-binding protein 2a. Antimicrob Agents Chemother. 1987;31:919–24.
15. Chambers HF. Methicillin resistance in staphylococci: molecular and biochemical basis and clinical implications. Clin Microbiol Rev. 1997;10:781–91.
16. Chambers HF. Penicillin-binding protein-mediated resistance in pneumococci andstaphylococci. J Infect Dis. 1999;179(Suppl. 2):S353–9.
17. Mohammad R, Mahmood Y, Au F. Comparison of different laboratory methods for detection of MRSA. Pak J Med Sci. 2006;22(4):442–5.
18. Matsuhashi M, Song MD, Ishino F, Wachi M, Doi M, Inoue M, Ubukata K, Yamashita N, Konno M. Molecular cloning of the gene of a penicillin-binding protein supposed to cause high resistance to P-lactam antibiotics in *Staphylococcus* aureus. J Bacteriol. 1986;167:975–80.
19. Hanssen A, Kjeldsen G, Sojlid JUE. Local variants of Staphylococcal Cassette chromosome *mec* in Sporadic methicillin-resistant *Staphylococcus aureus* and Methicillin-resistant coagulase-negative Staphylococci: evidence of horizontal gene transfer? Antimicrob Agents Chemother. 2004;48(1):285–96. doi:10.1128/AAC.48.1.285-296.2004.
20. Fowoyo PT, Ogunbanwo ST. Virulence and toxigenicity of coagulase-negative staphylococci in Nigerian traditional fermented foods. Can J Microbiol. 2016;62:1–7.
21. Bauer AW, Kirby WM, Sherris JC, Turck M. Antibiotic susceptibility testing by standardized single disc method. Am J Clin Pathol. 1996;44:493–6.
22. Clinical and Laboratory Standards Institute (CLSI). M100-S22. Performance standards for antimicrobial susceptibility testing; 22nd informational supplement. Clinical and Laboratory Standards Institute, Wayne, 2012.
23. Coelho SMO, Reinoso E, Pereira IA, Soares LC, Demo M, Bogni C, Souza MMS. Virulence factors and antimicrobial resistance of *Staphylococcus aureus* isolated from bovine mastitis in Rio de Janeiro. Pesq Vet Bras. 2009;29:369–74.
24. Gradelski E, Aleksunes L, Valera L, Bonner D, Fung- Tomc J. Correlation between genotype and phenotypic categorization of Staphylococci based on methicillin susceptibility and resistance. J Clin Microbiol. 2001;39(8):2961–3. doi:10.1128/JCM.39.8.2961-2963.2001.
25. Ingato SP, Kimangá N, Omuse G, Kariuki S, Gunturu R, Dinda V. Characteristics of archived coagulase negative staphylococci isolates at a University hospital, Nairobi, Kenya. Kenya. Open J Med Microbiol. 2014;4:236–41.
26. Procop GW, Shrestha NK, Tuohy MJ, Hall GS, Isada CM. Rapid identification of *Staphylococcus aureus* and the *mecA* Gene from BacT/ALERT blood culture bottles by using the light cycler system. J Clin Microbiol. 2002;40(7):2659–61. doi:10.1128/JCM.40.7.2659-2661.2002.
27. Han JE, Hwang SY, Kim JH, Shin SP, Jun JW, Chai JY, Park YH, Park SC. CPRMethicillin resistant coagulase-negative staphylococci isolated from South Korean ducks exhibiting tremor. Acta Vet Scand. 2013;55(1):88. doi:10.1186/1751-0147-55-88.
28. Suzuki E, Hiramatsu K, Yokota T. Survey of methicillin—resistant clinical strains of coagulase negative for *mecA* gene distribution. Antimicrob Agent Chemother. 1992;36:429–34.
29. Massida O, Montanari MP, Mingoia M, Viraldo PE. Borderline methicillin susceptible *Staphylococcus aureus* strains have more in common than reduced susceptibility to penicillase-resistant penicillins. Antimicrob Agents Chemother. 1996;40:2769–74.
30. Massida O, Mingoia M, Fadda D, Whalen MB, Montanari MP, Varaldo PE. Analysis of the beta lactamase plasmid of borderline methicillin susceptible *Staphylococcus aureus*: focus on *bla* complex genes and cadmium resistance determinants cadD and cadX. Plasmid. 2006;55:114–27.

5

Stryphnodendron adstringens and purified tannin on *Pythium insidiosum*: in vitro and in vivo studies

Rodrigo Trolezi[1], Juliana Maziero Azanha[1], Natália Rodrigues Paschoal[2], Jéssica Luana Chechi[1], Marcelo José Dias Silva[3], Viciany Eric Fabris[4], Wagner Vilegas[3], Ramon Kaneno[1], Ary Fernandes Junior[1] and Sandra de Moraes Gimenes Bosco[1*]

Abstract

Background: *Pythium insidiosum* is the etiological agent of pythiosis, an emerging life-threatening infectious disease in tropical and subtropical regions. The pathogen is a fungus-like organism resistant to antifungal therapy, for this reason, most cases need extensive surgical debridments as treatment, but depending on the size and anatomical region of the lesion, such approach is unfeasible. We investigate the fungicidal effect and toxicity of crude bark extract of *Stryphnodendron adstringens* and commercially available tannin on *Pythium insidiosum* both in vitro and in vivo.

Methods: Standardized fragments of mycelia of fifteen isolates of *P. insidiosum* were tested with different concentrations of bark extract (10 to 30% v/v) and tannin (0.5, 1.0 and 1.5 mg/mL). For in vivo study, fifteen rabbits were experimentally infected with zoospores of *P. insidiosum* and treated by oral and intralesional applications of bark extract and tannin. Acute toxicity tests with both substances were also performed in rats.

Results: In vitro studies showed fungicidal effect for both substances at different concentrations and the SEM showed alteration on the cell wall surface of the pathogen. All infected rabbits developed a firm nodular mass that reached around 90 mm^2 ninety days after inoculation, but neither the intralesional inoculation of tannin, nor the oral administration of crude extract and tannin were able to promote remission of the lesions.

Conclusions: Lesions developed by rabbits presented an encapsulated abscess being quite different of naturally acquired pythiosis, which is characterized by ulcerated lesions. Since no toxicity was observed in rats or rabbits inoculated with these products, while in vitro experiments showed direct antifungal effect, therapeutic activity of *S. adstringens* and tannin should be clinically tested as an alternative for healing wounds in naturally acquired pythiosis.

Keywords: *Pythium insidiosum*, Pythiosis, Susceptibility tests, Oomycete

Background

Pythiosis is caused by the oomycete *Pythium insidiosum* in different animal species mainly in tropical regions. One of the most important differences between oomycetes and true fungi is the absence of ergosterol in the cell membrane of oomycetes that may explain the failure of conventional therapy since most antifungal drugs acts on this cell compound [1].

Lack of an efficient treatment against this pathogen has stimulated the search for new potentially useful compounds including natural products. One of the pioneering studies using natural compounds against *P. insidiosum* was conducted by Zanette et al. [2], who showed that garlic extract is able to inhibit the zoopospores filamentation.

Stryphnodendron adstringens, popularly called barbatimão in Brazil, is a common medicinal plant found in Brazilian Cerrado region [3]. This species belongs to

*Correspondence: smgbosco@ibb.unesp.br
[1] Department of Microbiology and Immunology, Institute of Biosciences of Botucatu, UNESP Univ Estadual Paulista, Botucatu, SP 18618-970, Brazil
Full list of author information is available at the end of the article

the family Fabaceae and it is widely used in traditional medicine for diarrhoeas, gynaecological problems and for wound healing [4]. In addition, antimicrobial, anti-inflammatory, antiulcerogenic and wound cicatrizing properties of bark extract have been reported [5–8]. These effects are attributed to the major compound, tannin, found in the barks and leaves of this tree that shows fungicidal activity against *Candida albicans*, *Candida* spp., *Trichophyton rubrum* and *Cryptococcus neoformans* [3, 9, 10].

Based on these previous reports, we hypothesized that *S. adstringens* has bioactive compounds that could be able to fight *P. insidiosum*. Therefore, in this study we evaluated the effect of both crude bark extract of *S. adstringens* and commercially available tannin on the in vitro growth of *P. insidiosum*, as well as their in vivo activity in experimentally infected rabbits.

Methods

Bark extract of *Stryphnodendron adstringens*

Stryphnodendron adstringens barks were collected in Rubião Junior district (Botucatu, SP, Brazil, 22°52′60″S and 48°28′60″W), during the morning period. Voucher specimens were deposited at the Herbarium of the Department of Botany, Institute of Biosciences, UNESP, under the number 026633 BOTU. A crude extract was obtained according to Betoni et al. [11]. Briefly, *S. adstringens* barks were dried, ground and extracted with 70% methanol at 4–8 °C and filtered after 48 h. The residual plant material was re-extracted with methanol 70% and filtered after 24 h. The extract was concentrated in a rotary evaporator at 45 °C for elimination of methanol and kept in sterile flask under refrigeration until use. Levels of total tannin in the extract were measured according to Waterhouse [12], as follows: 10 mg of the extract were dissolved in 50 mL of distilled water, and a 2 mL aliquot was mixed with 2 mL of Folin–Ciocalteu reagent and homogenized. Three minutes later, 2 mL of 8% sodium carbonate solution were added to this mixture, stirred and kept for 2 h at room temperature. Then, centrifugated at 2000 rpm to measure total levels of tannin. The analytical calibration curve of commercially available tannin (Sigma-Aldrich) was estimated by the absorbance at 725 ηm of 10, 20, 30, 40, 60 and 80 μL/mL.

In vitro antimicrobial effect of bark extract of *S. adstringens* and tannin

Fifteen isolates, obtained from clinical cases in human (B-01) and equines (Eq-2 to Eq-15) occurred in São Paulo State, Brazil, were maintained in Sabouraud (SAB) Agar, at 37 °C/7 days. After this period standardized mycelia fragments of 5 mm of diameter were tested with different concentrations of bark extract and purified tannin. Ten to 30% of bark extract were added to 1.0 mL of SAB broth and *P. insidiosum* hyphae standardized fragments of mycelia were added to these solutions. These fragments were incubated under shaking (100 rpm) at 37 °C/24 h. After that, each fragment was placed individually in SAB agar plates and incubated at 37 °C/7 days in order to follow the hyphal growth and determine the minimal fungicidal concentration (MFC). All tests were performed in quintuplicate. Tannin was tested at concentrations of 0.5, 1.0 and 1.5 mg/mL using the same procedure described for bark extract. Control groups consisted of hyphae standardized fragments incubated in SAB broth and placed in SAB agar. Hyphae fragments at MFC, were cut and fixed with 2.5% glutaraldehyde and then routinely processed for analysis by scanning electron microscopy (SEM) aiming to evaluate the hyphal morphology.

In vivo acute toxicity test

In order to investigate whether bark extract and tannin administration by oral route would be toxic, we employed the test of acute toxicity, according to Loomis & Haynes [13]. Briefly, we administered 5 g/Kg of bark extract or tannin, by gavage, in male Wistar rats weighting 250 g. For this assay 15 rats were divided in 3 groups and treated with bark extract, tannin or saline solution (control). Animals were observed for five days, when they were anesthetized with zolazepan chloride (Zoletil® 50, Virbac) and euthanized by anesthetic overdose. Blood was used to analyse serum levels of liver and kidney biochemical markers (ALT, AST, alkaline phosphatasis and urea) and complete hemogram. Liver and kidney were also excised and fixed in 10% formaldehyde and routinely processed for histopathological analysis. Rats were kept in cages (5 animals/cage) in the animal facility of the Department of Microbiology and Immunology, Institute of Biosciences, UNESP, and all procedures were approved by the local Ethics Committee on Animal Use (protocol number 536).

In vivo experimental pythiosis

Fifteen New Zealand rabbits were inoculated with 2 mL of induction medium (as described according to Mendoza and Prendas [14] containing around 20.000 zoospores of *P. insidiosum*), in the occipital region, as described by Pereira et al. [15]. Thirty days after inoculation, the animals were separated into five different groups with 3 animals each for treatment as follows: *S. adst.* = bark extract by oral route (90 mg/day); TAN = intralesional tannin (30 mg/mL each 48 h); TAN-VO = tannin by oral route (60 mg/day); TAN-PRED = intramuscular injection of methylprednisolone (1 mg/Kg, once a week) and intralesional tannin (30 mg/mL, associated with 1% DMSO, each 48 h), and control group (no treatment). Association with DMSO aimed to enhance the tannin diffusion while methylprednisolone was administrated at anti-inflammatory dose. The treatments were followed by macroscopic visual inspection and palpation, and histopathology analysis of HE and Gomori-Grocott stained slides. Transverse and longitudinal lengths were also measured with a caliper to calculate the wound area (mm^2). Infected rabbits were also analyzed on hepatic and kidney functions through the quantification of biochemical parameters (AST, ALT, alkaline phosphatasis and urea), as well as complete hemogram. Stomach and duodenum of animals treated by oral route were histopatologically analyzed. Rabbits were kept in individual cages at the animal facility of the Departments of Microbiology and Immunology, Institute of Biosciences, UNESP, and all procedures were approved by the local Ethics Committee on Animal Use, UNESP (protocol number 370).

Results

Crude bark extract showed 46.14% of total tannin concentration, which amount was considered for the serial dilution to determine the MFC (Table 1). Three out of 15 *P. insidiosum* isolates (20%) required more than 1.5 mg/mL; ten (66.7%) showed MFC between 1 and 1.5 mg/mL, while only two isolates (13.3%) required less than 1.0 mg/mL of bark extract to be inhibited. In relation of commercially available tannin, six isolates were inhibited at 0.5 mg/mL (40%), three isolates were inhibited at 1.0 mg/mL (20%) and six at 1.5 mg/mL (40%). Figure 1 shows the morphological features of hyphae of control group (Fig. 1A) with cylindrical body and smooth surface. Changes induced by bark extracts at MFC are illustrated at Fig. 1B, showing rough surface, release of anamorphic content and numerous granular material on the cell wall surface.

Toxicity tests made in rats showed that *S. adstringens* extract, as well as tannin, presented no acute toxicity, since no changes were observed in biochemical parameters of liver and kidney functions or animal behavior. Erythrocytes and leukocytes countings were also similar to the control animals. Administration of bark extract or tannin solution in rabbits seems to be also free of toxic effects on liver, kidney and blood system (Table 2).

All rabbits developed lesions at the inoculation site. Overall, the lesions appeared 20–30 days after inoculation and were characterized by encapsulated abscess with a firm consistency. Table 3 shows the mean size of the lesions before and at the end of treatment, indicating that there were no differences between the control group and any therapeutic approach we used. Macroscopic evaluation showed large granulomatous lesion containing caseous necrotic material with yellowish-green pus (Fig. 2). Microscopically we observed the typical eosinophilic granuloma with abundance of fibrous connective tissue and numerous hyphal elements evidenced by silver staining (Fig. 3).

Table 1 Isolates of *Pythium insidiosum* obtained from clinical cases of pythiosis in human (B-01) and horses (Eq-2 to 15), evaluated for minimal fungicidal concentration (MFC) of bark extract (in percentage of v/v, mg/mL of dry weight of extract and mg/mL of total tannin quantification) and purified tannin (mg/mL)

Pythium insidiosum isolates	MFC of bark extract			MFC purified tannin (mg/mL)
	% (v/v)	mg/mL of extract, according to dry weight	Total tannins (mg/mL)	
B-01	14	2.80	1.29	1.00
Eq-2	12	2.40	1.10	1.50
Eq-3	20	4.00	1.84	1.50
Eq-4	16	3.20	1.48	1.50
Eq-5	26	5.20	2.40	0.50
Eq-6	17	3.40	1.57	1.00
Eq-7	16	3.20	1.48	1.50
Eq-8	11	2.20	1.01	1.50
Eq-9	16	3.20	1.48	1.00
Eq-10	16	3.20	1.48	1.50
Eq-11	11	2.20	1.01	0.50
Eq-12	10	2.00	0.92	0.50
Eq-13	12	2.40	1.10	0.50
Eq-14	11	2.20	1.01	0.50
Eq-15	10	2.00	0.92	0.50

Discussion

Antimicrobial activity of *S. adstringens* has been shown on *Candida* spp., *Cryptococcus neoformans*, some dermatophytes, viruses, bacteria and protozoa [3, 8–10, 16, 17].

It antimicrobial activity combined with the healing action leaded us to choose this medicinal plant to investigate its therapeutic potential against *P. insidiosum* and pythiosis.

We first evaluated the in vitro effect of bark extract and tannin on this pathogen and observed that both were effective in inhibiting the mycelial growth. The tannin content in the bark extract was 46.14% and it was enough to inhibit the in vitro growth of pathogen. It has been reported that tannin may promote the precipitation of protein and/or polysaccharides, leading to formation of tannin-protein and/or tannin-polysaccharides complexes, justifying its antimicrobial effect [18]. Morphological analysis by SEM revealed several granular precipitations on the cell wall surface that may be the polysaccharide complexes. Cell wall of this pathogen is composed mainly by β-glucan and cellulose (polysaccharides), which may be one of the targets for tannins.

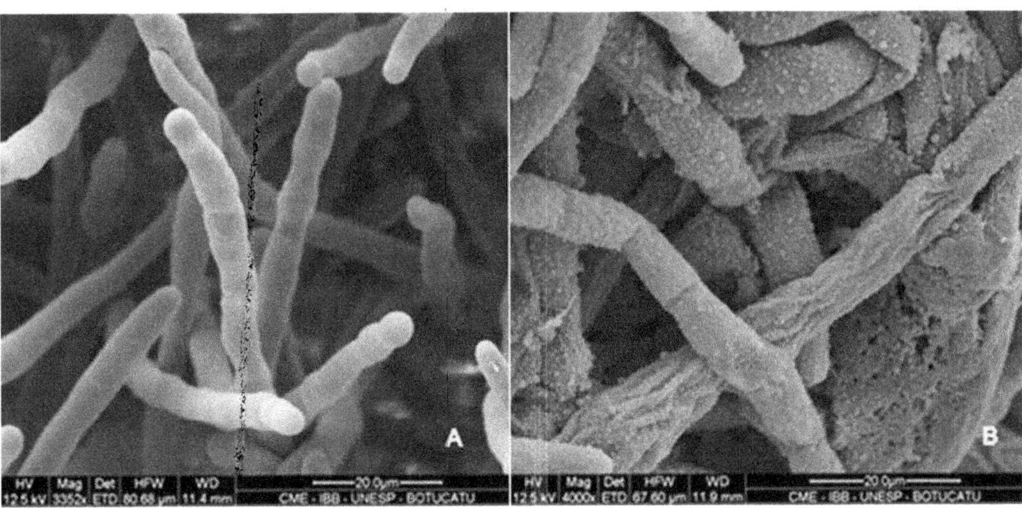

Fig. 1 Scanning electron microscopy of *Pythium insidiosum* from control group (**A**) and treated with MFC of bark extract of *S. adstringens* (**B**). Observe the cylindrical morphology of hyphae and smooth surface of cell wall from control group, while the hyphae treated with bark extract show rough surface of cell wall, high amount of granular material and release of anamorphic material

Table 2 Erythrocytes, white blood cells and plasma biochemical values of rats and rabbits from control and treatment groups (mean ± SD)

Animals	Treatments	RBC X10^6 cells/μL	WBC X10^6 cells/μL	ALT U/l	AST U/l	ALF U/l	Urea mg/dL	Creatinine mg/dL
Rats	Control	7.34 ± 0.47	3.1 ± 0.27	20.38 ± 1.41	125.00 ± 0.26	71.15 ± 0.31	71.30 ± 0.34	9.37 ± 0.57
	Bark extract	7.38 ± 0.47	2.96 ± 0.11	20.90 ± 1.61	123.8 ± 0.98	70.71 ± 0.58	71.12 ± 0.76	9.06 ± 0.29
	Tannin	7.35 ± 0.42	2.98 ± 0.16	20.04 ± 1.12	123.6 ± 0.89	70.62 ± 0.54	71.14 ± 0.86	9.30 ± 0.42
Rabbits	Control	5.63 ± 0.80	6.33 ± 1.06	71.39 ± 1.61	53.58 ± 0.76	25.27 ± 0.26	23.47 ± 1.20	1.22 ± 0.23
	S. adst	6.13 ± 1.06	6.46 ± 1.35	72.27 ± 2.07	53.53 ± 1.35	24.54 ± 0.61	23.17 ± 0.30	0.87 ± 0.14
	TAN	6.20 ± 1.11	6.70 ± 0.80	71.94 ± 1.99	53.14 ± 1.53	24.16 ± 1.09	23.13 ± 0.15	1.08 ± 0.12
	TAN-VO	6.53 ± 1.00	6.86 ± 1.30	71.66 ± 1.43	53.95 ± 1.39	23.74 ± 1.53	22.96 ± 0.42	0.96 ± 0.09
	TAN-PRED	6.23 ± 0.92	6.56 ± 0.85	72.16 ± 0.60	52.16 ± 0.60	23.46 ± 1.43	22.87 ± 1.07	0.97 ± 0.13

RBC red blood cells, *WBC* white blood cells, *ALT* alanine aminotransferase, *AST* aspartate aminotransferase, *ALF* alkaline phosphatasis

Table 3 Transverse and longitudinal lengths of the rabbit pythiosis lesions before and after 60 days of the different treatment protocols

Groups	Measurement before treatment (mm)	Measurement after treatment (mm)
S. adst.	16 × 20	85 × 88
TAN	25 × 26	90 × 91
TAN-VO	17 × 17	87 × 89
TAN-PRED	18 × 22	85 × 89
Control	21 × 17	89 × 89

There is no standardized technique for in vitro studies of *P. insidiosum* and the few studies reporting tests of susceptibility of this pathogen were carried out with the zoospores, a form found in the environment [15, 19, 20]. Studies on the hyphal form of the pathogen are scarce and should be more stimulated, since they are simple and reproducible [21]. Regarding the susceptibility of this pathogen to natural compounds, Zanette et al. [2] observed that garlic extracts inhibited the formation of germinative tube in the zoospores of seventeen isolates of *P. insdiosum*. Krajaejun et al. [22] observed that the volatile organic compound obtained from the endophytic fungus *Musdocor crispans* was able to inhibit the mycelia growth of thirty isolates of *P. insidiosum*. Sriphana et al. [23] evaluated the roots of a traditional medicinal plant in Thailand, *Alyxia schlechteri* and found three new lignan esters, called alyterinates A–C [1–3], which had an inhibitory effect on hyphal growth, while terbinafine and itraconazole failed to show antifungal effect. Additional study carried out by these authors also found that the alkaloid clauraila E, obtained from *Clauseana harmandiana* roots, another traditional medicinal plant in Thailand, was able to inhibit mycelia growth [24]. More

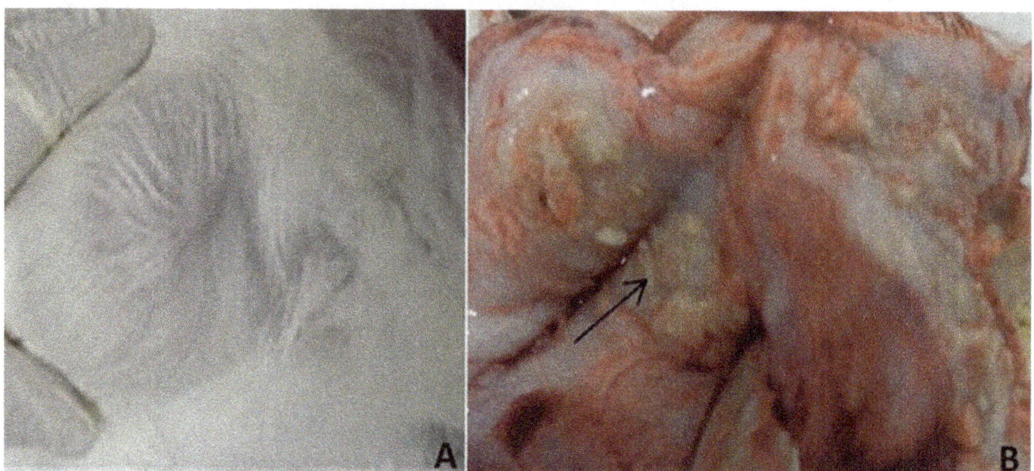

Fig. 2 Macroscopic aspect of encapsulated abscess in rabbit experimental model. **A** External view, **B** internal view of the abscess exhibiting caseous yellowish–green material in the center (*arrow*) surrounded by fibrous connective tissue

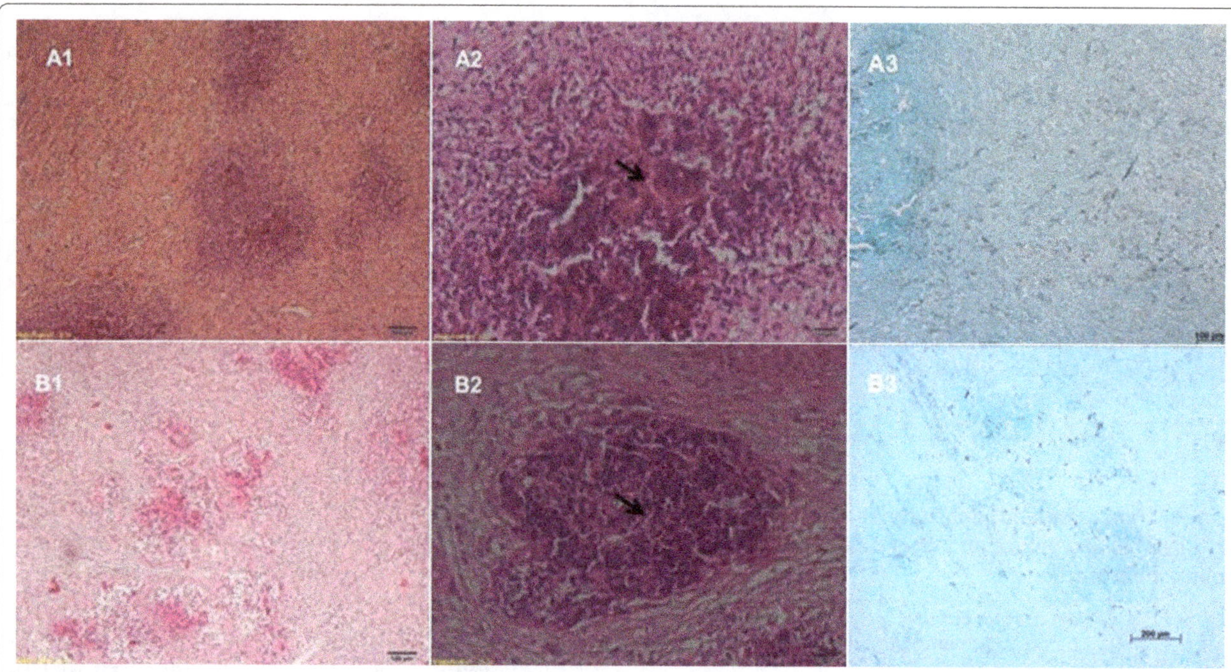

Fig. 3 Histological section of one animal from control group (**A**) and *S. adst.* group (**B**). *(1)* general view of both treatments (Hematoxilin–Eosin, 100×), *(2)* presence of hyphae and defense cells, with predominance of neutrophils and eosinophils (Hematoxilin–Eosin, 200×), *(3)* general view of granuloma showing high amounts of hyphae (Gomori-Grocott, 100×)

recently, Suthiwong et al. [25] found four new compounds from the fruits of *Micromelum falcatum* able to inhibit the mycelia growth of *P. insidiosum*. Fonseca et al. [26] evaluated the effect of essential oils of Lamiaceae Family and observed that *Origanum vulgare* showed the best performance in inhibiting the germination of zoospores of *P. insidiosum*. Therefore, it seems that new compounds with potential therapeutic activity against pythiosis may come from nature. In this sense, Fonseca et al. [27] showed that topical cream with essential oils of *O. vulgare* and *Mentha piperita* enhances the effect of immunotherapy to reduce the size of pythiosis lesions.

Few studies on pythiosis were conducted both in vitro and in vivo. Pereira et al. [15] evaluated the effect in vitro and in vivo of caspofungin, who administered it by intravenous rout and observed only fungistatic effect of this antifungal agent. Likewise, Loreto et al. [28] evaluated the effect of diphenyl diselenide in vitro and in vivo administrated by oral route, and also observed fungistatic effect of this compound and no toxicity.

Our in vivo toxicological evaluation of bark extract and purified tannin in Wistar rats showed no signs of toxicity in the histologic sections of liver and kidney or biochemical parameters of hepatic and renal functions. No hepatic or renal dysfunctions were observed in rabbits either. These results are a little bit different of those reported by Costa et al. [29] who evaluated the acute toxicity of different concentrations of bark extract in Swiss mice and rats, and observed more toxicological effects in mice than in rats.

Despite of being very effective in vitro and showed no toxicity in vivo, the application of bark extract or tannin in the experimental model of pythiosis were not as satisfactory as expected. In all rabbits the main macroscopic aspect of lesion was of encapsulated abscess, with very rigid fibrous connective tissue. At necropsy it was observed caseous necrotic material with focus of yellowish–green pus, in agreement with Miller and Campbel [30], pioneers of experimental studies on pythiosis. We believe that this encapsulated abscess is the most important reasons for low perfusion of tannin administrated intralesionally, which provides a physical barrier to medications, even when associated with dimethyl sulphoxide (DMSO, a potent organic solvent used to facilitate the perfusion) and systemic administration of methylpredinisolone (used in anti-inflammatory dose). Actually, this barrier had difficulted the needle insertion for in situ inoculation of the solutions and should also avoid the perfusion of orally administrated substances.

Therefore, an important difficulty for evaluating new approaches for treatment in vivo especially topical ones, is that lesions observed in experimental disease in rabbits is very different of naturally acquired disease. Horses and dogs, for example, develop ulcerated subcutaneous lesions, while in rabbits the lesions are well encapsulated in a fibrous abscess. Then, it is possible that the effectivity of *S. adstringens* extracts against *P. insidiosum* lesions would be observed in a more adequate model.

Conclusion

Our results allow us to conclude that both bark extract and purified tannin have direct fungicidal effect on hyphal growth of different isolates of *P. insidiosum*. Despite we were not able to demonstrate a therapeutic effect in our experimental model, the abcense of toxicity in addition to the lack of efficient conventional medications for pythiosis, it would be ethically acceptable to test these compounds topically as alternative treatment of naturally infected horses and dogs.

Abbreviations

SAB: Sabouraud (agar and broth); MFC: minimal fungicidal concentration; AST: aspartate aminotransferase; ALT: alanine aminotransferase; HE: Hematoxylin–Eosin stain.

Authors' contributions

RT carried out all experiments and data analysis. RT, RK, AFJr and SMGB participated in the design of the study and in the manuscript writing. JMA, NRP and JLC collaborated in in vitro and in vivo studies, manuscript writing. VEF conducted histopathological analysis, manuscript writing. MJDS and WV performed tannin quantification on bark extract, manuscript writing. All authors have read and approved the final manuscript.

Author details

[1] Department of Microbiology and Immunology, Institute of Biosciences of Botucatu, UNESP Univ Estadual Paulista, Botucatu, SP 18618-970, Brazil. [2] School of Veterinary Medicine and Animal Science, UNESP Univ Estadual Paulista, Botucatu, SP, Brazil. [3] Institute of Chemistry, UNESP Univ Estadual Paulista, Araraquara, SP, Brazil. [4] Department of Pathology, Botucatu School of Medicine, UNESP Univ Estadual Paulista, Botucatu, SP, Brazil.

Acknowledgements

The authors thank to Prof. Luiz Cláudio Di Stasi for suggesting the acute toxicity tests; to Carolina de Cássia Assumpção and Lara Vadrighi for lab assistance and animals care; to Ana Livia Ferreira Furtado for helping with quantification of tannin.

Competing interests

All authors declare that they have no competing interests.

Funding

The authors thank to São Paulo State Research Foundation (FAPESP, Grants: 2009/18466-0, 2011/14710-4 and 2011/21834-1) for the financial support and fellows granted.

References

1. Gaastra W, Lipman LJA, De Cock AWAM, Exel TK, Pegge RBG, Scheurwater J, Vilela R, Mendoza L. *Pythium insidiosum*: an overview. Vet Microbiol. 2010. doi:10.1016/j.vetmic.2010.07.019.
2. Zanette RA, Bittencourt PER, Weiblen C, Pilotto MB, Pigatto AS, Ceolin RB, Moretto MB, Alves SH, Santurio JM. *In vitro* susceptibility of *Pythium insidiosum* to garlic extract. J Afr Microbiol Res. 2011. doi:10.5897/AJMR11.821.
3. Melo Silva F, de Paula JE, Espindola LS. Evaluation of the antifungal potential of Brazilian Cerrado medicinal plants. Mycoses. 2009. doi:10.1111/j.1439-0507.2008.01647.x.
4. Nunes GP, Silva MF, Resende UM, Siqueira JM. Plantas medicinais comercializadas por raizeiros no Centro de Campo Grande, Mato Grosso do Sul. Rev Bras Farmacogn. 2003;13:83–92.
5. Audi EA, Toledo DP, Peres PG, Kimura E, Pereira WK, de Mello JC, Nakamura C, Alves-do-Prado W, Cuman RK, Bersani-Amado CA. Gastric antiulcerogenic effects of *Stryphnodendron adstringens* in rats. Phytother Res. 1999. doi:10.1002/(SICI)1099-1573(199905)13:3<264:AID-PTR443>3.0.CO;2-R.
6. Hernandes L, Pereira LMS, Palazzo F, Mello JCP. Wound-healing evaluation of ointment from *Stryphnodendron adstringens* (barbatimão) in rat skin. Braz J Pharmac Sci. 2010;46(3):431–6.

7. Pereira EM, Gomes RT, Freire NR, Aguiar EG, Brandão MD, Santos VR. *In vitro* antimicrobial activity of Brazilian medicinal plant extracts against pathogenic microorganisms of interest to dentistry. Planta Med. 2011. doi :10.1055/s-0030-1250354.
8. Fernandes A Jr, Albano M, Alves FCB, Andrade BFMT, Barbosa LN, Silva GS, Di Stasi LC. Medicinal plants from the Brazilian Savanna with antibacterial properties. Euro J Med Plants. 2014. doi:10.9734/EJMP/2014/5945.
9. Ishida K, Melo JCP, Cortez DAG, Dias Filho BP, Ueda-Nakamura T, Nakamura CV. Influence of tannins from *Stryphnodendron adstringens* on growth and virulence factors of *Candida albicans*. J Antimicrob Chemother. 2006. doi:10.1093/jac/dkl377.
10. Ishida K, Rozental S, de Mello JC, Nakamura CV. Activity of tannins from *Stryphnodendron adstringens* on *Cryptococcus neoformans*: effects on growth, capsule size and pigmentation. Ann Clin Microbiol Antimicrob. 2009. doi:10.1186/1476-0711-8-29.
11. Betoni JEC, Mantovani RP, Barbosa LN, Di Stasi LC, Fernandes Junior A. Synergism between plant extract and antimicrobial drugs used on *Staphylococcus aureus* diseases. Mem Inst Oswaldo Cruz. 2006. doi:10.1590/S0074-02762006000400007.
12. Waterhouse AL. Polyphenolics: Determination of total phenolics. In: Wrolstad RE, editor. Current protocols in food analytical chemistry. NewYork: John Wiley; 2002.
13. Loomis TA, Hayes AW. Loomis's essentials of toxicology. 4th ed. London: Academic Press Limited; 1996.
14. Mendoza L, Prendas J. A method to obtain rapid zoosporogenesis of *Pythium insidiosum*. Mycopathologia. 1988;104:59–62.
15. Pereira DIB, Santurio JM, Alves SH, Argenta JS, Pötter L, Spanamberg A, Ferreiro L. Caspofungin in vitro and in vivo activity against Brazilian *Pythium insidiosum* strains isolated from animals. J Antimicrob Chemoth. 2007. doi:10.1093/jac/dkm332.
16. Holetz FB, Ueda-Nakamura T, Dias Filho BP, Mello JCP, Morgado-Díaz JA, Toledo CEM, Nakamura CV. Biological effects of extracts obtained from *Stryphnodendron adstringens* on *Herpetomonas samuelpessoai*. Mem Inst Oswaldo Cruz. 2005. doi:10.1590/S0074-02762005000400010.
17. Felipe AM, Rincão VP, Benati FJ, Linhares RE, Galina KJ, de Toledo CE, Lopes GC, de Mello JC, Nozawa C. Antiviral effect of *Guazuma ulmifolia* and *Stryphnodendron adstringens* on poliovirus and bovine herpesvirus. Biol Pharm Bull. 2006. doi:10.1248/bpb.29.1092.
18. Santos SC, Costa WF, Ribeiro JP, Guimarães DO, Ferri PH, Ferreira HD, Seraphin JC. Tannin composition of barbatimão species. Fitoterapia. 2002. doi:10.1016/S0367-326X(02)00081-3.
19. Sekhon AS, Padhye AA, Garg AK. *In vitro* sensitivity of *Penicillium marneffei* and *Pythium insidiosum* to various antifungal agents. Eur J Epidemiol. 1992. http://www.jstor.org/stable/3520676.
20. Argenta JS, Santurio JM, Alves SH, Pereira DI, Cavalheiro AS, Spanamberg A, Ferreiro L. *In vitro* activities of voriconazole, itraconazole and terbinafine alone or in combination against *Pythium insidiosum* isolates from Brazil. Antimicrob Agents Chemother. 2008. doi:10.1128/AAC.01075-07.
21. Brown TA, Grooters AM, Hosgood GL. *In vitro* susceptibility of *Pythium insidiosum* and *Lagenidium* sp. to itraconazole, posaconazole, voriconazole, terbinafine, caspofungin, and mefenoxam. Am J Vet Res. 2008;69(11):1463–8.
22. Krajaejun T, Lowhnoo T, Yingyong W, Rujirawat T, Fucharoen S, Strobel GA. *In vitro* antimicrobial activity of volatile organic compounds from *Muscodor crispans* against the pathogenic oomycete *Pythium insidiosum*. SE Asian J Trop Med. 2012;43(6):1474–83.
23. Sriphana U, Thongsri Y, Ardwichai P, Poopasit K, Prariyachatigul C, Simasathiansophon S, Yenjai C. New lignan esters from *Alyxia schlechteri* and antifungal activity against *Pythium insidiosum*. Fitoterapia. 2013. doi:10.1016/j.fitote.2013.08.005.
24. Sriphana U, Thongsri Y, Prariyachatigul C, Pakawatchai C, Yenjai C. Clauraila E from the roots of *Clausena harmandiana* and antifungal activity against *Pythium insidiosum*. Arch Pharm Res. 2013. doi:10.1007/s12272-013-0115-5.
25. Suthiwong J, Sriphana U, Thongsri Y, Promsuwan P, Prariychatigul C, Yenjai C. Coumarinoid from the fruits of *Micromelum facatum*. Fitoterapia. 2014. doi:10.1016/j.fitote.2014.02.004.
26. Fonseca AOS, Pereira DIB, Botton SA, Pötter L, Sallis ESV, Júnior SFV, Filho FSM, Zambrano CG, Maroneze BP, Valente JSS, Baptista CT, Braga CQ, Dal Ben V, Meireles MCA. Treatment of experimental pythiosis with essential oils of *Origanum vulgare* and *Mentha piperita* singly, in association and in combination with immunotherapy. Vet Microbiol. 2015. doi:10.1016/j.vetmic.2015.05.023.
27. Fonseca AOS, Pereira DIB, Jacob RG, Maia Filho FS, Oliveira DH, Maroneze BP, Valente JSS, Osório LG, Botton SA, Meireles MCA. *In vitro* susceptibility of Brazilian *Pythium insidiosum* isolates to essential oils of some Lamiaceae Family species. Mycopathologia. 2015. doi:10.1007/s11046-014-9841-6.
28. Loreto ES, Alves SH, Santurio JM, Nogueira CW, Zeni G. Diphenyl diselenide in vitro and in vivo activity against the oomycete *Pythium insidiosum*. Vet Microbiol. 2012. doi:10.1016/j.vetmic.2011.10.008.
29. Costa MA, Mello JCP, Kaneshima EN, Ueda-Nakamura T, Dias Filho BP, Audi EA, Nakamura CV. Acute and chronic toxicity of an aqueous fraction of the stem bark of *Stryphnodendron adstringens* (barbatimão) in rodents. Evid Based Complement Alternat Med. 2013. doi:10.1155/2013/841580.
30. Miller RI, Campbell SF. Experimental pythiosis in rabbits. Sabouraudia. 1983;21:331–41.

6

Development of a fast and low-cost qPCR assay for diagnosis of acute gas pharyngitis

Mustafa Kolukirik[1*], Mesut Yılmaz[2], Orhan Ince[3], Canan Ketre[3], Ayşe Istanbullu Tosun[4] and Bahar K. Ince[5]

Abstract

Background: Group A streptococci (GAS) are the most common bacterial cause of acute pharyngitis and account for 15–30 % of cases of acute pharyngitis in children and 5–10 % of cases in adults. In this study, a real-time quantitative PCR (qPCR) based GAS detection assay in pharyngeal swab specimens was developed.

Methods: The qPCR assay was compared with the gold standard bacterial culture and a rapid antigen detection test (RADT) to evaluate its clinical performance in 687 patients. The analytical sensitivity of the assay was 240 cfu/swab. Forty-five different potential cross-reacting organisms did not react with the test. Four different laboratories for the reproducibility studies were in 100 % (60/60) agreement for the contrived GAS positive and negative swab samples.

Results: The relative sensitivities of the RADT and the qPCR test were 55.9 and 100 %; and the relative specificities were 100 and 96.3 %, respectively. Duration of the total assay for 24 samples including pre-analytical processing and analysis changed between 42 and 55 min depending on the type of qPCR instrument used. A simple DNA extraction method and a low qPCR volume made the developed assay an economical alternative for the GAS detection.

Conclusion: We showed that the developed qPCR test is rapid, cheap, sensitive and specific and therefore can be used to replace both antigen detection and culture for diagnosis of acute GAS pharyngitis.

Keywords: Group A streptococci, Acute pharyngitis, qPCR, Rapid antigen detection test

Background

Acute pharyngitis is a nonspecific symptom that can result from a number of viral or bacterial infections. Group A streptococci (GAS) are the most common bacterial cause of acute pharyngitis and account for 15–30 % of cases of acute pharyngitis in children and 5–10 % of cases in adults [1]. The cost per case of GAS pharyngitis was estimated to be approximately $205, with about half of the costs attributed to nonmedical costs such as missed days of work by parents for child care [2].

GAS pharyngitis is usually self-limited and resolves without the need for antibiotic treatment [3]; however, a minority of patients develop severe complications such as scarlet fever and peritonsillar cellulitis, as well as immune-mediated complications, including post-streptococcal glomerulonephritis and acute rheumatic fever. Early treatment of GAS pharyngitis with appropriate antibiotics is known to reduce symptom severity and duration, decrease transmission of the organism, and reduce the risk of acute rheumatic fever [4]. Incidence of the rheumatic heart disease changes between 0.03 and 2.1 % based on the development status of the countries [5].

As most pharyngitis is viral in origin, accurate diagnosis can reduce the unnecessary use of antibiotics and potential development of antibiotic resistance [6, 7]. However, accurate diagnosis of GAS pharyngitis is difficult for a number of reasons. First, diagnosis of GAS pharyngitis using clinical signs alone is unreliable due to the broad overlap in symptoms between the viral and bacterial etiologies [4]; physicians miss up to 50 % of GAS pharyngitis cases and identify 20–40 % of non-GAS sore

*Correspondence: mustafa.kolukirik@engy.com.tr
[1] ENGY Environmental and Energy Technologies Biotechnology Research and Development Limited Company, Istanbul, Turkey
Full list of author information is available at the end of the article

throat cases as requiring antibiotics [8]. Second, many children are asymptomatic carriers of GAS, with the prevalence of GAS throat carriage estimated at 12 % [9]. Third and the most important, the standard procedure for laboratory detection of GAS, culture on blood agar, typically requires 24–48 h [10], which is problematic for physicians to provide the diagnosis on the same day of patients office visit.

Value of rapid testing for the GAS pharyngitis diagnosis in directing clinical management and reducing unnecessary antibiotic prescription has been documented [11, 12]. The fast diagnosis methods include rapid antigen detection tests (RADTs) and nucleic acid-based methodologies. RADTs provide results within minutes, but exhibit only 72–90 % sensitivity compared to that of a culture [13]. Polymerase chain reaction (PCR) [14, 15], real-time quantitative PCR (qPCR) [16, 17] and loop-mediated isothermal amplification (LAMP) [18, 19] based tests for the detection of GAS have been described. These tests have high sensitivity (>93 %) and good specificity (>95 %). The PCR and qPCR based tests have not been found wide application due to insufficient clinical evaluation [14, 16], high cost [17] and labor intensive laboratory work [15]. A LAMP based method, the Illumigene group A Streptococcus assay, has been developed by Meridian Bioscience and cleared by the FDA. Henson et al. [19] and Anderson et al. [18] evaluated its clinical performance and reported that the assay is rapid (<1 h), easy to perform and highly sensitive and specific.

Current Infectious Diseases Society of America (IDSA) guidelines state that a clinical diagnosis of GAS pharyngitis must be confirmed [4]. Reimbursement for the culture and the molecular based analyses are 9.12$ and 48.24$ respectively in USA, which makes the Illumi-gene group A Streptococcus assay (28$/test), an economically feasible tool for diagnosis of GAS pharyngitis (Sales Sheet: Illumigene Group A Streptococcus). On the other hand, there is no reimbursement for the molecular detection of GAS pharyngitis in most of the developing countries due to the very high costs of the tests. Furthermore, the clinical signs have been the major diagnostic tools in developing countries like Turkey where the cost of antibiotic treatment is very low (3–10$). This has resulted in considerable social burden [20] and unnecessary antibiotic prescriptions in up to 75 % of patients with acute tonsillopharyngitis [21] and a total (outpatients and hospital care) antibiotic use of 42.3 defined daily doses/1000 inhabitants per day (DID) for Turkey which has made Turkey the first among 40 countries in Europe in the calculation of unit ranks for antibiotic usage [22].

In this study, we aimed to develop a qPCR based GAS detection assay in pharyngeal swab specimens that is as rapid as the previous molecular tests, as sensitive and specific as the culture test and as economical as the low-cost antibiotic treatments.

Methods

Study participants and collection of specimens

The study was conducted in accordance with the Declaration of Helsinki and approved by Istanbul Medipol University (IMU) Research Ethics Committee. The throat swab specimens were collected at IMU Hospital from 687 patients aged between 5 and 12 years presenting acute sore throat over the winter/spring of 2012 and 2013. The study population included 356 (51.8 %) female and 331 (48.2 %) male patients. No restrictions were placed on gender, medications or known pharmaceutical therapies.

Two blind samples were collected using the BBL CultureSwab EZ II—Double Swab (Becton–Dickinson, USA) according to the standard methods [4]. One swab was used for the RADT and culture and the other was used for the qPCR assay. The samples for the culture and antigen tests were transported to Istanbul Medipol University Laboratory at ambient temperature and processed on the day of sample collection. The samples for the molecular analysis were transported to Istanbul Technical University Molecular Biology, Genetics and Biotechnology Research Center (ITU MOBGAM) at +2 to 8 °C and analyzed on the day of sample collection.

Culture and antigen test

The swabs were inoculated on BBL strep selective agar (Becton–Dickinson, USA) plates and incubated at 35 °C for 16–18 h. Catalase negative colonies with a morphology of β-hemolytic streptococcus were transferred to 5 % sheep blood agar and subjected to bacitracin, sulfamethoxazole–trimethoprim (SXT) susceptibility test, BBL DrySlide PYR and BBL Streptocard Enzyme Latex Test Kit (Becton–Dickinson, USA) for GAS confirmation.

After inoculation of the SSA plate, the same swab was used for evaluation with the Clearview® Strep A Exact II Cassette test (Inverness Medical Professional Diagnostics, USA). The procedure was performed according to the instructions provided by the manufacturer.

Molecular analyses

The swabs were cut and placed into 1.5 ml microcentrifuge tubes containing 400 μl of 0.1 M Tris–HCl pH 8.0. The tubes were placed in TSS-2000 turbo thermal shaker & heater (Inovia Technology, Turkey), shaken for 20 s at 3000 rpm, incubated at +95 °C for 10 min and shaken for 20 s at 3000 rpm. The swabs were removed from the sample tubes and discarded. The samples were immediately used in qPCRs and stored at −20 °C after the qPCR set up.

Two different qPCRs (qPCR-GAS and qPCR-PC) were set up by combining 5 μl of the supernatant with 5 μl of two different 2x qPCR master mix in 0.1 ml reaction tubes. The qPCR-GAS and qPCR-PC contained primers targeting *Streptococcus pyogenes* pyrogenic exotoxin B (speB) and *Bacillus thermocatenulatus* triacylglycerol lipase (BTL2) genes respectively. The qPCR-PC also contained BTL2 gene. The qPCR-PC was set up as a positive control reaction to evaluate inhibitory effect of the sample on the DNA amplification. Five microlitre DNase free molecular grade water was combined with 5 µl of 2x qPCR-GAS master mix as a negative control (qPCR-NC).

Biospeedy EvaGreen Real-Time PCR 2x premix (Bioeksen R&D Technologies, Turkey) was used for qPCR. The premix contains 12 mg/ml bovine serum albumin (BSA), 40 mg/ml PEG 400, %0.5 Tween 20, 40 mM Tris–HCl pH 8.0, 100 mM KCl, 3 mM $MgCl_2$, 0.4 mM dNTP mix, 0.2U Hot-Start Taq DNA Polymerase and 0.2x EvaGreen Dye. The 2x qPCR-GAS master mix was prepared by adding 200 nM of the each speB1166-F (5′-AAAGTAGGCGG ACATGCCTTTG-3′) and speB1268-R (5′-CAAGACGG AAGAAGCCGTCAG-3′) primers to the premix. The 2x qPCR-PC master mix was prepared by adding 200 nM of the each BTL908-F (5′-CGACGGATACTGCCCGC TAC-3′) and BTL1014-R (5′-CCGTTCGGTGGAAAAG CTCA-3′) primers and 5 ng of their target BTL2 gene to the premix.

QPCR cycling conditions were an initial 3 min at 95 °C step, followed by 35 amplification cycles of 95 °C for 5 s and 60 °C for 25 s. A melt-curve analysis with a temperature transition rate of 0.5 °C/s was performed from 60 to 90 °C to determine if only one amplified product was generated during qPCR. The qPCR was carried out using four different Real-Time PCR system: Biorad CFX Connect (Bio-Rad Laboratories, USA), LightCycler 480 (Roche Applied Science, USA), StepOne Plus (Life Technologies, USA) and Xxpress (BJS Biotechnologies, UK). The samples which had a melting temperature (Tm) of qPCR-GAS between 80 and 81 °C and no specific amplification in qPCR-NC were considered positive. The samples that had no specific amplification in the qPCR-GAS and qPCR-NC were considered negative for GAS. Threshold cycle (Ct) of the qPCR-PC was lower than 25 with a Tm between 80 and 81 °C. The qPCR-PC Ct values higher than 25 were considered an indicator of PCR inhibitor interference.

The amplified DNA fragments in positive qPCR-GAS reactions from the tested 687 patients and the contrived positive (*S. pyogenes* ATCC 19615) swab samples were purified using High Pure PCR Product Purification Kit (Roche Applied Science, USA) and sequenced using the ABI prism Big Dye Terminator Cycle Sequencing Ready Reaction Kit on an ABI Prism 377 DNA sequencer (Life Technologies, USA). The sequences were analyzed in Chromas software package version 2.0 (Technelysium, Australia) and manually checked for the reading errors. The sequences were aligned with *S. pyogenes* strain ATCC 19615 whole genome region from 849512 to 849614 (Access# CP008926.1) coding speB gene using Clustal Omega (http://www.ebi.ac.uk/Tools/msa/clustalo/).

Analytical sensitivity

Twenty replicates of the BBL CultureSwab EZ—Single Swab (Becton–Dickinson, USA) were spiked with 10^1–10^4 CFU *S. pyogenes* ATCC 19615 in 100 µl Buffer1 (0.1 M Tris–HCl pH 8.0). Following determination of a detection limit in a wide range, e.g. between 2×10^2 and 3×10^2 CFU, five more dilutions were prepared within this range. Limit of detection (LOD) stated a 95 % (19/20) probability of obtaining the reference samples positive for GAS. *S. pyogenes* ATCC 49399 and 12344 strains were also tested at the determined LOD. Interferences of 5 mg/mL mucus and 10 % v/v human saliva in Buffer1 were tested with contrived positive (ATCC 19615) samples prepared at the determined LOD. Analytical sensitivity studies were carried out using Biorad CFX Connect qPCR instrument.

Analytical specificity

In-Silico PCR with speB1166-F and speB1268-R primers was carried out using the Primer Blast tool (http://www.ncbi.nlm.nih.gov/tools/primer-blast/) to test the cross reactivity among all available sequences in DNA databases. 55 bp fragment of *Bacillus* sp. GL1 unsaturated glucuronyl hydrolase gene (AB019619) and 1217 bp fragment of *Myxococcus stipitatus* DSM 14675 long-chain-fatty-acid-CoA ligase gene (CP004025) were amplified with total mismatches of 7 and 9 bases respectively. *Myxococcus stipitatus* DSM 14675 and chemically synthesized 55 base fragment of the *Bacillus* sp. GL1 DNA (Macrogen Inc., Europe) were included in the analytic specifity tests.

The BBL CultureSwab EZ—Single Swab (Becton–Dickinson, USA) were spiked with 10^6 CFU bacterial or fungal organisms in 100 µl Buffer1. 20 ng/µl human DNA, 20 ng/µl *Bacillus* sp. GL1 DNA and the following organisms were tested for the cross reactivity:

Acinetobacter baumannii, Aeromonas hydrophila, Arcanobacterium haemolyticum, Bordetella bronchiseptica, Burkholderia cepacia, Campylobacter jejuni, Candida albicans, Citrobacter freundii, Corynebacterium diphtheria, Corynebacterium pseudodiphtheriticum, Enterococcus faecalis, Enterococcus faecium, Escherichia coli, Haemophilus influenzae, Klebsiella oxytoca, Klebsiella pneumoniae, Lactococcus lactis, Legionella pneumophila, Listeria monocytogenes, Moraxella catarrhalis,

Morganella morganii, Myxococcus stipitatus, Neisseria pharyngis, Neisseria meningitidis, Proteus mirabilis, Pseudomonas aeruginosa, Staphylococcus aureus, Staphylococcus epidermidis, Stenotrophomonas maltophilia, Streptococcus agalactiae, Streptococcus anginosus, Streptococcus bovis, Streptococcus canis, Streptococcus dysgalactiae (subspecies equisimilis), Streptococcus equinus, Streptococcus intermedius, Streptococcus mitis, Streptococcus mutans, Streptococcus pneumoniae, Streptococcus salivarius, Streptococcus suis, Streptococcus uberis, Streptococcus sp. *viridans type.*

Reproducibility

Contrived high positive (10^5 CFU ATCC 19615), positive (240 CFU ATCC 19615), low negative (10^5 CFU non-target organism mix) and negative (without any organism) swab samples were prepared using Buffer1. Five sets of blind-coded panels of 12 samples (three replicates of the four swab types) were supplied to four independent laboratories each having a different qPCR instrument (Biorad CFX Connect, LightCycler 480, StepOne Plus and Xxpress). Samples were randomly sorted within each panel to mask sample identities. Different operators at each site performed testing on the same day (intra-assay variability) for 5 days (inter-assay variability). Duration of the total assay for 12 samples was also measured each day.

Statistical analysis

After assessment of normality of data, differences between the replicate samples in terms of Ct and Tm values were evaluated using the Student's t test. Analyses were performed using the software MINITAB 17 (Minitab Ltd., England).

The sample size to show that the developed assay is not worse than the culture was calculated based on 5 % non-inferiority limit as described by Blackwelder [23]. It was estimated that "If there is a true 5 % difference between the developed assay and the culture, then 375 patients are required to be 90 % sure that the upper limit of a one-sided 95 % confidence interval (or equivalently a 90 % two-sided confidence interval) will exclude a difference in favour of the standard group of more than 5 %".

Results

LOD of the qPCR test was 240 CFU/Test for *S. pyogenes* ATCC 19615. The swabs containing 240 CFU *S. pyogenes* ATCC 49399 or 12344 strains also produced positive reactions. The qPCRs at the stated LOD were positive for all of the replicates with Ct value of 25.9 ± 1.2 and a single Tm peak at 80.3 ± 0.2 °C. The qPCR product sequences matched 100 % with *S. pyogenes* strain ATCC 19615 speB gene.

Human DNA, *Bacillus* sp. GL1 DNA and the potential cross-reacting microorganisms did not react with the test. Some of the negative control organisms gave a Ct value between 30 and 35, but the Tm was not consistent with the target amplification (80–81 °C). 5 mg/mL mucus and 10 % v/v human saliva did not interfere with the test results at the stated LOD. There were no statistically important Ct differences between the samples with and without interfering substances ($t > 2.02$, $df = 38$, $p < 0.05$).

All of the sites for the reproducibility studies were in 100 % agreement (60/60) for the contrived positive and negative samples. There were no statistically important Ct and Tm differences between the positive tests carried out in the different qPCR instruments ($t > 2.00$, $df = 58$, $p < 0.05$). Biorad CFX Connect, LightCycler 480, StepOne Plus and Xxpress produced Tm values of 80.3 ± 0.2, 80.3 ± 0.1, 80.2 ± 0.2 and 80.2 ± 0.1 °C respectively. Duration of the total assay for 24 samples including pre-analytical processing and analysis was 50 ± 2, 51 ± 3, 55 ± 3 and 42 ± 3 min for Biorad CFX Connect, LightCycler 480, StepOne Plus and Xxpress respectively.

Table 1 compares the results for the developed qPCR method and the RADT, to those of the conventional culture method that is well known as a gold standard for GAS detection [10]. The four different qPCR instruments produced the same test results for the clinical performance evaluation. The qPCR product sequences from the positive 222 throat swabs matched 100 % with *S. pyogenes* strain ATCC 19615 speB gene. PCR inhibition was not detected by means of a lack of internal control (BTL2 gene) amplification for all of the samples.

In no case was a throat swab negative by the qPCR method but positive by culture. However, positive results occurred by the qPCR method for some samples that were negative by culture. All of the discordant results by the RADT method versus the results of culture were positive by culture.

Table 1 Performance characteristics comparison of the developed qPCR method to those of the rapid antigen test (RAT) and the gold standard culture method for detection of GAS from the 687 throat swabs

Results	Culture	RAT	QPCR
Positive	204	114	222
Negative	483	573	465
Prevalence	29.7 %	16.6 %	32.3 %
Sensitivity		69.4 %	100 %
Specificity		100 %	96.4 %
Positive predictive value		100 %	92.9 %
Negative predictive value		84.3 %	100 %

Discussion

Sensitivity and specificity of the DNA amplification based GAS detection tests have already been reported to be 100 and 95 % for PCR [15], 100 and 100 % for qPCR [16] and 100 and 98 % for LAMP [18]. The approximate times required to complete these tests including pre-analytical processing and analysis are as follows: PCR, 3–4 h; qPCR, 1.5–3 h; LAMP, 50–60 min. We showed that the developed qPCR test is rapid (42–55 min), sensitive (100 %) and specific (96.4 %) and therefore can be used to replace both antigen detection and culture for diagnosis of acute GAS pharyngitis. With the speed of the qPCR assay, results can be relayed to health care providers and patients in less than 2 h after the test is ordered.

The high speed of the developed qPCR test was mainly because of the rapid DNA extraction method that can be completed in less than 15 min for 24 samples. The extraction method did not eliminate the possible PCR inhibitors such as collagen [24]. The DNA amplification facilitators, betaine and BSA, were included in the qPCRs to compensate the possible effects of the inhibitors [25]. This application resulted in no PCR inhibition in the clinical performance studies.

In this study, RADT provided the fastest results, but exhibited only 69.4 % sensitivity compared to that of culture. Due to difficulties in the sampling from children, the swab used for RADT was first used to inoculate an agar plate in the clinical performance evaluation studies. This is one of the limitations of the study since some of the bacterial content might have been removed from the swab and affected sensitivity of RADT. The low sensitivity problem of the antigen tests has frequently been reported [13]. If RADTs are performed routinely, culture must be applied to the all RADT-negative specimens. The non-GAS acute pharyngitis accounts for 70–95 % of the cases [1] and only 70 % of the true-positive samples are expected to be detected using RADTs. If culture is performed after RADT, more than 70 % of the patients should have a throat culture.

There are no methods defined in the literature to distinguish GAS carriage from actual streptococcal pharyngitis. All the patients in our study had presented with acute sore throat and up to 12 % of these may actually be carriers [9].

The qPCR product sequences of 18 samples that were culture negative but qPCR positive matched with *S. pyogenes* speB gene. Although throat culture was considered as the gold standard, the detected GAS DNA may be associated with the following: First, some of the patients might have taken antibiotics at the time throat swabs were taken. This would restrict growth on a culture but not the qPCR results. Second, errors of sampling may always be an issue. Third, qPCR may be more sensitive than standard culture. All of the positive patients by qPCR were treated with antibiotics effective against GAS, even though the health care providers responsible for these patients were unaware of the qPCR result. Uhl et al. [17] also reported that all discordant positive results for the qPCR method versus the results of culture were believed to be associated with the disease when they evaluated the GAS test results along with the medical history recorded by the health care provider. On the other hand, the qPCR assay does not distinguish between DNA from viable and non-viable organisms. In order to prevent the false positive results, DNA from the non-viable GAS can be eliminated via pretreatment of the specimens with propidium monoazide [26] or DNase-I [27]. Since the specificity of the developed qPCR test was high enough, we do not recommend application of these pretreatment strategies avoid increase in total analysis time and cost.

The simple DNA extraction using only the Tris–HCl buffer and the low qPCR volume (10 μl) makes the developed assay a very economical alternative for GAS detection. Based on the outcomes of this study, "Republic of Turkey Social Security Institution Health Applications Notification" has recently been updated and "*S. pyogenes* fast PCR test" was added to the reimbursement list [28]. Reimbursement for the *S. pyogenes* fast PCR test is 1.95$ that was calculated based on a testing potential of 2 million tests per year.

Conclusion

Our rapid, cheap, sensitive and specific qPCR test can replace both antigen detection and culture for diagnosis of acute GAS pharyngitis.

Authors' contributions

MK and MY ideated the study and conceived the data. MK, MY, and BKI drafted manuscript. AIT performed microbiological analyses and gathered the study data; OI, MK and CK performed qPCR analyses. MK and CK analyzed and MY and AIT provided interpretation of the study data. All authors read and approved the final manuscript.

Author details

[1] ENGY Environmental and Energy Technologies Biotechnology Research and Development Limited Company, Istanbul, Turkey. [2] Infectious Diseases and Clinical Microbiology, Istanbul Medipol University, Istanbul, Turkey. [3] Istanbul Technical University, Istanbul, Turkey. [4] Microbiology, Istanbul Medipol University, Istanbul, Turkey. [5] Bogazici University, Istanbul, Turkey.

Acknowledgements

"Turkish Public Health Institution" and "Trakya University, Department of Pharmaceutical Microbiology" supplied organisms for the analytical specificity studies.

Competing interests

The authors declare that they have no competing interests.

Funding

The study was funded by ENGY Environmental and Energy Technologies Biotechnology Research and Development Limited Company and Istanbul Medipol University Research Fund.

Informed consent

Informed consent was obtained from all individual participants included in the study.

References

1. Bisno AL. Acute pharyngitis. N Engl J Med. 2001;344:205–11.
2. Pfoh E, Wessels MR, Goldmann D, Lee GM. Burden and economic cost of group A streptococcal pharyngitis. Pediatrics. 2008;121:229–34.
3. Centor RM. Expand the pharyngitis paradigm for adolescents and young adults. Ann Intern Med. 2009;151:812–5.
4. Shulman ST, Bisno AL, Clegg HW, Gerber MA, Kaplan EL, Lee G, et al. Clinical practice guideline for the diagnosis and management of group A streptococcal pharyngitis: 2012 update by the Infectious Diseases Society of America. Clin Infect Dis. 2012;55:e86–102.
5. Sainani GS, Sainani AR. Rheumatic fever—how relevant in India today? J Assoc Physicians India. 2006;54(Suppl):42–7.
6. Joachim L, Campos D Jr, Smeesters PR. Pragmatic scoring system for pharyngitis in low-resource settings. Pediatrics. 2010;126:e608–14.
7. Smeesters PR, Campos D Jr, Van Melderen L, de Aguiar E, Vanderpas J, Vergison A. Pharyngitis in low-resources settings: a pragmatic clinical approach to reduce unnecessary antibiotic use. Pediatrics. 2006;118:e1607–11.
8. McIsaac WJ, White D, Tannenbaum D, Low DE. A clinical score to reduce unnecessary antibiotic use in patients with sore throat. CMAJ. 1998;158:75–83.
9. Shaikh N, Leonard E, Martin JM. Prevalence of streptococcal pharyngitis and streptococcal carriage in children: a meta-analysis. Pediatrics. 2010;126:e557–64.
10. Langlois DM, Andreae M. Group A streptococcal infections. Pediatr Rev. 2011;32:423–9 **(quiz 30)**.
11. Mainous AG 3rd, Zoorob RJ, Kohrs FP, Hagen MD. Streptococcal diagnostic testing and antibiotics prescribed for pediatric tonsillopharyngitis. Pediatr Infect Dis J. 1996;15:806–10.
12. Needham CA, McPherson KA, Webb KH. Streptococcal pharyngitis: impact of a high-sensitivity antigen test on physician outcome. J Clin Microbiol. 1998;36:3468–73.
13. Forward KR, Haldane D, Webster D, Mills C, Brine C, Aylward D. A comparison between the Strep A Rapid Test Device and conventional culture for the diagnosis of streptococcal pharyngitis. Can J Infect Dis Med Microbiol. 2006;17:221–3.
14. Kumar A, Bhatnagar A, Gupta S, Khare S, Suman R. sof gene as a specific genetic marker for detection of *Streptococcus pyogenes* causing pharyngitis and rheumatic heart disease. Cell Mol Biol (Noisy-le-grand). 2011;57:26–30.
15. Thenmozhi R, Balaji K, Kanagavel M, Karutha Pandian S. Development of species-specific primers for detection of *Streptococcus pyogenes* from throat swabs. FEMS Microbiol Lett. 2010;306:110–6.
16. Dunne EM, Marshall JL, Baker CA, Manning J, Gonis G, Danchin MH, et al. Detection of group a streptococcal pharyngitis by quantitative PCR. BMC Infect Dis. 2013;13:312.
17. Uhl JR, Adamson SC, Vetter EA, Schleck CD, Harmsen WS, Iverson LK, et al. Comparison of LightCycler PCR, rapid antigen immunoassay, and culture for detection of group A streptococci from throat swabs. J Clin Microbiol. 2003;41:242–9.
18. Anderson NW, Buchan BW, Mayne D, Mortensen JE, Mackey TL, Ledeboer NA. Multicenter clinical evaluation of the illumigene group A Streptococcus DNA amplification assay for detection of group A Streptococcus from pharyngeal swabs. J Clin Microbiol. 2013;51:1474–7.
19. Henson AM, Carter D, Todd K, Shulman ST, Zheng X. Detection of *Streptococcus pyogenes* by use of Illumigene group A Streptococcus assay. J Clin Microbiol. 2013;51:4207–9.
20. Ozkaya-Parlakay A, Uysal M, Kara A. Group A streptococcal tonsillopharyngitis burden in a tertiary Turkish hospital. Turk J Pediatr. 2012;54:474–7.
21. Ovet G, Balci YI, Polat Y, Ersoy E, Covut IE. Akut tonsillofarenjit tanısı alarak antibiyotik başlanan hastaların ne kadarından A Grubu Beta Hemolitik Streptokoklar sorumludur? Tıp Araştırmaları Dergisi. 2009;7:122–5.
22. Versporten A, Bolokhovets G, Ghazaryan L, Abilova V, Pyshnik G, Spasojevic T, et al. Antibiotic use in eastern Europe: a cross-national database study in coordination with the WHO Regional Office for Europe. Lancet Infect Dis. 2014;14:381–7.
23. Blackwelder WC. "Proving the null hypothesis" in clinical trials. Control Clin Trials. 1982;3:345–53.
24. Radstrom P, Knutsson R, Wolffs P, Lovenklev M, Lofstrom C. Pre-PCR processing: strategies to generate PCR-compatible samples. Mol Biotechnol. 2004;26:133–46.
25. Abu Al-Soud W, Radstrom P. Effects of amplification facilitators on diagnostic PCR in the presence of blood, feces, and meat. J Clin Microbiol. 2000;38:4463–70.
26. Kobayashi H, Oethinger M, Tuohy MJ, Hall GS, Bauer TW. Improving clinical significance of PCR: use of propidium monoazide to distinguish viable from dead *Staphylococcus aureus* and *Staphylococcus epidermidis*. J Orthop Res. 2009;27:1243–7.
27. Villarreal JV, Jungfer C, Obst U, Schwartz T. DNase I and Proteinase K eliminate DNA from injured or dead bacteria but not from living bacteria in microbial reference systems and natural drinking water biofilms for subsequent molecular biology analyses. J Microbiol Methods. 2013;94:161–9.
28. Official Gazette of the Republic of Turkey, 24 December 2014, #29215.

7

Systematic review and meta-analysis of mortality of patients infected with carbapenem-resistant *Klebsiella pneumoniae*

Liangfei Xu, Xiaoxi Sun and Xiaoling Ma*

Abstract

Purpose: Carbapenem resistant *K. pneumoniae* (CRKP) has aroused widespread attention owing to its very limited therapeutic options, and this strain has increased rapidly in recent years. Although it is accepted that drug resistance is associated with increased mortality in general, but some other studies found no such relationship. To estimate mortality of patients infected with CRKP in general and analyze factors for mortality of this infection, thus, we conducted this systematic review and meta-analysis.

Methods: A systematic literature review of relevant studies published until December 2015 was conducted. We selected and assessed articles reporting mortality of patients infected with CRKP.

Results: Pooled mortality was 42.14% among 2462 patients infected with CRKP versus 21.16% in those infected with carbapenem-susceptible *K. pneumoniae* (CSKP). The mortality of patients with bloodstream infection (BSI) or urinary tract infection was 54.30 and 13.52%, respectively, and 48.9 and 43.13% in patients admitted to the intensive care unit (ICU) or who underwent solid organ transplantation (SOT). Mortality was 47.66% in patients infected with *K. pneumoniae* carbapenemase-producing *K. pneumoniae* and 46.71% in those infected with VIM-producing *K. pneumoniae.* Geographically, mortality reported in studies from North America, South America, Europe, and Asia was 33.24, 46.71, 50.06, and 44.82%, respectively.

Conclusions: Our study suggests that patients infected with CRKP have higher mortality than those infected with CSKP, especially in association with BSI, ICU admission, or SOT. We also considered that patients' survival has a close relationship with their physical condition. Our results imply that attention should be paid to CRKP infection, and that strict infection control measures and new antibiotics are required to protect against CRKP infection.

Keywords: CRKP, Carbapenem-resistant, *K. pneumoniae*, Mortality

Background

It is well known that *Klebsiella pneumoniae* is ubiquitous in nature, one of the most relevant opportunistic pathogens, and causes various human infections such as bloodstream infection (BSI), urinary tract infection (UTI), surgical-site infection, and pneumonia [1–3]. Resistance can develop in *K. pneumoniae* isolates, notably producing extended-spectrum β-lactamases (ESBLs). ESBL-producing strains of *K. pneumoniae* are currently found throughout the world and have caused numerous outbreaks of infection [4, 5]. Carbapenems represent the first-line therapy for severe infection by ESBL-producing *K. pneumoniae* [6]. However, since Yigit et al. [7, 8] reported the first *K. pneumoniae* carbapenem (KPC)-producing *K. pneumoniae* isolate in North Carolina in 1996, carbapenem-resistant strains have increased rapidly, rising from 1.6 to 10.4% associated with central line blood-stream infections between 2001 and 2011 in the

*Correspondence: xiaolingma@126.com
Department of Laboratory Medicine, Anhui Provincial Hospital, Anhui Medical University, Hefei 230001, Anhui, China

United States, and have aroused widespread attention, presenting a challenge because the antimicrobial treatment options remain very restricted [7, 9].

Carbapenem-resistant *K. pneumoniae* (CRKP) deactivates the carbapenems through two main mechanisms: (1) acquisition of carbapenemase genes that encode for enzymes capable of hydrolyzing carbapenems—the three most important carbapenemase types being KPC-type enzymes, metallo-β-lactamases (VIM, IMP, NDM), and OXA-48 type enzymes; and (2) reduction in the accumulation of antibiotics by a quantitative and/or qualitative deficiency of porin expression in combination with overexpression of β-lactamases that possess weak affinity for carbapenems [10].

Most researchers reported higher mortality rates among persons infected with CRKP isolates [11–30] while others reported contrary results [31, 32]. In recent years, many studies from single medical centers or individual countries have reported mortality rates in patients infected with CRKP, but until now there has been no systematic review focusing on mortality resulting from carbapenem-resistant infections in general. Although in a recent meta-analysis Falagas et al. [33] reported a higher all-cause mortality among patients infected with carbapenem-resistant Enterobacteriaceae than in those with carbapenem-susceptible infections, but their research included only nine studies. Considering this scenario, we conducted a systematic review and meta-analysis to estimate the mortality of patients infected with CRKP, and analyzed mortality resulting from multiple infection types and patients conditions.

Methods

Search strategy

Two independent examiners (LF.X. and XX.S.) searched entries in the PubMed and EMBASE databases from their inception until December 22, 2015 to identify potentially relevant studies. The search terms included "*Klebsiella pneumoniae*" AND resistance AND ("carbapenem" OR "imipenem" OR "meropenem" OR "ertapenem"). The language was restricted to English.

Inclusion and exclusion criteria

Studies were considered in accordance with inclusion criteria if articles reported mortality of patients infected with CRKP. Research that focused on children, did not differentiate mortality between infection and colonization, did not define the strains that were carbapenem resistant, and did not present the exact death toll were excluded. In this analysis, carbapenem resistance was defined as resistance to carbapenems such as imipenem, meropenem, and ertapenem, irrespective of susceptibility to other antibiotics.

Assessment of study quality

The articles were assessed for quality of the cohort or case–control studies included in the systematic analysis according to the Newcastle-Ottawa scale (NOS) score [34], ranging from 0 to 9. Studies with a NOS score of 5 or greater were included in this analysis.

Data extraction

Two independent investigators (LF.X. and XX.S.) extracted information from eligible articles. Divergences were solved by discussion and consultation of the relevant literature. The information extracted from original publications included title, first author, year of publication and experiment, type of study, sample size, characteristics of the study population (mean age, sex, type of infection, mean severity of underlying disease), and crude mortality rates in patients infected with CRKP and carbapenem-susceptible *K. pneumoniae* (CSKP). If articles reported mortality from both infection and colonization, we extracted information only regarding infections.

Statistical analysis

We calculated the pooled odds ratio (OR) and 95% confidence interval (CI) by comparing crude mortality in patients with CRKP with that in patients with CSKP. Between-study heterogeneity was assessed by the χ^2 test ($p < 0.10$ was selected to indicate the presence of heterogeneity, in which case a random-effects model was adopted; otherwise a fixed-effects model was applied) and I^2 test (to assess the degree of heterogeneity) [35, 36]. We then calculated pooled rates of mortality in patients infected with CRKP, and stratified analyses with respect to geographic location, infection types, carbapenemase types, and patients conditions performed. Freeman–Tukey arcsine transformations were used to stabilize the variances, and after the meta-analysis we transformed the summary estimates and the CI boundaries back to proportions using the sine function [37]. We used Stata version 12.0 software for all statistical calculations.

Results

Results of the systematic literature search

We identified and screened 3168 articles. After exclusion by title and abstract, the remaining 87 articles were subjected to full-text assessment for eligibility. Among these articles, 12 were duplicates, seven did not differentiate between infection- and colonization-related mortality, and six did not report valid data. Ultimately, 62 studies were analyzed based on the inclusion and exclusion criteria (Fig. 1).

The basic characteristics of these 62 studies are summarized in Table 1 [11–32, 38–77]. These articles were published from 1999 to 2015 and the sample size varied

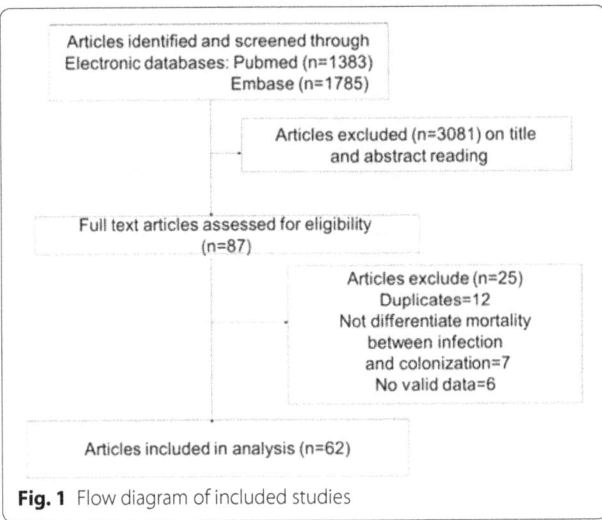

Fig. 1 Flow diagram of included studies

across studies, ranging from 7 to 1022. The total number of patients in this systematic review was 4701, of whom 2462 had CRKP infection and the remainder CSKP infection. Among these patients, the reported death was 1018 among the CRKP patients and 398 among the CSKP patients. In the pooled analysis, the overall mortality was 42.14% (95% CI 37.06–47.31) in patients infected with CRKP and 21.16% (95% CI 16.07–26.79) in CSKP patients (Table 2).

Comparison of mortality in CRKP and CSKP patients

Among the included articles, 22 compared mortality between patients infected with CRKP and CSKP. The summary estimate of these studies from the random-effects model suggested that patients with CRKP had a significantly higher mortality than those with CSKP in the univariate analysis (pooled crude OR 2.80; 95% CI 2.15–3.65) with a moderate heterogeneity I^2 of 33.9% ($p = 0.031$) (Fig. 2).

Mortality in multiple patient conditions

As shown in Table 2, 722 patients had BSI and 284 had UTI, 479 were in an intensive care unit (ICU), and 362 underwent solid organ transplantation (SOT). In the pooled analysis, the mortality was 54.30% (95% CI 47.51–61.02), 13.52% (95% CI 7.50–20.92), 48.9% (95% CI 44.47–53.46), and 43.13% (95% CI 32.40–54.16) in BSI, UTI, ICU-admission, and SOT patients, respectively.

Mortality in multiple carbapenemase types

In this subgroup analysis, we mainly analyzed the mortality of patients infected with KPC-producing *K. pneumoniae* and VIM-producing *K. pneumoniae.* In the articles included, 302 patients were infected with KPC-producing *K. pneumoniae* and 73 were infected with VIM-producing *K. pneumoniae.* The mortality among these two types of carbapenemases was 47.66% (95% CI 38.61–56.79) and 46.71% (95% CI 35.81–57.73), respectively (Table 2).

Mortality in different geographic locations

Twenty-three studies were carried out in North America, eight in South America, twenty-one in Europe, and ten in Asia. The rate of mortality was 33.24% (95% CI 25.08–42.00) of 980 patients in North America, 46.71% (95% CI 39.83–53.66) of 191 in South America, 50.06% (95% CI 41.45–58.62) of 860 in Europe, and 44.82% (95% CI 37.83–51.91) of 431 in Asia (Table 2).

Discussion

ESBL-producing *K. pneumoniae* as an opportunistic pathogen is becoming more challenging to treat because of the emergence of carbapenem resistance, and has a significant influence on patient mortality. The primary result of this analysis was the pooled crude mortality of 42.14% among patients with CRKP, which is intimately connected with patients' health and physical status.

Although it is accepted that drug resistance is associated with increased mortality because patients tend to receive inappropriate empiric therapy in general [4, 78], other studies have found no such relationship. Bhavnani et al. [79] reported that clinical success was similar between patients with ESBL and those with non-ESBL-producing *K. pneumoniae*, and ESBL production alone did not appear to be an independent risk factor for treatment failure. Kim et al. [80] also found that ESBL production was not significantly associated with death. In addition, García-Sureda et al. [81] reported that CRKP isolates are less virulent and fit than CSKP isolates in an antibiotic-free environment. We conducted this systematic review and meta-analysis to estimate the mortality of patients infected with CRKP in general and to study the factors related to mortality resulting from this infection. We found that patients infected with CRKP had significantly higher mortality in comparison with CSKP (crude OR 2.80). To identify risk factors associated with the higher mortality of CRKP infections, we conducted a stratified analysis of patient condition, carbapenemase types, and study location.

Based on multiple patient conditions, our analysis confirmed that patients with CRKP in association with BSI, ICU admission, or SOT have a higher mortality than the pooled mortality, although UTI patients have a lower mortality than the pooled overall mortality, even lower than that of CSKP patients. From this result, we assumed that patient survival has a close relationship with patients' underlying illness and comorbidities. Mouloudi et al. [26] reported that BSI, ICU admission, and recent receipt of a

Table 1 Characteristics of the eligible studies

Author, year	Study type	Region/ study year	Resistance	CRKP mortality (%)	CSKP mortality (%)	P value	Carbapenemases	Infection type	ICU	SOT
Vardakas (2015) [11]	Retrospective cohort study	Greece 2006.1–2009.10	CLSI 2010	58/80 (72.5)	14/24 (58.3)	0.19	NA	BSI:44/65	80	0
Brizendine (2015) [16]	Retrospective cohort study	USA 2011.12–2013.10	CLSI 2012	16/157 (10.2)	NA	NA	NA	UTI:16/157	0	0
Pouch (2015) [12]	Nested case–control study	USA 2007.1–2010.12	CLSI 2009	6/20 (30)	8/80 (10)	0.03	NA	UTI:6/20	0	20
Ny (2015) [13]	Retrospective cohort study	USA 2011.1–2013.12	NA	7/48 (14.6)	5/48 (10.4)	0.76	NA	UTI:2/27	0	0
Girmenia (2015) [39]	Retrospective cohort study	Italy 2010.1–2013.7	NA	65/112 (58.1)	NA	NA	NA	Any infection:65/112	0	112
Hoxha (2015) [14]	Prospective matched cohort study	Italy 2012.11–2013.7	Eucast Guideline	30/49 (61)	10/49 (20)	NA	NA	Any infection:30/49	0	0
Cubero (2015) [15]	Retrospective cohort study	Spain 2010.10–2012.12	EUCAST 2015	8/20 (40)	1/9 (11.1)	NA	NA	Any infection:8/20	0	0
Chang (2015) [40]	Retrospective study	Taiwan 2012.1–2012.12	CLSI 2012	21/41 (51.2)	NA	NA	KPC:6/8	Any infection:21/41	41	0
Chen (2015) [68]	Retrospective study	Taiwan 2014.4–10	NA	12/41 (29.3)	NA	NA	NA	Any infection:12/41	0	0
Madrigal (2015) [66]	Retrospective study	Spain 2014.5–9	NA	2/5 (40)	NA	NA	NA	Any infection:2/5	0	0
Bias (2015) [70]	Retrospective, observational cohort study	USA –2014.8	NA	5/30 (16.7)	NA	NA	NA	Any infection:5/30	0	30
Katsiari (2015) [67]	Prospective, observational study	Greece 2010.4–2012.3	CLSI 2012	14/32 (43.8)	NA	NA	KPC:11/28VIM:3/5	BSI:9/16	32	0
Maristela Freire (2015) [69]	Retrospective cohort study	Brazil 2009.1–2013.12	CLSI 2012	13/31 (41.9)	NA	NA	KPC:13/31	BSI:7/11 UTI:1/10	0	31
Brizendine (2015) [16]	Retrospective cohort study	USA 2006–2012	NA	4/22 (18)	1/64 (1.5)	NA	NA	UTI:4/22	0	22
Sarah Welch (2015) [65]	Retrospective cohort study	USA	NA	19/51 (37.3)	NA	NA	NA	Pneumonia:19/51	0	0
van Duin (2014) [16]	Prospective, multi-center, observational study	USA 2011.12–2013.3	CLSI	26/114 (22.8)	NA	NA	NA	BSI:5/26	0	0
Simkins (2014) [17]	Retrospective case–control study	USA 2006.1–2010.12	NA	6/13 (46.2)	3/39 (7.7)	0.005	NA	Any infection:6/13	0	13
Viviana Gómez Rueda (2014) [18]	Case–case–control study	Colombia 2008.1–2011.1	CLSI	31/61 (50.8)	20/61 (32.8)	NA	NA	Any infection:31/61	0	0
Christoph Lübbert (2014) [71]	Retrospective study	Germany 2010.9–2011.9	NA	7/8 (87.5)	NA	NA	KPC:7/8	Any infection:7/8	0	8
Qureshi (2014) [42]	Retrospective cohort study	USA 2009.1–2012.10	NA	0/21 (0.00)	NA	NA	NA	UTI:0/21	0	0

Table 1 continued

Author, year	Study type	Region/ study year	Resistance	CRKP mortality (%)	CSKP mortality (%)	P value	Carbapenemases	Infection type	ICU	SOT
Mouloudi (2014) [43]	Retrospective cohort study	Greece 2008.1–2011.12	EUCAST 2012	14/17 (82.4)	NA	NA	NA	BSI:14/17	17	17
Bulent Aydinl (2014) [72]	Retrospective analysis	Turkey 2012.1–2013.11	NA	2/5 (40)	NA	NA	NA	Any infection:2/5	0	5
Gallagher (2014) [44]	Retrospective case–case–control study	USA 2005.6–2010.10	CLSI 2009	19/43 (44.2)	NA	NA	NA	BSI:19/43	0	0
Graziella Hanna Pereira (2013) [47]	Retrospective cohort study	Brazil 2008.10–2010.10	CLSI 2010	16/33 (48)	NA	NA	NA	BSI:9/11 UTI:3/21 Pneumonia:3/7	0	0
Orsi (2013) [19]	Case–case–control study	Italy 2008.7–2011.6	EUCAST	25/65 (38.5)	12/43 (27.9)	NA	KPC:14/36	Any infection:25/65	0	0
Kontopidou (2013) [48]	Retrospective cohort study	Greece 2009.9–2010.6	CLSI 2010	29/127 (22.8)	NA	NA	NA	Any infection:29/127	127	0
Hussein (2013) [20]	Retrospective case control study	Israel 2006.1–2008.12	CLSI 2006	45/103 (43.7)	62/214 (29)	NA	NA	BSI:45/103	0	0
Luci Correa (2013) [22]	Matched case–control study	Brazil 2006.1–2008.8	CLSI 2009	10/20 (50)	11/40 (27.5)	0.085	NA	Any infection:10/20	0	0
Clancy (2013) [49]	Single-center, retrospective study	USA 2008.8–2011.7	CLSI 2012	3/17 (17.6)	NA	NA	NA	BSI:3/17	0	17
Cober (2013) [21]	Retrospective cohort study	USA 2006–2009	NA	8/19 (42.1)	7/46	0.005	NA	BSI:8/19	0	19
Grossi (2013) [73]	Retrospective cohort study	Italy 2009.1–2012.10	NA	11/36 (30.6)	NA	NA	NA	Any infection:11/36	0	36
Cicora (2013) [50]	Observational, retrospective study	Argentina 2011.4–2012.6	CLSI 2010	2/6 (33.3)	NA	NA	KPC:2/6	UTI:2/6	0	6
Paola Di Carlo (2013) [46]	Prospective case series study	Italy 2011,8–2012.8	EUCAST	12/30 (40)	NA	NA	KPC:12/30	Any infection:12/30	30	0
Fligou (2013) [88]	Retrospective cohort study	Greece	CLSI	21/48 (43.8)	NA	NA	KPC:21/48	BSI:21/48	48	0
Rose (2012) [74]	Retrospective, cohort study	USA 2006–2011	NA	20/44 (45.5)	NA	NA	NA	BSI:20/44	0	0
Sanchez-Romero (2012) [51]	Retrospective cohort study	Spain 2009.1–2009.12	CLSI 2011	13/28 (46.4)	NA	NA	VIM:13/28	Any infection:13/28	28	0
Liu (2012) [23]	Matched case–control study	Taiwan 2007.1–2009.12	CLSI 2009	15/25 (60)	20/50	0.102	NA	BSI:15/25	0	0
Kalpoe (2012) [52]	Retrospective cohort study	USA 2005.1–2006.10	NA	10/14 (71.4)	NA	NA	NA	Any infection:10/14	0	14
Borer (2012) [53]	Retrospective case control study	Israel 2007.5–2010.1	CLSI 2006	13/42 (31)	NA	NA	NA	Any infection:13/42	0	0
Bergamasco (2012) [54]	Retrospective cohort study	Brazil 2009.7–2010.2	CLSI 2009	5/12 (41.7)	NA	NA	KPC:2/12	Any infection:5/12	0	12

Table 1 continued

Author, year	Study type	Region/ study year	Resistance	CRKP mortality (%)	CSKP mortality (%)	P value	Carbapenemases	Infection type	ICU	SOT
Ben-David (2012) [24]	Retrospective cohort study	Israel 2006.1–2006.12	CLSI 2006	29/42 (69.1)	45/150 (30)	<0.001	NA	BSI:29/42	0	0
Balkhy (2012) [55]	Retrospective/prospective surveillance study	Saudi Arabia 2009.9–2010.8	CLSI 2009	8/20 (40)	NA	NA	NA	Any infection:8/20	0	0
Jason Gallagher (2011) [75]	A retrospective, cohort study	USA 2006–2011	NA	24/44 (54.5)	NA	NA	NA	BSI:24/44	0	0
Pereira (2011) [56]	Retrospective cohort study	Brazil 2008.10–2010.8	CLSI 2010	9/22 (40.9)	NA	NA	NA	Any infection:9/22	0	0
Orsi (2011) [25]	Retrospective case control study	Italy 2008.7–2009.12	EUCAST	11/28 (39.3)	12/43	NA	NA	Any infection:11/28	0	0
Neuner (2011) [57]	Retrospective cohort study	USA 2007.1–2009.5	CLSI 2009	35/60 (58.3)	NA	NA	NA	BSI:35/60	0	0
Diana Gaviria (2011) [31]	Retrospective matched case–control study	USA 2009.4–2011.12	CLSI	1/19 (5.3)	3/38 (7.9)	NA	NA	Any infection:1/19	0	0
Cuzon (2011) [59]	Retrospective cohort study	France 2010.4–2010.6	CLSI 2010	5/7 (71.4)	NA	NA	NA	Any infection:5/7	0	0
Elisa Maria Beirão (2011) [58]	Retrospective cohort study	Brazil 2008.1–2008.12	CLSI 2009	3/6 (50)	NA	NA	KPC:3/6	Any infection:3/6	0	0
Nguyen (2010) [60]	Retrospective cohort study	USA 2004.1–2008.9	CLSI	29/48 (60.4)	NA	NA	NA	BSI:29/48	0	0
Vardakas (2010) [76]	Retrospective cohort study	Greece 2006.1–2009.9	NA	42/56 (75)	NA	NA	NA	Any infection:42/56	56	0
Mouloudi (2010) [26]	Retrospective nested case–control study	Greece 2007.1–2008.12	CLSI 2007	25/37 (67.6)	9/22 (40.9)	0.03	KPC: 15/19 VIM:10/18	BSI:25/37	0	0
Gregory (2010) [61]	Retrospective case–control study	Puerto Rico 2008.2–2008.9	CLSI 2009	7/19 (36.8)	NA	NA	NA	Any infection:7/19	0	0
Balandin Moreno (2010) [77]	Retrospective cohort study	Spain 2009.7–2010.4	NA	2/8 (25)	NA	NA	VIM:2/8	Any infection:2/8	8	0
Gasink (2009) [27]	Case–control study	USA 2006.10–2008.4	NA	18/56 (32.1)	85/863 (9.8)	NA	KPC:18/56	Any infection:18/56	0	0
Daikos (2009) [28]	Prospective observational study	Greece 2005.2–2006.3	CLSI 2004	6/14 (42.9)	25/148 (16.9)	NA	VIM:6/14	BSI:6/14	0	0
Borer (2009) [62]	Matched retrospective, historical cohort study	Israel 2005.10–2008.10	CLSI 2006	30/64 (46.9)	NA	NA	NA	BSI:23/32	0	0
Schwaber (2008) [29]	Retrospective cohort study	Israel 2003–2006	CLSI 2005	21/48 (43.8)	7/56 (12.5)	NA	NA	Any infection:21/48	0	0
Patel (2008) [30]	Retrospective matched case–control	USA 2004.7–2006.6	CLSI 2006	48/99 (48.5)	20/99 (20.2)	<0.001	NA	Any infection:48/99	0	0

Table 1 continued

Author, year	Study type	Region/ study year	Resistance	CRKP mortality (%)	CSKP mortality (%)	P value	Carbapenemases	Infection type	ICU	SOT
Falagas (2007) [32]	Retrospective matched case–control study	Greece 2000.10–2006.5	NA	16/53 (30.2)	18/53 (34)	0.83	NA	Any infection:16/53	0	0
Woodford (2004) [63]	Retrospective cohort study	USA 2000.4–2001.4	CLSI	8/14 (57.1)	NA	NA	KPC:8/14	Any infection:8/14	14	0
Muhammad Ahmad. (1999) [64]	Retrospective cohort study	USA 1994.12–1995.11	CLSI 1994	6/8 (75)	NA	NA	NA	Any infection:6/8	8	0

CLSI Clinical and Laboratory Standards Institute, *CRKP* carbapenem-resistant *K. pneumoniae*, *CSKP* carbapenem-susceptible *K. pneumonia*, *BSI* bloodstream infection, *UTI* urinary tract infection

Table 2 Mortality of patients based on patient condition, carbapenemases type, study region

Subgroup	Number of studies	Sample size	Mortality Rate %(95% CI)	Statistical model
Pooled mortality	P < 0.001			
CRKP	62	2462	42.14 (37.06–47.31)	Random
CSKP	22	2239	21.12 (16.07–26.79)	Random
Patient conditions	P < 0.001			
Bloodstream infections	20	722	54.30 (47.51–61.02)	Random
Urinary tract infections	8	284	13.52 (7.50–20.92)	Random
Intensive care unit	12	479	53.90 (39.44–68.00)	Random
Solid organ transplantation	15	362	43.13 (32.40–54.16)	Random
Carbapenemases type	P = 0.645			
KPC-producing *Klebsiella pneumoniae*	13	302	47.66 (38.61–49.51)	Random
VIM-producing *Klebsiella pneumoniae*	5	73	46.71 (35.81–57.73)	Random
Region	P = 0.062			
North America	23	980	33.24 (25.08–42.00)	Random
South America	8	191	46.71 (39.83–53.66)	Fixed
Europe	21	860	50.06 (41.45–58.62)	Random
Asia	10	431	44.82 (37.83–51.91)	Random

CRKP Carbapenem-resistant *K. pneumoniae*, *CSKP* carbapenem-susceptible *K. pneumonia*

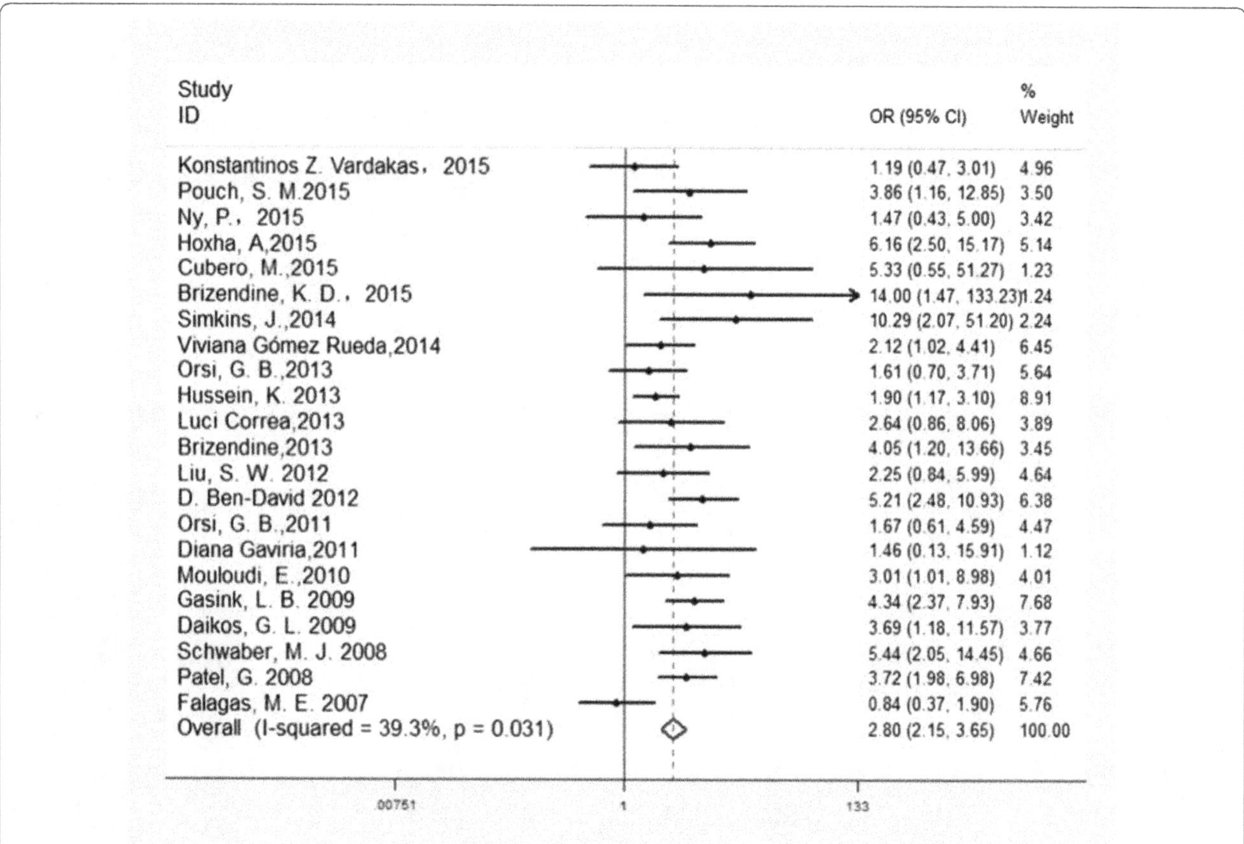

Fig. 2 Crude odds ratio (OR) for the association between carbapenem resistance and mortality of patients with *K. pneumoniae* infection

SOT were associated with ICU and in-hospital mortality in patients infected with CRKP. In addition, patients who had undergone organ transplantation or ICU admission were always subjected to surgical procedures, prolonged ICU stay, preexisting immunosuppression, and the use of invasive devices, which contributed to patients' poor physical condition and resultant higher mortality. In contrast, Daikos et al. suggested that UTI is a relatively mild infection that has only a slight influence on the general condition of patients, and carries a low mortality in general [25]. It has been shown that factors such as underlying illness and comorbidities have a more important influence on mortality than appropriate empiric treatment with multidrug-resistant Gram-negative bacteria [82]. Although the underlying patient's condition is important for the outcome of such patients, meanwhile a timely effective treatment can also help to improve the survival rate. Patients in a poor state of health with CRKP were subjected to pathogens longer compared to CSKP infection due to lack of an effective therapy, ultimately, led to a higher mortality.

In the present analysis, patients infected with KPC-producing *K. pneumoniae* have a higher mortality than pooled overall mortality (47.66 vs 42.14%). This result may contribute to KPC-producing *K. pneumoniae* having stronger invasiveness, and the KPC-encoding *blaKPC* always carry other drug-resistant genes, leading to a pronounced drug resistant [83]. Previous studies have demonstrated *K. pneumoniae*-encoding *blaKPC* to be an independent risk factor in patient mortality [26, 27]. In addition, KPC-producing *K. pneumoniae* is considered a successful pathogen because of its ability to persist and spread, causing nosocomial outbreaks. Bratu et al. [84] reported that KPC-producing *K. pneumoniae* isolates are resistant to not only all β-lactam antimicrobials but also frequently other classes of antimicrobials, such as aminoglycosides and fluoroquinolones. In this systematic review, the patients from North America have lower mortality in comparison with the other three locations. This phenomenon may be attributed to a higher level of medical care and different treatment methods in North America, such as combination antibiotics, treatment with polymyxins and tigecycline, and adjunctive procedures (e.g., catheter removal, drainage, or debridement). There is evidence that tigecycline and polymyxins have activity against many CRKP isolates in vitro, and there have been cases reported of successful treatment of CRKP infection with polymyxins and tigecycline [85–87]. Patel et al. [30] also reported that removal of the focus of infection (i.e., debridement) was independently associated with patient survival.

There are several limitations to this analysis. First, as the included studies reported only unadjusted data on mortality, we analyzed only crude mortality among patients with CRKP. Second, most studies may have lacked power in differentiating death caused by CRKP from any other factors, and it is difficult to draw definitive conclusions from current evidence because of the residual confounding factors and small sample sizes in many studies. Third, some studies included in our meta-analysis did not define a cutoff value to judge the susceptibility of *K. pneumoniae* to carbapenems, and when defined the cutoff value varied among studies owing to different reference criteria. Thus, there exists the potential for heterogeneity. Fourth, most studies were retrospective in nature and thus susceptible to selection bias. Last, we selected only English-language articles, thus limiting the scope of our analysis.

Conclusions

Our study suggests that patients infected with CRKP have a higher mortality than those infected with CSKP, especially patients with BSI, ICU admission, or SOT intervention. We suggest that the survival of patients has a close relationship with their physical condition. Thus, our results imply that attention should be paid to CRKP infection in patients in a poor state of health, and that strict infection control measures and new antibiotics are required to protect against CRKP infection.

Abbreviations

CRKP: carbapenem-resistant *Klebsiella pneumoniae*; CSKP: carbapenem-susceptible *Klebsiella pneumoniae*; BSI: bloodstream infection; UTI: urinary tract infection; ICU: intensive care unit; SOT: solid organ transplantation.

Authors' contributions

LX and XS designed the study, performed the articles search and screen. LX wrote the paper. LX and XS performed the Statistical analysis. XM reviewed the manuscript. All authors read and approved the final manuscript.

Acknowledgements

Not applicable.

Competing interests

The authors declare that they have no competing interests.

Consent for publication

Informed consent was obtained from all individual participants included in the review.

References

1. Podschun R, Ullmann U. *Klebsiella* spp. as nosocomial pathogens: epidemiology, taxonomy, typing methods, and pathogenicity factors. Clin Microbiol Rev. 1998;11:589–603.

2. Daikos GL, Markogiannakis A, Souli M, Tzouvelekis LS. Bloodstream infections caused by carbapenemase-producing *Klebsiella pneumoniae*: a clinical perspective. Expert Rev Anti Infect Ther. 2012;10(12):1393–404.
3. Broberg CA, Palacios M, Miller VL. Klebsiella: a long way to go towards understanding this enigmatic jet-setter. F1000prime Rep. 2014;6:64.
4. Tumbarello M, Spanu T, Sanguinetti M, Citton R, Montuori E, Leone F, Fadda G, Cauda R. Bloodstream infections caused by extended-spectrum-beta-lactamase-producing *Klebsiella pneumoniae*: risk factors, molecular epidemiology, and clinical outcome. Antimicrob Agents Chemother. 2006;50(2):498–504.
5. Paterson DL, Yu VL. Editorial response: extended-spectrum β-lactamases: a call for improved detection and control. Clin Infect Dis. 1999;29:1419–22.
6. Pitout JDD, Laupland KB. Extended-spectrum β-lactamase-producing Enterobacteriaceae: an emerging public-health concern. Lancet Infect Dis. 2008;8(3):159–66.
7. Yigit H, Queenan AM, Anderson GJ, Domenech-Sanchez A, Biddle JW, Steward CD, Alberti S, Bush K, Tenover FC. Novel carbapenem-hydrolyzing beta-lactamase, KPC-1, from a carbapenem-resistant strain of Klebsiella pneumoniae. Antimicrob Agents Chemother. 2001;45(4):1151–61.
8. Jacob JT, Klein E, Laxminarayan R, Beldavs Z, Lynfield R, Kallen AJ, Ricks P, Edwards J, Srinivasan A, Fridkin S, et al. Vital signs: carbapenem-resistant Enterobacteriaceae. Morb Mortal Wkly Rep. 2013;62(9):165–70.
9. Nordmann P, Cuzon G, Naas T. The real threat of Klebsiella pneumoniae carbapenemase-producing bacteria. Lancet Infect Dis. 2009;9(4):228–36.
10. Nordmann P, Dortet L, Poirel L. Carbapenem resistance in Enterobacteriaceae: here is the storm! Trends Mol Med. 2012;18(5):263–72.
11. Vardakas KZ, Matthaiou DK, Falagas ME, Antypa E, Koteli A, Antoniadou E. Characteristics, risk factors and outcomes of carbapenem-resistant *Klebsiella pneumoniae* infections in the intensive care unit. J Infect. 2015;70(6):592–9.
12. Pouch SM, Kubin CJ, Satlin MJ, Tsapepas DS, Lee JR, Dube G, Pereira MR. Epidemiology and outcomes of carbapenem-resistant *Klebsiella pneumoniae* bacteriuria in kidney transplant recipients. Transpl Infect Dis. 2015;17(6):800–9.
13. Ny P, Nieberg P, Wong-Beringer A. Impact of carbapenem resistance on epidemiology and outcomes of nonbacteremic *Klebsiella pneumoniae* infections. Am J Infect Control. 2015;43(10):1076–80.
14. Hoxha A, Karki T, Giambi C, Montano C, Sisto A, Bella A, D'Ancona F, Study Working G. Attributable mortality of carbapenem-resistant *Klebsiella pneumoniae* infections in a prospective matched cohort study in Italy, 2012–2013. J Hosp Infect. 2015;92(1):61–6.
15. Cubero M, Cuervo G, Dominguez MA, Tubau F, Marti S, Sevillano E, Gallego L, Ayats J, Pena C, Pujol M, et al. Carbapenem-resistant and carbapenem-susceptible isogenic isolates of Klebsiella pneumoniae ST101 causing infection in a tertiary hospital. BMC Microbiol. 2015;15:177.
16. Brizendine KD, Richter SS, Cober ED, van Duin D. Carbapenem-resistant *Klebsiella pneumoniae* urinary tract infection following solid organ transplantation. Antimicrob Agents Chemother. 2015;59(1):553–7.
17. Simkins J, Muggia V, Cohen HW, Minamoto GY. Carbapenem-resistant *Klebsiella pneumoniae* infections in kidney transplant recipients: a case-control study. Transpl Infect Dis. 2014;16(5):775–82.
18. Rueda VG. Risk factors for infection with carbapenem-resistant *Klebsiella pneumoniae*: a case–case–control study. Colomb Méd. 2014;45(2):54–60.
19. Orsi GB, Bencardino A, Vena A, Carattoli A, Venditti C, Falcone M, Giordano A, Venditti M. Patient risk factors for outer membrane permeability and KPC-producing carbapenem-resistant *Klebsiella pneumoniae* isolation: results of a double case–control study. Infection. 2013;41(1):61–7.
20. Hussein K, Raz-Pasteur A, Finkelstein R, Neuberger A, Shachor-Meyouhas Y, Oren I, Kassis I. Impact of carbapenem resistance on the outcome of patients' hospital-acquired bacteraemia caused by *Klebsiella pneumoniae*. J Hosp Infect. 2013;83(4):307–13.
21. Cober E, Brizendine K, Richter S, Koval C, Van Duin D. Impact of carbapenem resistance in *Klebsiella pneumoniae* blood stream infection in solid organ transplantation. Am J Transpl. 2013;13(SUPPL. 5):186.
22. Correa L, Martino MDV, Siqueira I, Pasternak J, Gales AC, Silva CV, Camargo TZS, Scherer PF, Marra AR. A hospital-based matched case–control study to identify clinical outcome and risk factors associated with carbapenem-resistant *Klebsiella pneumoniae* infection. BMC Infect Dis. 2013;13(1):80.
23. Liu SW, Chang HJ, Chia JH, Kuo AJ, Wu TL, Lee MH. Outcomes and characteristics of ertapenem-nonsusceptible *Klebsiella pneumoniae* bacteremia at a university hospital in Northern Taiwan: a matched case–control study. J Microbiol Immunol Infect. 2012;45(2):113–9.
24. Ben-David D, Kordevani R, Keller N, Tal I, Marzel A, Gal-Mor O, Maor Y, Rahav G. Outcome of carbapenem resistant *Klebsiella pneumoniae* bloodstream infections. Clin Microbiol Infect. 2012;18(1):54–60.
25. Orsi GB, Garcia-Fernandez A, Giordano A, Venditti C, Bencardino A, Gianfreda R, Falcone M, Carattoli A, Venditti M. Risk factors and clinical significance of ertapenem-resistant *Klebsiella pneumoniae* in hospitalised patients. J Hosp Infect. 2011;78(1):54–8.
26. Mouloudi E, Protonotariou E, Zagorianou A, Iosifidis E, Karapanagiotou A, Giasnetsova T, Tsioka A, Roilides E, Sofianou D, Gritsi-Gerogianni N. Bloodstream infections caused by metallo-beta-lactamase/*Klebsiella pneumoniae* carbapenemase-producing *K. pneumoniae* among intensive care unit patients in Greece: risk factors for infection and impact of type of resistance on outcomes. Infect Control Hosp Epidemiol. 2010;31(12):1250–6.
27. Gasink LB, Edelstein PH, Lautenbach E, Synnestvedt M, Fishman NO. Risk factors and clinical impact of *Klebsiella pneumoniae* carbapenemase-producing *K. pneumoniae*. Infect Control Hosp Epidemiol. 2009;30(12):1180–5.
28. Daikos GL, Petrikkos P, Psichogiou M, Kosmidis C, Vryonis E, Skoutelis A, Georgousi K, Tzouvelekis LS, Tassios PT, Bamia C, et al. Prospective observational study of the impact of VIM-1 metallo-beta-lactamase on the outcome of patients with *Klebsiella pneumoniae* bloodstream infections. Antimicrob Agents Chemother. 2009;53(5):1868–73.
29. Schwaber MJ, Klarfeld-Lidji S, Navon-Venezia S, Schwartz D, Leavitt A, Carmeli Y. Predictors of carbapenem-resistant *Klebsiella pneumoniae* acquisition among hospitalized adults and effect of acquisition on mortality. Antimicrob Agents Chemother. 2008;52(3):1028–33.
30. Patel G, Huprikar S, Factor SH, Jenkins SG, Calfee DP. Outcomes of carbapenem-resistant *Klebsiella pneumoniae* infection and the impact of antimicrobial and adjunctive therapies. Infect Control Hosp Epidemiol. 2008;29(12):1099–106.
31. Gaviria D, Bixler D, Thomas CA, Ibrahim SM. Carbapenem-resistant *Klebsiella pneumoniae* associated with a long-term-care facility—West Virginia, 2009–2011. Morb Mortal Wkly Rep. 2011;60:1418–20.
32. Falagas ME, Rafailidis PI, Kofteridis D, Virtzili S, Chelvatzoglou FC, Papaioannou V, Maraki S, Samonis G, Michalopoulos A. Risk factors of carbapenem-resistant *Klebsiella pneumoniae* infections: a matched case control study. J Antimicrob Chemother. 2007;60(5):1124–30.
33. Falagas ME, Tansarli GS, Karageorgopoulos DE, Vardakas KZ. Deaths attributable to carbapenem-resistant Enterobacteriaceae infections. Emerg Infect Dis. 2014;20(7):1170–5.
34. Wells, G. A. et al. The Newcastle-Ottawa Scale (NOS) for assessing the quality of nonrandomised studies in meta-analyses. (2014). Available at: http://www.ohri.ca/programs/clinical_epidemiology/oxford.asp. Accessed 15 Feb 2015.
35. Higgins JP, Thompson SG. Quantifying heterogeneity in a meta-analysis. Stat Med. 2002;21(11):1539–58.
36. DerSimonian R, Laird N. Meta-analysis in clinical trials. Control Clin Trials. 1986;7(3):177–88.
37. Freeman MF, Tukey JW. Transformations related to the angular and the square root. Ann Math Stat. 1950;21(4):607–11.
38. van Duin D, Cober E, Richter SS, Perez F, Kalayjian RC, Salata RA, Evans S, Fowler VG Jr, Kaye KS, Bonomo RA. Impact of therapy and strain type on outcomes in urinary tract infections caused by carbapenem-resistant *Klebsiella pneumoniae*. J Antimicrob Chemother. 2015;70(4):1203–11.
39. Girmenia C, Rossolini GM, Piciocchi A, Bertaina A, Pisapia G, Pastore D, Sica S, Severino A, Cudillo L, Ciceri F, et al. Infections by carbapenem-resistant *Klebsiella pneumoniae* in SCT recipients: a nationwide retrospective survey from Italy. Bone Marrow Transplant. 2015;50(2):282–8.
40. Chang YY, Chuang YC, Siu LK, Wu TL, Lin JC, Lu PL, Wang JT, Wang LS, Lin YT, Huang LJ, et al. Clinical features of patients with carbapenem nonsusceptible *Klebsiella pneumoniae* and *Escherichia coli* in intensive care units: a nationwide multicenter study in Taiwan. J Microbiol Immunol Infect. 2015;48(2):219–25.
41. van Duin D, Perez F, Rudin SD, Cober E, Hanrahan J, Ziegler J, Webber R, Fox J, Mason P, Richter SS, et al. Surveillance of carbapenem-resistant *Klebsiella pneumoniae*: tracking molecular epidemiology and outcomes through a regional network. Antimicrob Agents Chemother. 2014;58(7):4035–41.

42. Qureshi ZA, Syed A, Clarke LG, Doi Y, Shields RK. Epidemiology and clinical outcomes of patients with carbapenem-resistant *Klebsiella pneumoniae* bacteriuria. Antimicrob Agents Chemother. 2014;58(6):3100–4.
43. Mouloudi E, Massa E, Papadopoulos S, Iosifidis E, Roilides I, Theodoridou T, Piperidou M, Orphanou A, Passakiotou M, Imvrios G, et al. Bloodstream infections caused by carbapenemase-producing *Klebsiella pneumoniae* among intensive care unit patients after orthotopic liver transplantation: risk factors for infection and impact of resistance on outcomes. Transplant Proc. 2014;46(9):3216–8.
44. Gallagher JC, Kuriakose S, Haynes K, Axelrod P. Case-case-control study of patients with carbapenem-resistant and third-generation-cephalosporin-resistant *Klebsiella pneumoniae* bloodstream infections. Antimicrob Agents Chemother. 2014;58(10):5732–5.
45. Shilo S, Assous MV, Lachish T, Kopuit P, Bdolah-Abram T, Yinnon AM, Wiener-Well Y. Risk factors for bacteriuria with carbapenem-resistant *Klebsiella pneumoniae* and its impact on mortality: a case–control study. Infection. 2013;41(2):503–9.
46. Di Carlo P, Gulotta G, Casuccio A, Pantuso G, Raineri M, Farulla CA, Bonventre S, Guadagnino G, Ingrassia D, Cocorullo G, Mammina C, Giarratano A. KPC-3 *Klebsiella pneumoniae* ST258 clone infection in postoperative abdominal surgery patients in an intensive care setting: analysis of a case series of 30 patients. BMC Anesthesiol. 2013;13(1):13.
47. Pereira GH, Garcia DO, Mostardeiro M, Fanti KS, Levin AS. Outbreak of carbapenem-resistant *Klebsiella pneumoniae*: two-year epidemiologic follow-up in a tertiary hospital. Mem Inst Oswaldo Cruz. 2013;108(1):113–5.
48. Kontopidou F, Giamarellou H, Katerelos P, Maragos A, Kioumis I, Trikka-Graphakos E, Valakis C, Maltezou HC. Infections caused by carbapenem-resistant *Klebsiella pneumoniae* among patients in intensive care units in Greece: a multi-centre study on clinical outcome and therapeutic options. Clin Microbiol Infect. 2013;20(2):O117–23.
49. Clancy CJ, Chen L, Shields RK, Zhao Y, Cheng S, Chavda KD, Hao B, Hong JH, Doi Y, Kwak EJ, et al. Epidemiology and molecular characterization of bacteremia due to carbapenem-resistant *Klebsiella pneumoniae* in transplant recipients. Am J Transplant. 2013;13(10):2619–33.
50. Cicora F, Mos F, Paz M, Allende NG, Roberti J. Infections with blaKPC-2-producing *Klebsiella pneumoniae* in renal transplant patients: a retrospective study. Transplant Proc. 2013;45(9):3389–93.
51. Sanchez-Romero I, Asensio A, Oteo J, Munoz-Algarra M, Isidoro B, Vindel A, Alvarez-Avello J, Balandin-Moreno B, Cuevas O, Fernandez-Romero S, et al. Nosocomial outbreak of VIM-1-producing *Klebsiella pneumoniae* isolates of multilocus sequence type 15: molecular basis, clinical risk factors, and outcome. Antimicrob Agents Chemother. 2012;56(1):420–7.
52. Kalpoe JS, Sonnenberg E, Factor SH, del Rio Martin J, Schiano T, Patel G, Huprikar S. Mortality associated with carbapenem-resistant *Klebsiella pneumoniae* infections in liver transplant recipients. Liver Transplant. 2012;18(4):468–74.
53. Borer A, Saidel-Odes L, Eskira S, Nativ R, Riesenberg K, Livshiz-Riven I, Schlaeffer F, Sherf M, Peled N. Risk factors for developing clinical infection with carbapenem-resistant *Klebsiella pneumoniae* in hospital patients initially only colonized with carbapenem-resistant *K. pneumoniae*. Am J Infect Control. 2012;40(5):421–5.
54. Bergamasco MD, Barroso Barbosa M, de Oliveira Garcia D, Cipullo R, Moreira JC, Baia C, Barbosa V, Abboud CS. Infection with *Klebsiella pneumoniae* carbapenemase (KPC)-producing K. pneumoniae in solid organ transplantation. Transpl Infect Dis. 2012;14(2):198–205.
55. Balkhy HH, El-Saed A, Al Johani SM, Francis C, Al-Qahtani AA, Al-Ahdal MN, Altayeb HT, Arabi Y, Alothman A, Sallah M. The epidemiology of the first described carbapenem-resistant *Klebsiella pneumoniae* outbreak in a tertiary care hospital in Saudi Arabia: how far do we go? Eur J Clin Microbiol Infect Dis. 2012;31(8):1901–9.
56. Pereira GH, Garcia DO, Mostardeiro M, Ogassavara CT, Levin AS. Spread of carbapenem-resistant *Klebsiella pneumoniae* in a tertiary hospital in Sao Paulo, Brazil. J Hosp Infect. 2011;79(2):182–3.
57. Neuner EA, Yeh JY, Hall GS, Sekeres J, Endimiani A, Bonomo RA, Shrestha NK, Fraser TG, van Duin D. Treatment and outcomes in carbapenem-resistant *Klebsiella pneumoniae* bloodstream infections. Diagn Microbiol Infect Dis. 2011;69(4):357–62.
58. Beirão EM, Furtado JJD, Girardello R, Ferreira H, Gales AC. Clinical and microbiological characterization of KPC-producing *Klebsiella pneumoniae* infections in Brazil. Braz J Infect Dis. 2011;15(1):69–73.
59. Cuzon G, Ouanich J, Gondret R, Naas T, Nordmann P. Outbreak of OXA-48-positive carbapenem-resistant *Klebsiella pneumoniae* isolates in France. Antimicrob Agents Chemother. 2011;55(5):2420–3.
60. Nguyen M, Eschenauer GA, Bryan M, O'Neil K, Furuya EY, Della-Latta P, Kubin CJ. Carbapenem-resistant *Klebsiella pneumoniae* bacteremia: factors correlated with clinical and microbiologic outcomes. Diagn Microbiol Infect Dis. 2010;67(2):180–4.
61. Gregory CJ, Llata E, Stine N, Gould C, Santiago LM, Vazquez GJ, Robledo IE, Srinivasan A, Goering RV, Tomashek KM. Outbreak of carbapenem-resistant *Klebsiella pneumoniae* in Puerto Rico associated with a novel carbapenemase variant. Infect Control Hosp Epidemiol. 2010;31(5):476–84.
62. Borer A, Saidel-Odes L, Riesenberg K, Eskira S, Peled N, Nativ R, Schlaeffer F, Sherf M. Attributable mortality rate for carbapenem-resistant *Klebsiella pneumoniae* bacteremia. Infect Control Hosp Epidemiol. 2009;30(10):972–6.
63. Woodford N, Tierno PM Jr, Young K, Tysall L, Palepou MF, Ward E, Painter RE, Suber DF, Shungu D, Silver LL, et al. Outbreak of *Klebsiella pneumoniae* producing a new carbapenem-hydrolyzing class A beta-lactamase, KPC-3, in a New York Medical Center. Antimicrob Agents Chemother. 2004;48(12):4793–9.
64. Ahmad M, Urban C, Mariano N, Bradford PA, Calcagni E, Projan SJ, Bush K, Rahal JJ. Clinical characteristics and molecular epidemiology associated with imipenem-resistant *Klebsiella pneumoniae*. Clin Infect Dis. 1999;29(2):352–5.
65. Welch S, Neuner E, Lam S, Bauer S, van Duin D, Eric C, Bass S. Antimicrobial treatment and mortality risk for carbapenem-resistant *Klebsiella pneumonia*. Crit Care Med. 2015;43(12 suppl 1):115–6.
66. Madrigal MD, Blazquez C, Saldana R, Rubio V. Infection and colonization by carbapenem resistant *Klebsiella pneumoniae* in haematology patients. Haematologica. 2015;100(SUPPL 1):471.
67. Katsiari M, Panagiota G, Likousi S, Roussou Z, Polemis M, Alkiviadis Vatopoulos C, Evangelia Platsouka D, Maguina A. Carbapenem-resistant *Klebsiella pneumoniae* infections in a Greek intensive care unit: molecular characterisation and treatment challenges. J Glob Antimicrob Resist. 2015;3(2):123–7.
68. Chen I-L, Huang H-J, Toh H-S. Outbreak of carbapenem-resistant *Klebsiella pneumoniae* in a regional hospital of southern Taiwan. J Microbiol Immunol Infect. 2015;48(2):S151.
69. Freire MP, Abdala E, Moura ML, de Paula FJ, Spadao F, Caiaffa-Filho HH, David-Neto E, Nahas WC, Pierrotti LC. Risk factors and outcome of infections with *Klebsiella pneumoniae* carbapenemase-producing *K. pneumoniae* in kidney transplant recipients. Infection. 2015;43(3):315–23.
70. Bias T, Sharma A, Malat G, Lee D. Doyle A (2015) Outcomes associated with carbapenem-resistant *Klebsiella pneumoniae* (CRKP) in solid organ transplant (SOT) recipients. Am J Transpl. 2015;15(Suppl 3):1.
71. Lübbert C, Rodloff AC, Laudi S, Simon P, Busch T, Mössner J, Bartels M, Kaisers UX. Sa1016 lessons learned from excess mortality due to kpc-producing *Klebsiella pneumoniae* in liver transplant recipients. Gastroenterology. 2014;46(5):S-938.
72. Ozden K, Ozturk G, Aydinli B, Uyanik MH, Albayrak A, Arslan S. Carbapenem resistant *Klebsiella pneumoniae* infection in liver transplant recipients. Liver Transplant. 2014;20(Suppl 1):S-292.
73. Grossi P, Mularoni A, Campanella M, Vizzini G, Conaldi P, Gridelli B. Carbapenem resistant *Klebsiella pneumoniae* (CRKP) infection in solid organ transplant recipients (SOT): a single center analysis. Am J Transplant. 2013;13:343.
74. Rose CKS, Bhatt P, MacDougall C, Gallagher I. A cohort study of patients with klebsiella bacteremia with carbapenem resistance compared to those with third-generation cephalosporin resistance. Crit Care Med. 2012;40(12 SUPPL 1):84.
75. Gallagher J, Bhatt PD, Marino E. A comparison of patients with *Klebsiella bacteremia* with imipenem-resistance to those with 3rd generation cephalosporin resistance. Pharmacotherapy. 2011;31(10):346e–7e.
76. Vardakas K, Matthaiou D, Antupa E, Pappas E, Kechagioglou G, Koteli A. Antoniadou E (2010) Characteristics and outcomes of intensive care unit patients with carbapenem-resistant Klebsiella pneumoniae bacteraemia. Clin Microbiol Infect. 2010;16(Suppl 2):S358.
77. Balandin Moreno B, Isidoro Fernandez B, Vazquez Grande G, Ortega MA, Alcantara Carmona S, Alvarez Martinez L. Infections with metallo-b-lactamase (MBL)-producing *Klebsiella pneumoniae:* clinical features of a

nosocomial oubreak in a spanish intensive care unit. Intensive Care Med. 2010;36(SUPPL 2):S256.
78. Cordery RJ, Roberts CH, Cooper SJ, Bellinghan G, Shetty N. Evaluation of risk factors for the acquisition of bloodstream infections with extended-spectrum beta-lactamase-producing *Escherichia coli* and *Klebsiella* species in the intensive care unit; antibiotic management and clinical outcome. J Hosp Infect. 2008;68(2):108–15.
79. Bhavnani SM, Ambrose PG, Craig WA, Dudley MN, Jones RN, Program SAS. Outcomes evaluation of patients with ESBL- and non-ESBL-producing *Escherichia coli* and *Klebsiella* species as defined by CLSI reference methods: report from the SENTRY Antimicrobial Surveillance Program. Diagn Microbiol Infect Dis. 2006;54(3):231–6.
80. Kim BN, Woo JH, Kim MN, Ryu J, Kim YS. Clinical implications of extended-spectrum β-lactamase-producing *Klebsiella pneumoniae* bacteraemia. J Hosp Infect. 2002;52(2):99–106.
81. Garcia-Sureda L, Domenech-Sanchez A, Barbier M, Juan C, Gasco J, Alberti S. OmpK26, a novel porin associated with carbapenem resistance in *Klebsiella pneumoniae*. Antimicrob Agents Chemother. 2011;55(10):4742–7.
82. Vardakas KZ, Rafailidis PI, Konstantelias AA, Falagas ME. Predictors of mortality in patients with infections due to multi-drug resistant Gram negative bacteria: the study, the patient, the bug or the drug? J Infect. 2013;66(5):401–14.
83. Villegas MV, Lolans K, Correa A, Kattan JN, Lopez JA, Quinn JP, Colombian Nosocomial Resistance Study G. First identification of *Pseudomonas aeruginosa* isolates producing a KPC-type carbapenem-hydrolyzing beta-lactamase. Antimicrob Agents Chemother. 2007;51(4):1553–5.
84. Bratu S, Landman D, Haag R, Recco R, Eramo A, Alam M, Quale J. Rapid spread of carbapenem-resistant *Klebsiella pneumoniae* in New York City: a new threat to our antibiotic armamentarium. Arch Intern Med. 2005;165(12):1430–5.
85. Bratu S, Tolaney P, Karumudi U, Quale J, Mooty M, Nichani S, Landman D. Carbapenemase-producing *Klebsiella pneumoniae* in Brooklyn, NY: molecular epidemiology and in vitro activity of polymyxin B and other agents. J Antimicrob Chemother. 2005;56(1):128–32.
86. Karabinis A, Paramythiotou E, Mylona-Petropoulou D. Colistin for Klebsiella pneumoniae—associated sepsis. Clin Infect Dis. 2004;38(1):e7–9.
87. Daly MW, Riddle DJ, Ledeboer NA, Dunne WM, Ritchie DJ. Tigecycline for the treatment of pneumonia and empyema caused by carbapenemase producing *Klebsiella pneumoniae*. Pharmacotherapy. 2007;27(7):1052–7.
88. Fligou F, Papadimitriou-Olivgeris M, Sklavou C, Anastassiou ED, Marangos M, Filos K. Risk factors and predictors of mortality for KPC-producing *Klebsiella pneumoniae* bactereamia during intensive care unit stay. Eur J Anaesthesiology. 2013;30(suppl 51):187.

8

Brucella melitensis VirB12 recombinant protein is a potential marker for serodiagnosis of human brucellosis

Shiva Mirkalantari[1], Amir-Hassan Zarnani[2,3], Mahboobeh Nazari[4], Gholam Reza Irajian[1] and Nour Amirmozafari[1*]

Abstract

Background: The numerous drawbacks of current serological tests for diagnosis of brucellosis which mainly results from cross reactivity with LPS from other gram-negative bacteria have generated an increasing interest to find more specific non-LPS antigens. Previous studies had indicated that Brucella VirB12 protein, a cell surface protein and component of type IV secretion system, induces antibody response during animal infection. However, this protein has not yet been tested as a serological diagnostic marker in human brucellosis.

Methods: Recombinant VirB12 protein was prepared and evaluated the efficacy of it in an indirect enzyme-linked immunosorbent assay (ELISA) for brucellosis with sera collected from different region of Iran and the results were compared with a commercial ELISA kit.

Results: Sera from human brucellosis patients strongly reacted to the purified recombinant VirB12. The sensitivity, specificity, accuracy, negative predictive value and positive predictive value of recombinant VirB12-based ELISA related to the commercial-ELISA method were 87.8, 94, 90, 80 and 96.6% respectively.

Conclusions: We concluded that antigenic VirB12 have a property value that can be considered as a candidate for using in serodiagnostic tests for human brucellosis.

Keywords: Brucellosis, VirB12, Recombinant proteins, Enzyme-linked immunosorbent assay, *Brucella melitensis*

Background

Brucella spp. is a facultative intracellular pathogen that can be involved with many tissues and organs leading to a chronic infection, Brucellosis, in animals and humans [1–5]. Brucellosis is caused by several species of the genus Brucella including *Brucella abortus, Brucella melitensis, Brucella suis, Brucella canis, Brucella ovis*, and *Brucella neotomae* [6–9]. *B. melitensis* is the most frequently isolated species which is endemic in many developing countries [10, 11]. Clinical manifestations of brucellosis are very similar to other febrile diseases; therefore, the clinical diagnosis of this disease remains a challenge [12]. Common laboratory tests include either bacteriological culture of the pathogen or serological titration of anti-Brucella antibody. Although the gold standard test is said to be bacteriological isolation, the success rate of blood cultures is around 70–80% of cases in acute disease produced by *B. melitensis* [13]. This rate is very much lower in chronic cases. Various factors including disease duration, isolation method, and prior antibiotic intake can drastically impact the bacteriological diagnosis [2]. Serum agglutination serological tests often rely on detection of antibody against smooth lipoplysaccharide (LPS) present on bacterial cell surface. Due to existence of extensive cross reactivity with LPS from other gram negative bacteria, the specificity of these approaches are poorly suited for use in general diagnostic laboratories [2, 14–18]. The drawbacks of these classical serological tests have generated an increasing interest in finding more

*Correspondence: amirmozafari@yahoo.com
[1] Microbiology Department, Faculty of Medicine, Iran University of Medical Sciences, Tehran, Iran
Full list of author information is available at the end of the article

specific non-LPS based antigen candids [2, 19, 20]. In this regard, the outer membrane proteins of Brucella species have been proposed as appropriate candidate for antigenic component. Rolan et al. [21] noted that Brucella VirB12 protein, a component of type IV secretion system, which is situated on bacterial cell surface, is expressed during infection and induces an antibody response in cattle. However, they had not looked at any possible humoral response in humans during active or chronic infections. In a previous communicate we reported cloning of the virB12 gene of *B. melitensis* [22]. In the present study, we are reporting expression and purification of the recombinant VirB12 protein. Furthermore, the seroreactivity of the purified recombinant virB12 of *B. melitensis* was evaluated with human serum samples in an indirect enzyme-linked immunosorbent assay (ELISA) for brucellosis.

Methods

Preparation and recognition of Brucella VirB12 recombinant protein

The plasmid construct pET28a-VirB12 was purified from an overnight culture of *Escherichia coli* DH5α cell. The construct was transformed into competent *E. coli* Bl21 (ED3) cells. The cell harboring recombinant plasmid was spread on Luria-Bertani (LB) agar culture medium containing kanamycin. After verification, the transformed *E. coli* BL21 cells harboring the PET28a-VirB12 plasmid were used in the expression study. A single colony of the transformed cell was incubated overnight in 2 ml LB broth medium containing kanamycin (100 μl/ml) at 37 °C with constant shaking (200 rpm). The next day, 500 μl of culture materials was removed and incubated in 200 ml LB broth. The culture was grown to an OD_{600} nm of 0.6 with vigorous shaking (200 rpm) at 37 °C. Isopropyl-β-D-thiogalactopyranoside (IPTG) was added to a final concentration of 1 mM for expression of VirB12 recombinant protein. The incubated period was continued for another 4 h at 37 °C with shaking at 200 rpm. For analysis of production of the expressed protein, bacterial suspension were tested at 2 and 4 h intervals and analyzed on 12% SDS-PAGE. Following the fermentation process, cells were harvested by centrifugation at 6000×*g* for 15 min at 4 °C. Supernatants were discarded and cell pellets were frozen at −70 °C. The cell pellets were suspended with 10 mM Na_2HPO_4, 10 mM NaH_2PO_4 and 500 mM NaCl (pH, 7.4) and disrupted by sonication for 2 min. After sonication, the mixture was centrifuged at 15.200×*g* for 15 min at 4 °C. The pellet containing insoluble recombinant VirB12 protein (inclusion bodies) was washed three times with 50 mM Tris-Hcl, 10 mM EDTA, 100 mM NaCl and 0.5% Triton–X100 (pH 8). The pellet was resuspended in buffer containing 8 M urea, 10b mM TrisHcl (pH 7.4) and solubilized for 4 h by stirring at room temperature. The solubilized inclusion body was centrifuged at 15.200×*g* for 40 min at 4 °C, and the supernatant was collected. Affinity chromatography Ni-NTA column was used to purify VirB12. Were loaded onto Ni2—charged Hitrap column pre-equilibrated with 8 M urea in 20 mM sodium phosphate buffer, pH 7.4. VirB12 was eluted using a linear gradient with imidazol (10-500 mM) in 8 M urea, pH 7.4. Protein purification was monitored by 280 nm absorbance. Recombinant protein was analyzed by 12% sodium–dodecyl sulfate polyacrylamide gel electrophoresis, followed by coomassie Brilliant Blue 250 staining. Refolding was performed with cheotropic agent concentration gradient dialysis. The solution of denatured protein was dialyzed against 2 lit of freshly prepared 6, 4, 2, 1, 0 M urea with 5 mMTris (pH 7.4). With each concentration, the protein was dialyzed 12 h at 4 °C. Bradford method with bovine serum albumin (BSA) as a standard was used to assay protein concentration. Purified protein was evaluated by western blot using an anti His-tag-HRP antibody.

Immunoreactivity of recombinant Brucella purified rVirB12 to human sera using western blotting

Recombinant protein was subjected to 12% gradient SDS-PAGE with the molecular protein marker and was transferred from the unstained polyacrylamide gel onto 0.45 μm nitrocellulose membrane. The blotted membrane blocked using 5% skim milk in TSBST 1%. After washing with TSBT, transferred proteins were immunostained with serum obtained from human brucellosis infection at a dilution of 1/1000. Secondary antibody conjugated to horseradish peroxidase was used in the assay. The reaction was visualized with enhanced chemiluminescence (ECL) and ECL system (GE Healthcare. Uppsala, Sweden).

Production of polyclonal anti-virB12 recombinant protein in rabbit

A mature white New Zealand rabbit was immunized with purified VirB12 recombinant protein. Immunization was performed according to the protocol of Hay et al. [23]. In the first i.m injection, mixture of 250 μg recombinant protein with the same volume of Freund's complete adjuvant was injected. For second injection the rabbit was injected with 125 μg recombinant protein with the same volume of Freund's incomplete adjuvant, 1, 2 weeks later. Finally, 2 weeks after the last immunization, blood was collected and sera separated.

ELISA test with commercial kit

To investigate the serological status of the samples from human and evaluate the quality of the detection method, all of 100 serum samples were subjected to ELISA kit (IBL, Germany). The plate wells of IBL ELISA kit were coated with a bacterial lysate of B.abortus strain w99 as the antigen. Ref comparsion of four commercial IgM and IgG ELISA kits for diagnosing brucellosis.

Immunoreactivity of recombinant Brucella virB12 to human sera using ELISA

Positive samples were from the patients with a positive ELISA test. Clinical sera from human were analyzed by indirect ELISA using recombinant VirB12 as antigen. The immunoassay plates (Maxisorp, nunc, Denmark) were coated with purified recombinant VirB12 protein at a concentration of 5 μg/ml in PBS and incubated at 4 °C, overnight. The wells emptied and washed three times with phosphate buffer saline-Tween20 (PBST) and then blocked with 5% skim milk for 2 h at 37 °C. Plates were filled with sera at a dilution of 1/100 and incubated at 37 °C for 1 h. After washing with PBST for five times the plates were incubated with HRP conjugates for 1 h at 37 °C. After washing with PBST, the wells of plates were charged with substrate solution containing TMB (3,3′,5,5′-tetra methyl benzidine). Color development was stopped by adding H_2SO_4 20%, after 10 min of incubation of the plates in dark at room temperature. Absorbance was measured at 450 nm wavelength in an ELISA reader. Each samples run in duplicate. Additionally, as a control for each serum, wells were left uncoated. To determine the cut off value for ELISA 60 known positive and 40 known negative sera for human brucellosis were used.

Evaluation of ELISA method against commercial ELISA

The sensitivity, specificity, positive predictive value and negative predictive value of recombinant VirB12 ELISA for serodiagnosis of brucellosis were evaluated in comparison to commercial ELISA kit.

Results

Preparation and recognition of Brucella VirB12 recombinant protein

The pET28a-VirB12 recombinant plasmid was transformed in Bl21 (DE3) *E. coli* cells. Bacteria harboring recombinant plasmid were grown in LB medium. They were induced with 1 mM IPTG to express target recombinant protein. Samples were taken before and at 1 h intervals after induction. Total protein was electrophoresed on 12% SDS PAGE gel. SDS-PAGE analyses showed the expected molecular mass of approximately 25 kDa fusion recombinant protein. The recombinant VirB12 was mostly accumulated in the cytoplasm of *E. coli* transformant as inclusion bodies which could only by extracted and purified under denaturing condition using 8 M urea (Fig. 1). The recombinant VirB12 was mostly accumulated in the cytoplasm of *E. coli* transformant as inclusion bodies, which could only by extracted and purified under denaturing condition using 8 M urea. Following purification of rViB12 by Ni-NTA affinity chromatography, the yield of the purified protein was estimated by Bradford method to be about 0.6 mg/ml of culture (Fig. 2).

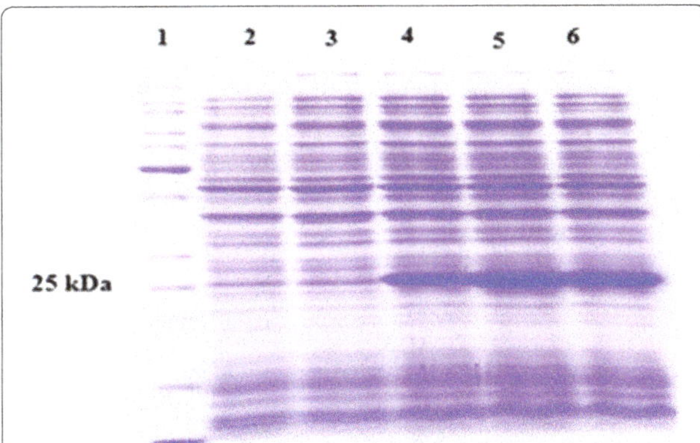

Fig. 1 Analysis of expressed VirB12 recombinant protein at different times after induction on SDS-PAGE (12% w/v). *Lane 1* protein molecular mass marker (KDa). *Lane 2* protein expression in Bl21 (DE3) with pET28a vector 1 h after adding IPTG. *Lane 3* protein expression in transformed Bl21 (DE3) with pET28a-VirB12 recombinant vector before adding IPTG. *Lane 4* protein expression in transformed Bl21 (DE3) with pET28a-VirB12 recombinant vector 1 h after adding IPTG. *Lane 5* protein expression in transformed Bl21 (DE3) with pET28a-VirB12 recombinant vector 2 h after adding IPTG. *Lane 6* protein expression in transformed Bl21 (DE3) with pET28a-VirB12 recombinant vector 4 h after adding IPTG

Immunoreactivity of recombinant Brucella purified rVirB12 to human sera using western blotting

To evaluate immune reactivity of the purified protein, western blot was performed with sera (1/1000 dilution) from *Brucella* infected human. The sera from human reacted to purified recombinant VirB12. Antigenicity of the expressed protein was confirmed by western blot analysis using patient sera. The specific antibody response from five patient sera was observed. Serum samples from normal individual was also tested as negative control and no anti VirB12 antibodies were detected. Additionally, there was no reactivity between the expressed pET28a in *E. coli* Bl21 (DE3) with patient serum (Fig. 3).

Production of polyclonal anti-virB12 recombinant protein in rabbit

Increasing the antibody titers to high level after third boost was confirmed the good immunogenicity of VirB12. The rabbit antiserum was able to recognize the virB12 in Brucella lysate and the purified recombinant VirB12.

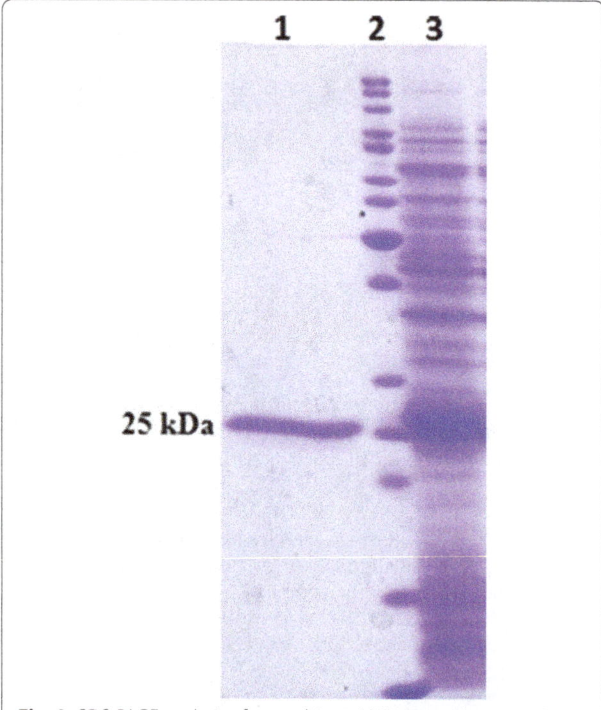

Fig. 2 SDS-PAGE analysis of recombinant VirB12 protein expression and its purification. *Lane 1* elution of recombinant VirB12 protein through Ni-NTA column. *Lane 2* protein molecular mass marker (KDa). *Lane 3* protein protein expression in transformed Bl21 (DE3) with pET28a-VirB12 recombinant vector 3 h after adding IPTG

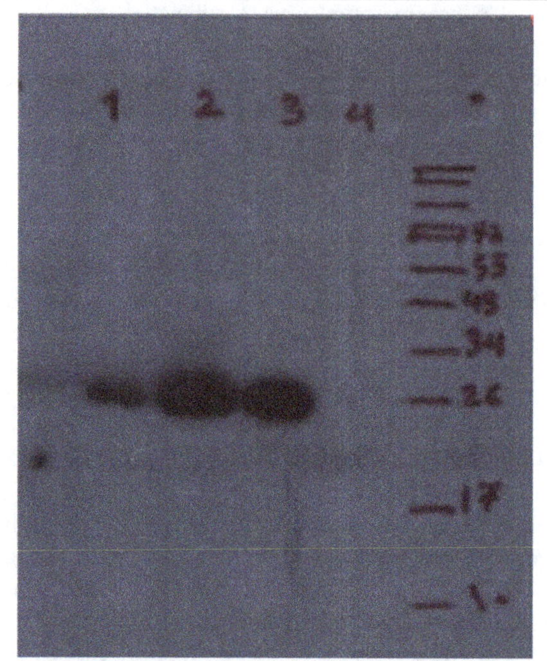

Fig. 3 Western blot analysis against recombinant VirB12 protein by infect patient sera. *Lane 1* western blotting with patient positive Brucella serum (1/500 diluation). *Lane 2, 3* western blotting with patient positive Brucella serum (1/100 diluation). *Lane 4* western blotting with normal individual

Evaluation of recombinant VirB12 ELISA

Immune reactivity of recombinant virB12 was determined using an indirect ELISA. A total 100 serum samples (66 commercial-ELISA positive and 34 commercial-ELISA negative) were collected from different region of the country and were tested by indirect ELISA against the recombinant VirB12 antigen. The VirB12 ELISA was considered positive only if the mean absorbance value was greater than two SDS above the mean value for healthy serum samples. The cut of value was 0.325 (mean, 0.17 SD, 0.077). Out of 100 serum samples tested, 60 (60%) were positive and 40 (40%) were negative by ELISA. The sensitivity, specificity, accuracy, negative predictive value and positive predictive value of recombinant VirB12-based ELISA related to the commercial-ELISA method are shown in Table 1.

Table 1 Evaluation of diagnostic value of recombinant VirB12 antigen-based ELISA against commercial ELISA

	Commercial ELISA positive	Commercial ELISA negative	Total
ELISA-virB12 positive	58	2	60
ELISA-VirB12 negative	8	32	40
Total	66	34	100

Sensitivity: true positive/true positive + false negative*100 = 87.8%

Specificity: true negative/true negative + false positive*100 = 94%

Positive predictive value: true positive/true positive + false positive*100 = 96.6%

Negative predictive value: true negative/true Negative + False positive*100 = 80%

Accuracy: true positive + true negative/total number*100 = 90%

Discussion

Despite using vaccination in livestocks, brucellosis remains as an endemic infection in many developing countries such as Iran. Human and animal infection with *Brucella* inflicts an enormous cost to people and government [24]. Since culture method for diagnosis of Brucellosis is time consuming and has infection risk for laboratory workers, serological tests are commonly used for clinical diagnosis [25]. Due to cross reactions with many other Gram negative bacteria in most routinely used LPS-based serological tests, identification of more specific *Brucella* spp. protective antigens can be useful for developing serological tests which avoid the drawbacks of classical ones. The outer membrane proteins in Gram negative bacteria have particular significance as a potential immunity target [26]. Brucella VirB12 is one of these structural protein which is expressed during Brucellosis infection. Investigators had demonstrated that VirB12 protein acts as an immunogen and induces partial immunity in animal models [27]. However, there is not any report concerning antigenicity of the recombinant VirB12 protein in human. VirB12 protein is located on the bacterial cell surface and is highly conserved among Brucella isolates. Therefore, VirB12 can be considered as an antigenic candidate for serological diagnosis of brucellosis. Use of recombinant VirB12 instead of extracted VirB12, is less time consuming, has a high yield and avoids handling with live pathogenic *Brucella*. In the present study, high level expression of VirB12 protein was carried out by the means of pET28a based on T7 promoter transcription translation signals in conjunction with suitable host cell *E. coli* Bl21 (DE3). The results of SDS-PAGE demonstrated that an IPTG concentration of 1 mM and 4 h of incubation under shaking condition was optimum for expression of protein. The cloning of *VirB12* gene in the pET28 system led to expression of a protein with size of approximately 25 kDa. The expressed protein contained 6 His Tag which is linked to the C-terminal of protein. These additional amino acids increase the size of expressed protein by 8 KDa. The presence of His tag sequence in the target protein also provides the possibility for purification through Ni-NTA affinity chromatography. Metal affinity chromatography was subsequently performed to purify VirB12, producing amount 3 mg of pure recombinant protein per liter of bacterial culture. Antigenicity of the purified protein component was evaluated in immunoblotting with human brucellosis sera. Data showed that the recombinant VirB12 protein could be detected as an antigenic component by sera from acute phase of human brucellosis. By using western blot analysis, we showed that the recombinant VirB12 did not shown any cross reactivity with normal human sera. There was also no serological interference related to the fused amino acids. The results, in consist of other researcher showed that there was no interference related to fused amino acids [12]. To examine the practical value of VirB12, 100 positive and negative serum samples from different part of country used in virB12 antigen based indirect ELISA for detection of antibody response against *Brucella*. The finding demonstrated that the virB12 recombinant protein had good immunogenicity and indicates that the availability of virB12 to the immune system. The Pearson correlation coefficient of the virB12 antigen-based indirect ELISA against commercial ELISA, a test based on LPS antigen was 0.73 ($P < 0.001$). The sensitivity of the virB12-ELISA was 87.8% and specificity was 94%. The accuracy in all samples reached 90%. The sensitivity and specificity of virB12 ELISA in comparison with commercial ELISA confirmed the fact this system comparable to the commercial assay available as a potential immunogenic marker for screening of brucellosis and needs further evaluation.

Conclusions

In summary, our results showed that VirB12 was expressed at high amounts in *E. coli* Bl21 and could be purified by Ni-NTA affinity chromatography. This recombinant protein reacted strongly with sera from patient with brucellosis by western blot. Thus we concluded that VirB12 is antigenic and has property to be considered as a suitable candidate for development of more specific diagnostic tests.

Abbreviations

ELISA: enzyme-linked immunosorbent assay; LPS: lipopolysaccharide; LB: Luria-Bertani; IPTG: isopropyl-β-D- thiogalactopyranoside; BSA: bovine serum albumin; ECL: enhanced chemiluminescence; PBST: phosphate buffer saline-Tween; TMB: 3,3′,5,5′-tetra methyl benzidine.

Authors' contributions

SM and NA designed the study, AHZ writing the article, SM and MN performed the laboratory tests, GRI statistical analysis and writing the study. All authors read and approved the final manuscript.

Author details

[1] Microbiology Department, Faculty of Medicine, Iran University of Medical Sciences, Tehran, Iran. [2] Dept. of Immunology, School of Public Health, Tehran University of Medical Sciences, Tehran, Iran. [3] Immunology Research Center, Iran University of Medical Sciences, Tehran, Iran. [4] Monoclonal Antibody Reaserch Center, Avicenna Research Institute, ACECR, Tehran, Iran.

Acknowledgements

Not applicable.

Competing interests

The authors declare that they have no competing interests.

Funding

The study was supported by Iran University of Medical Sciences.

References

1. Abbas B, Aldeewan A. Occurrence and epidemiology of *Brucella* spp. in raw milk samples at Basrah province, Iraq. Bulg J Vet Med. 2009;12(2):136–42.
2. Thavaselvam D, Kumar A, Tiwari S, Mishra M, Prakash A. Cloning and expression of the immunoreactive *Brucella melitensis* 28 kDa outer-membrane protein (Omp28) encoding gene and evaluation of the potential of Omp28 for clinical diagnosis of brucellosis. J Med Microbiol. 2010;59(4):421–8.
3. Delpino MV, Estein SM, Fossati CA, Baldi PC, Cassataro J. Vaccination with *Brucella* recombinant DnaK and SurA proteins induces protection against

Brucella abortus infection in BALB/c mice. Vaccine. 2007;25(37–38):6721–9. doi:10.1016/j.vaccine.2007.07.002.

4. Roset MS, Ibanez AE, de Souza Filho JA, Spera JM, Minatel L, Oliveira SC, et al. Brucella cyclic β-1,2-glucan plays a critical role in the induction of splenomegaly in mice. PLoS ONE. 2014;9(7):e101279. doi:10.1371/journal.pone.0101279.
5. Kahl-McDonagh MM, Ficht TA. Evaluation of protection afforded by *Brucella abortus* and *Brucella melitensis* unmarked deletion mutants exhibiting different rates of clearance in BALB/c mice. Infect Immun. 2006;74(7):4048–57. doi:10.1128/IAI.01787-05.
6. Zhao Z, Yan F, Ji W, Luo D, Liu X, Xing L, et al. Identification of immunoreactive proteins of *Brucella melitensis* by immunoproteomics. Sci China Life Sci. 2011;54(9):880–7. doi:10.1007/s11427-011-4218-2.
7. Tiwari AK, Kumar S, Pal V, Bhardwaj B, Rai GP. Evaluation of the recombinant 10-kilodalton immunodominant region of the BP26 protein of *Brucella abortus* for specific diagnosis of bovine brucellosis. Clin Vaccine Immunol. 2011;18(10):1760–4. doi:10.1128/CVI.05159-11.
8. Zygmunt MS, Baucheron S, Vizcaino N, Bowden RA, Cloeckaert A. Single-step purification and evaluation of recombinant BP26 protein for serological diagnosis of *Brucella ovis* infection in rams. Vet Microbiol. 2002;87(3):213.
9. Mirkalantari S. Optimizing of *Brucella* oprF recombinant protein expression as a soluble protein in *Escherichia coli*. Focus Sci. 2016;2:1.
10. Seleem MN, Boyle SM, Sriranganathan N. Brucellosis: a re-emerging zoonosis. Vet Microbiol. 2010;140(3–4):392–8. doi:10.1016/j.vetmic.2009.06.021.
11. Renukaradhya GJ, Isloor S, Crowther JR, Robinson M, Rajasekhar M. Development and field validation of an avidin-biotin enzyme-linked immunosorbent assay kit for bovine brucellosis. Rev Sci Tech. 2001;20(3):749–56.
12. Araj GF. Human brucellosis: a classical infectious disease with persistent diagnostic challenges. Clin Lab Sci. 1999;12(4):207–12.
13. Cassataro J, Delpino MV, Velikovsky CA, Bruno L, Fossati CA, Baldi PC. Diagnostic usefulness of antibodies against ribosome recycling factor from *Brucella melitensis* in human or canine brucellosis. Clin Diagn Lab Immunol. 2002;9(2):366–9.
14. Nielsen K. Diagnosis of brucellosis by serology. Vet Microbiol. 2002;90(1–4):447–59.
15. Contreras-Rodriguez A, Seleem MN, Schurig GG, Sriranganathan N, Boyle SM, Lopez-Merino A. Cloning, expression and characterization of immunogenic aminopeptidase N from *Brucella melitensis*. FEMS Immunol Med Microbiol. 2006;48(2):252–6. doi:10.1111/j.1574-695X.2006.00145.x.
16. Chaudhuri P, Prasad R, Kumar V, Gangaplara A. Recombinant OMP28 antigen-based indirect ELISA for serodiagnosis of bovine brucellosis. Mol Cell Probes. 2010;24(3):142–5. doi:10.1016/j.mcp.2009.12.002.
17. Nielsen K, Smith P, Widdison J, Gall D, Kelly L, Kelly W, et al. Serological relationship between cattle exposed to *Brucella abortus*, *Yersinia enterocolitica* O: 9 and *Escherichia coli* O157: H7. Vet Microbiol. 2004;100(1):25–30.
18. Pardon P, Sanchis R, Molenat G, Marly J, Renard D. Serological and allergic reactions of ewes after simultaneous vaccinations with two living attenuated strains of *Brucella* and *Salmonella*. Ann Rech Vet. 1990;21(2):153–60.
19. Tan W, Wang XR, Nie Y, Wang C, Cheng LQ, Wang XC, et al. Recombinant VirB5 protein as a potential serological marker for the diagnosis of bovine brucellosis. Mol Cell Probes. 2012;26(3):127–31.
20. Tiwari S, Kumar A, Thavaselvam D, Mangalgi S, Rathod V, Prakash A, et al. Development and comparative evaluation of a plate enzyme-linked immunosorbent assay based on recombinant outer membrane antigens Omp28 and Omp31 for diagnosis of human brucellosis. Clin Vaccine Immunol. 2013;20(8):1217–22. doi:10.1128/CVI.00111-13.
21. Sun YH, Rolan HG, den Hartigh AB, Sondervan D, Tsolis RM. *Brucella abortus* virB12 is expressed during infection but is not an essential component of the type IV secretion system. Infect Immun. 2005;73(9):6048–54. doi:10.1128/IAI.73.9.6048-6054.2005.
22. Mirkalantari S, Amirmozafari N, Kazemi B, Irajian G. Molecular cloning of virB12 gene of *Brucella melitensis* 16M strain in pET28a vector. Asian Pac J Trop Med. 2012;5(7):511–3. doi:10.1016/S1995-7645(12)60089-3.
23. Hey F, Westwood O, Nelson P. Practical immunology. West sussex: Wiley; 2002.
24. Kazak E, Oliveira SC, Goral G, Akalin H, Yilmaz E, Heper Y, et al. *Brucella abortus* L7/L12 recombinant protein induces strong Th1 response in acute brucellosis patients. Iran J Immunol. 2010;7(3):132.
25. Ko J, Splitter GA. Molecular host-pathogen interaction in brucellosis: current understanding and future approaches to vaccine development for mice and humans. Clin Microbiol Rev. 2003;16(1):65–78.
26. Galdiero S, Falanga A, Cantisani M, Tarallo R, Della Pepa ME, D'Oriano V, et al. Microbe-host interactions: structure and role of gram-negative bacterial porins. Curr Protein Pept Sci. 2012;13(8):843–54.
27. Rolan HG, den Hartigh AB, Kahl-McDonagh M, Ficht T, Adams LG, Tsolis RM. VirB12 is a serological marker of *Brucella* infection in experimental and natural hosts. Clin Vaccine Immunol. 2008;15(2):208–14. doi:10.1128/CVI.00374-07.

9

Activity of AMP2041 against human and animal multidrug resistant *Pseudomonas aeruginosa* clinical isolates

Clotilde Silvia Cabassi[1], Andrea Sala[1], Davide Santospirito[1], Giovanni Loris Alborali[2], Edoardo Carretto[3], Giovanni Ghibaudo[4] and Simone Taddei[1*]

Abstract

Background: Antimicrobial resistance is a growing threat to public health. *Pseudomonas aeruginosa* is a relevant pathogen causing human and animal infections, frequently displaying high levels of resistance to commonly used antimicrobials. The increasing difficulty to develop new effective antibiotics have discouraged investment in this area and only a few new antibiotics are currently under development. An approach to overcome antibiotic resistance could be based on antimicrobial peptides since they offer advantages over currently used microbicides.

Methods: The antimicrobial activity of the synthetic peptide AMP2041 was evaluated against 49 *P. aeruginosa* clinical strains with high levels of antimicrobial resistance, isolated from humans ($n = 19$) and animals ($n = 30$). In vitro activity was evaluated by a microdilution assay for lethal dose 90% (LD_{90}), while the activity over time was performed by time-kill assay with 12.5 µg/ml of AMP2014. Evidences for a direct membrane damage were investigated on *P. aeruginosa* ATCC 27853 reference strain, on animal isolate PA-VET 38 and on human isolate PA-H 24 by propidium iodide and on *P. aeruginosa* ATCC 27853 by scanning electron microscopy.

Results: AMP2041 showed a dose-dependent activity, with a mean (SEM) LD_{90} of 1.69 and 3.3 µg/ml for animal and human strains, respectively. AMP2041 showed microbicidal activity on *P. aeruginosa* isolates from a patient with cystic fibrosis (CF) and resistance increased from first infection isolate ($LD_{90} = 0.3$ µg/ml) to the mucoid phenotype ($LD_{90} = 10.4$ µg/ml). The time-kill assay showed a time-dependent bactericidal effect of AMP2041 and LD_{90} was reached within 20 min for all the strains. The stain-dead assay showed an increasing of membrane permeabilization and SEM analysis revealed holes, dents and bursts throughout bacterial cell wall after 30 min of incubation with AMP2041.

Conclusions: The obtained results assessed for the first time the good antimicrobial activity of AMP2041 on *P. aeruginosa* strains of human origin, including those deriving from a CF patient. We confirmed the excellent antimicrobial activity of AMP2041 on *P. aeruginosa* strains derived from dog otitis. We also assessed that AMP2041 antimicrobial activity is linked to changes of the *P. aeruginosa* cell wall morphology and to the increasing of membrane permeability.

Keywords: Antimicrobial peptide, Pseudomonas aeruginosa, Cinical isolates, Multidrug resistance, Bacterial membrane damage

Background

Pseudomonas aeruginosa is a relevant pathogen causing human and animal infections. In humans, severe *P. aeruginosa* infections usually occur in immunocompromised patients and in nosocomial setting. *P. aeruginosa* infection often follow surgery or invasive procedures and causes mainly pneumonia and septicaemia. *P. aeruginosa* may also cause mild illnesses in healthy people, in which skin, ear and eye infections can occur. Moreover, *P. aeruginosa* is the major pathogen in the cystic fibrosis (CF). In CF, chronic *P. aeruginosa* infections occur in up to

*Correspondence: simone.taddei@unipr.it
[1] Department of Veterinary Science, University of Parma, Via del Taglio 10, 43126 Parma, Italy
Full list of author information is available at the end of the article

85% of CF patients and the *P. aeruginosa* strains involved develop antibiotic resistance and phenotypic changes, from first infection to chronic infection and mucoid phenotype. These phenotypical changes could play a major role in the persistence of *P. aeruginosa* infections in CF patients [1]. Antibiotic resistance and the persistence of the organisms despite therapy once chronic infection has been established, is leading to the search for more effective therapeutic approaches [1].

Pseudomonas aeruginosa also cause diseases in both livestock and companion animals, including otitis and urinary tract infections in dogs, mastitis in dairy cows and endometritis in horses [2]. Resistance phenotypes are more frequent in dogs and multi-drug resistant (MDR) *P. aeruginosa* seem to emerge mainly in those suffering from otitis. Antimicrobial resistance in animal *P. aeruginosa* infections should be closely monitored in the future, in line with possible animal-to-human transfers between pets and owners [2]. *P. aeruginosa* is naturally resistant to many classes of drugs and its capacity to rapidly develop resistance during treatment is a frequent source of therapeutic failures. *P. aeruginosa* is one of the six ESKAPE pathogens, reported by the Infectious Diseases Society of America, that urgently require novel therapies [3]. Rates of antibiotic resistance in *P. aeruginosa* are increasing worldwide even if the true frequency of infections caused by MDR *P. aeruginosa* is difficult to estimate. A review of studies reporting on MDR, extensively-drug resistant (XDR) and pan-drug resistant (PDR) *P. aeruginosa* infections revealed that aminoglycosides, antipseudomonal penicillins, cephalosporins, carbapenems and fluoroquinolones [4] have become ineffective as first line agents. The multidrug resistance of *P. aeruginosa* could be mediated by several mechanisms including multidrug efflux systems, enzyme production, outer membrane protein loss and target mutations [5]. The spread of antimicrobial resistance increase human and animal health hazard worldwide, thus makes mandatory the investigation of novel approaches to cover the therapeutic shortfall. In this view, one of the actions put forward in the European Commission Action Plan is to develop effective antimicrobials or alternatives for treatment of human and animal infections and to reinforce research to develop innovative means to combat antimicrobial resistance [6]. Antimicrobial peptides offer potential advantages over currently used classes of drugs. They may counteract pathogenic challenge by rapid, broad spectrum, microbicidal activity [7], targeting multiple pathogens with one treatment. Moreover, antimicrobial peptides may have the potential to ultimately reduce the rate of emergence of resistant microorganisms, since selective pressure is not focused to a single specific molecular target. Further, antimicrobial peptides could also be potentially used in conjunction with conventional antibiotics as part of a "combination therapy" to create an additive or synergistic effect.

The antimicrobial peptide AMP2041 is a cyclic antimicrobial peptide, belonging to a novel family of antimicrobial cationic peptides, which showed good antimicrobial activity against a panel of different Gram-positive and Gram-negative bacterial pathogens of animal origin [8]. The activity of AMP2041 against *P. aeruginosa* ATCC 27853 was also demonstrated, as well as additivity in combination with levofloxacin [9]. We hypothesized that the reported antimicrobial activity derived from a bacterial membrane damage, but a direct membrane damage was not previously investigated for *P. aeruginosa*.

The aim of the present work was to evaluate the antimicrobial activity of AMP2041 on different MDR, PDR and XDR *P. aeruginosa* clinical isolates of human origin, including five different phenotypes of *P. aeruginosa* derived from a single patient with cystic fibrosis, and on clinical MDR *P. aeruginosa* clinical isolates deriving from animals, mainly dogs with otitis. Further, we investigated the evidence for a direct membrane damage on *P. aeruginosa* ATCC 27853 reference strain.

Methods

Bacterial strains and antibiotic susceptibility

Isolates and their biochemical profiles, obtained by API System (bioMérieux, Marcy l'Etoile, France), are reported in Tables 1, 2 and 3. Antibiotic susceptibility tests were performed using the system Vitek2 (bioMérieux, Marcy l'Etoile, France) and/or the Kirby–Bauer method (antibiotic disks provided by Mast Diagnostics Germany, Oxoid, UK). *P. aeruginosa* drug-resistant strains were defined following the European Centre for Disease Prevention and Control (ECDC) guidelines [10]. The following

Table 1 *Pseudomonas aeruginosa* human clinical isolates

Reference number	ID number	Source	API20E	Sample	Resistance profile
[1]	PA-H 1	Human	2216004	Urine	XDR
[2]	PA-H 10	Human	2217046	Blood	MDR
[3]	PA-H 24	Human	2216046	Blood	XDR
[4]	PA-H 25	Human	2206046	Urine	MDR
[5]	PA-H 37	Human	2206046	Blood	MDR
[6]	PA-H 45	Human	2210004	Urine	MDR
[7]	PA-H 47	Human	2217046	Blood	MDR
[8]	PA-H 52	Human	2206006	Blood	MDR
[9]	PA-H 56	Human	2206046	Blood	XDR
[10]	PA-H 58	Human	2206006	Blood	MDR
[11]	PA-H 71	Human	2206046	Blood	MDR
[12]	PA-H 37/2	Human	2206006	Blood	MDR
[13]	PA-H 45/2	Human	2206006	Urine	MDR
[14]	PA-H 14	Human	2206046	Blood	MDR

Table 2 ***Pseudomonas aeruginosa*** **clinical isolates obtained from a single cystic fibrosis (CF) patient**

Reference number	ID number	Source	API20E	Sample	Resistance profile
[1]	PA-H 1PE (first infection)	Human	2206006	Sputum	Non-MDR
[2]	PA-H 2PCa (mucoid phenotype)	Human	2216004	Sputum	Non-MDR
[3]	PA-H 3BFa (chronic infection)	Human	2206046	Sputum	XDR
[4]	PA-H 3BFb (chronic infection)	Human	2217046	Sputum	XDR
[5]	PA-H 3BFc (chronic infection)	Human	2206046	Sputum	XDR

Table 3 ***Pseudomonas aeruginosa*** **animal clinical isolates**

Reference number	ID number	Source	API20E	Sample	Resistance profile
[1]	PA-VET 7	Dog	2206006	Auricular swab	MDR
[2]	PA-VET 9	Dog	2202001	Auricular swab	MDR
[3]	PA-VET 10	Dog	2216046	Auricular swab	MDR
[4]	PA-VET 11	Dog	2206046	Auricular swab	MDR
[5]	PA-VET 13	Dog	2206046	Liver	MDR
[6]	PA-VET 15A	Dog	2206006	Auricular swab	MDR
[7]	PA-VET 15B	Dog	2212004	Auricular swab	MDR
[8]	PA-VET 16	Dog	2206046	Auricular swab	MDR
[9]	PA-VET 17	Dog	2206046	Urine	MDR
[10]	PA-VET 18	Dog	2206046	Auricular swab	MDR
[11]	PA-VET 19	Dog	2206046	Auricular swab	MDR
[12]	PA-VET 20A	Dog	2206006	Urine	MDR
[13]	PA-VET 20B	Dog	2216004	Auricular swab	MDR
[14]	PA-VET 22	Dog	2206046	Auricular swab	MDR
[15]	PA-VET 23	Dog	2206006	Auricular swab	MDR
[16]	PA-VET 24	Dog	2206046	Foreskin swab	MDR
[17]	PA-VET 26	Dog	2216046	Auricular swab	MDR
[18]	PA-VET 27	Dog	2217046	Auricular swab	MDR
[19]	PA-VET 28	Dog	2206046	Auricular swab	MDR
[20]	PA-VET 29	Dog	2206046	Auricular swab	MDR
[21]	PA-VET 30	Dog	2206006	Auricular swab	MDR
[22]	PA-VET 31	Dog	2206046	Auricular swab	MDR
[23]	PA-VET 32	Dog	2206006	Auricular swab	MDR
[24]	PA-VET 33	Dog	2212046	Auricular swab	MDR
[25]	PA-VET 34	Dog	2206006	Auricular swab	MDR
[26]	PA-VET 35A	Dog	2212046	Foreskin swab	MDR
[27]	PA-VET 35B	Dog	2210004	Auricular swab	MDR
[28]	PA-VET 36	Dog	2206006	Auricular swab	MDR
[29]	PA-VET 37	Dog	2206006	Auricular swab	MDR
[30]	PA-VET 38	Dog	2210004	Auricular swab	MDR

classes of antimicrobials were tested: aminoglycosides, carbapenems, cephalosporins, fluoroquinolones, penicillins, monobactams, phosphonic acids, polymyxins. The resistance profiles of the isolates are reported in Tables 1, 2 and 3.

Peptide

The peptide AMP2041 used in this study was developed as described elsewhere [9], and synthesized from SelleckChem (Houston, TX, USA). The purity (>98%), sequence and concentration of the peptide were determined and verified by SelleckChem by using high pressure liquid chromatography (HPLC) and mass spectroscopy. The peptide was dissolved in phosphate buffer (PB) (10 mM, 0.8709 g/l K_2HPO_4, 0.6804 g/l KH_2PO_4, pH 7.0) at the concentration of 1 mg/ml.

Antibacterial activity evaluation

Methods were described in detail elsewhere [9]. Briefly, bacterial suspension was prepared in PB 10 mM measuring spectrophotometrically the absorbance at 600 nm to a concentration of 10^8 colony-forming units (CFU)/ml. The adjusted bacterial suspension was then diluted to obtain a final concentration of bacteria of approximately 5×10^5 CFU/ml. Serial dilutions of peptide were performed in a microtiter plate so that final concentrations were within the range 0.4–100 μg/ml. After bacterial suspension addition, microtiter plates were incubated for 2 h at 37 °C. Then, 20 μl of each dilution were plated onto tryptose agar containing 5% bovine erythrocytes. After 24 h of incubation at 37 °C, the colonies were counted. The minimal bactericidal concentration (MBC) was the lowest concentration of peptide that killed >99.9% of bacteria, while lethal dose 90% (LD_{90}) was the concentration of peptide that killed 90% of bacteria.

Time-kill assay

To evaluate the bactericidal kinetic, 5×10^5 CFU/ml of *P. aeruginosa* were incubated with 12.5 μg/ml of AMP2041 at 37 °C in PB. The concentration of 12.5 μg/ml was chosen because it represents the minimal concentration of peptide capable to kill all the tested bacterial strains. Moreover, the same concentration was used for the time-kill assay performed in a previous work on *P. aeruginosa* ATCC 27853 [9]. Aliquots of 20 μl were withdrawn at different intervals (every 5 min until 30 min, then every 10 min until 60 min, then every 30 min until 120 min) and plated onto tryptose agar containing 5% bovine erythrocytes. After overnight incubation at 37 °C, the CFU were counted. Controls were performed in PB without peptide.

Permeation of the bacterial inner membrane

To assess the ability of antimicrobial peptides to alter the permeability of the inner membrane (IM) of *P. aeruginosa*, a dead-cell stain procedure, using the cationic DNA-staining dye propidium iodide (PI) (Invitrogen, Carlsbad, CA, USA), was performed. PI is unable to permeate the membranes and therefore does not enter viable cells with intact membranes. In dead cells PI gain access to nucleic acids, intercalates between the bases and red fluorescence increases. The stain-dead assay was performed as described in a previous work [11] using 10^9 CFU/ml log-phase cultures of *P. aeruginosa* ATCC 27853, PA-H 24 and PA-VET 38 in the presence of 12.5 μg/ml of AMP2041 and of 3 μM PI. After peptide addition, the fluorescence emission of PI was measured every 5 min up to 25 min, by a fluorescence microscope (Nikon Eclipse 50i) at 1000×. 4′,6-diamidino-2-phenylindole (DAPI) (Invitrogen, Carlsbad, CA, USA) was used for counterstaining (blue fluorescence). Negative and positive controls (not shown) were obtained in absence of peptide and in presence of 1 mM ethylenediaminetetraacetic acid and 0.5% Triton X-100, respectively.

Scanning electron microscopy analysis

The test was performed on the *P. aeruginosa* ATCC 27853 reference strain. The cell/peptide ratio used for the scanning electron microscopy (SEM) assay was at least 20 times higher than in the conditions used to determine the MBC. After a contact time of 30 min with AMP2041, the bacterial pellet was obtained by centrifugation at 4000*g* for 5 min and washed twice in PB, pH 7.2. Bacteria were then fixed in a solution of 1% glutaraldehyde in 0.1 M sodium cacodylate (Santa Cruz Biotech, Santa Cruz, CA) for 1 h and washed with water for 1 h. Then, the bacteria were soaked again in water, and the pellet after centrifugation was dehydrated in a series of ethanol washes. Ten microliters of the bacterial suspension were then mounted and imaged.

Results

Antibacterial activity evaluation

The antibacterial activity of AMP2041 on the 49 clinical isolates of *P. aeruginosa* is shown in Fig. 1a, b. AMP2041 showed antibacterial activity against the tested clinical strains with an LD_{90} ranging from 1.69 to 3.3 μg/ml for animal and human strains, respectively (Table 4). The LD_{90} confidence interval 95% estimated for animal isolates was more narrow (1.14–2.25 μg/ml) compared to human strains (1.75–4.31 μg/ml). The activity of AMP2041 against *P. aeruginosa* strains derived from a single patient affected by CF is reported in Table 4 and Fig. 1b.

For first infection strain (PA-H 1PE) we observed a value of LD_{90} less than 1 μg/ml. For chronic infection strains (PA-H 3BFa, PA-H 3BFb and PA-H 3BFc) and mucoid phenotype strain (PA-H 2PCa), we observed a shift of LD_{90} towards higher values, ranging from 2.25 to 10.4 μg/ml. In particular, the highest LD_{90} was observed for the mucoid phenotype (10.4 μg/ml). For chronic infection strains as well as for the mucoid phenotype strain, AMP2041 was able to kill all the bacteria at a concentration of 12.5 μg/ml (Fig. 1b).

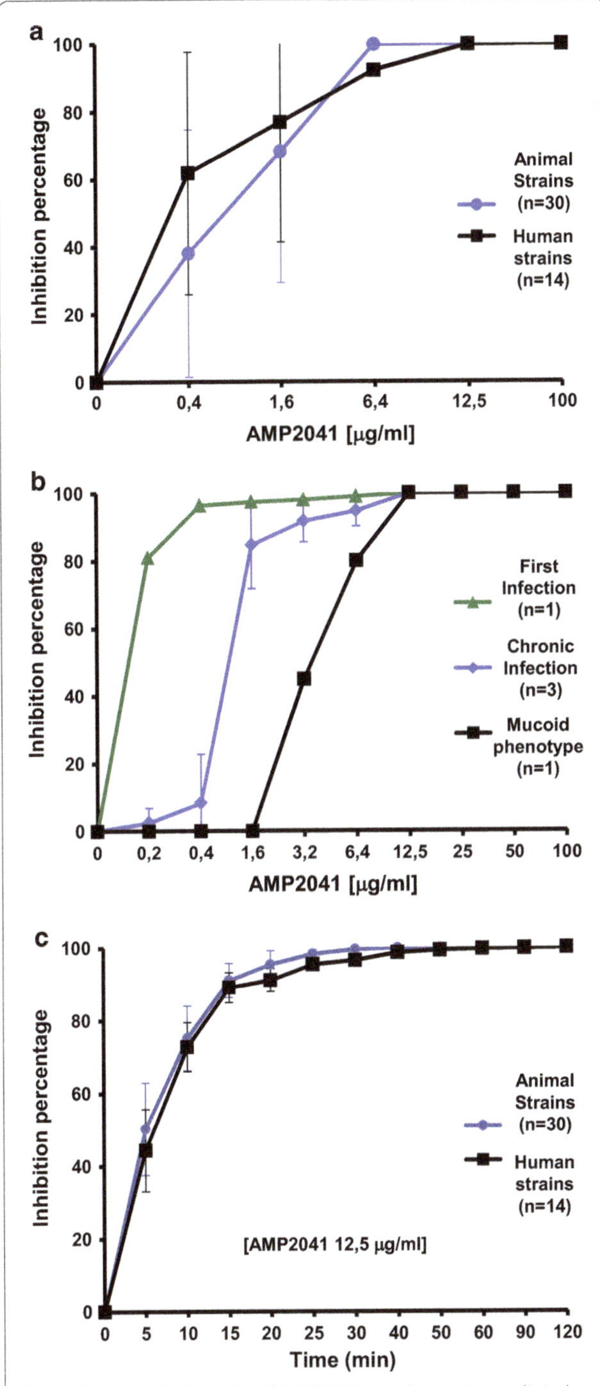

Fig. 1 Antimicrobial activity of AMP2041 on **a** *P. aeruginosa* clinical isolates and **b** *P. aeruginosa* isolates from a patient with cystic fibrosis. **c** Time-kill assay

Table 4 Antimicrobial activity of AMP2041 against PA isolates

Reference number	Human clinical isolates LD_{90} [μg/ml]	Cystic fibrosis isolates LD_{90} [μg/ml]	Animal clinical isolates LD_{90} [μg/ml]
[1]	3.02	0.3	1.09
[2]	1.03	10.4	8.30
[3]	0.6	4.5	0.77
[4]	1.14	3.8	0.93
[5]	0.18	3.2	2.91
[6]	6.07	–	2.87
[7]	7.78	–	2.94
[8]	3.77	–	1.75
[9]	3.63	–	1.75
[10]	0.97	–	0.94
[11]	2.14	–	2.80
[12]	6.15	–	0.99
[13]	0.95	–	2.33
[14]	5.04	–	1.41
[15]	–	–	1.06
[16]	–	–	1.16
[17]	–	–	1.01
[18]	–	–	0.56
[19]	–	–	0.77
[20]	–	–	0.63
[21]	–	–	1.39
[22]	–	–	0.98
[23]	–	–	1.14
[24]	–	–	0.36
[25]	–	–	2.15
[26]	–	–	0.53
[27]	–	–	2.87
[28]	–	–	2.80
[29]	–	–	0.51
[30]	–	–	0.83
Mean ± SD [95% CI]	3.3 ± 2.44 [1.75–4.31]	4.44 ± 3.31 [1.54–7.34]	1.69 ± 1.5 [1.14–2.25]

LD_{90} lethal dose 90%, *SD* standard deviation, *95% CI* 95% confidence interval

Time-kill assay

Inhibition percentages of AMP2041 over time on the 14 *P. aeruginosa* clinical human isolates and on the 30 *P. aeruginosa* clinical animal isolates are shown in Fig. 1c. A reduction of CFU count >90% was observed within 20 min of incubation with peptide.

Permeation of the bacterial inner membrane

The stain-dead assay showed a clear red fluorescence after 10 min for *P. aeruginosa* ATCC 27853 and for the animal isolate PA-VET 38, whilst the presence of fluorescence for the human isolate PA-H 24 was not clearly evident before 15 min of incubation (Fig. 2).

Scanning electron microscopy analysis

The SEM analysis was performed on the *P. aeruginosa* ATCC 27853 reference strain. The untreated bacteria displayed a smooth and intact surface (Fig. 3a) with typical rod morphology about 2 μm long and 0.5 μm wide. After incubation with AMP2041, bacteria showed several holes, multiple dents and bursts with deep craters throughout cell wall (Fig. 3b, c). Lysed cells and debris were also observed.

Discussion

Pseudomonas aeruginosa is an ubiquitous organism. Its ability to survive on minimal nutritional requirements and to tolerate a variety of physical conditions allows its persistence in both community and hospital settings [12]. *P. aeruginosa* is a serious therapeutic challenge for treatment of both community-acquired and nosocomial infections, due to the ability of this microorganism to develop resistance to multiple classes of antibacterial agents, even during the course of therapy [13, 14]. The increasing frequency of MDR or XDR *P. aeruginosa* strains is of concern as effective antimicrobial options are limited [15, 16]. Moreover, only a few new antibiotics are currently under development [6]. An increase in MDR bacterial infections among companion animals has been documented in multiple veterinary hospital settings [17]. This is of particular importance due to the risk of transmission to humans and other companion animals in close contact with infected animals, even because in our countries the pet population continues to rise and the contacts between people and their companion animals grows stronger [18–20]. Therefore, the discover of new agents or innovative approaches able to counteract the growing problem of antimicrobial resistance become crucial.

The synthetic peptide AMP2041 is a cationic peptide and possesses a significant proportion of hydrophobic or non-polar residues. These structural features are common to many antimicrobial peptides [9, 21]. The hydrophobic core is essential for the antimicrobial peptide to effectively permeate the bacterial membrane. The hydrophobic core is flanked at both ends by cationic and polar residues that help to solubilize the peptides in aqueous solution. Cationic and polar residues are also important for the initial electrostatic attraction of antimicrobial peptides to negatively charged phospholipid membranes of bacteria. Also the conformation assumed by AMP2041 might be responsible for the observed antimicrobial activity [8, 9, 22].

Antimicrobial activity of AMP2041 on human clinical isolates was never investigated before. In this study we evaluated the activity of AMP2041 on 19 MDR or XDR *P. aeruginosa* strains isolated from different pathological conditions of humans, among which five deriving from a CF patient. Moreover, the activity of AMP2041 was tested on a sample of 30 MDR *P. aeruginosa* strains derived from dog otitis. AMP2041 showed an excellent activity against all the examined strains. In particular, on average, it was more effective against animals strains, with an LD_{90} of 1.69 μg/ml and an MBC of 6.4 μg/ml (3.2 μM), compared with human strains, LD_{90} of 3.3 μg/ml, MBC of 12.5 μg/ml (6.2 μM). The antimicrobial activity found here for AMP2041 against *P. aeruginosa* is comparable or better than many highly-active antimicrobial peptides. Zhou et al. have found MIC values against *P. aeruginosa* ranging from 31 to >256 μg/ml for peptides synthesized via ring-opening polymerization of α-amino acid *N*-carboxyanhydrides [23]. Regarding the activity of Cecropin A, an insect antimicrobial peptide, against *P. aeruginosa*, a MIC value of 64 μg/ml is reported by Zhou et al. [23] and a lethal concentration of 3.5 μM by Andreu et al. [24]. For PR-39, an antimicrobial peptide from pig intestine, a lethal concentration of 200 μM against *P. aeruginosa* was reported [25]. Very recently, minimum lethal concentrations ranging from 3 to 100 μM were reported for *E. coli* MreB derived antimicrobial peptides against *P. aeruginosa* [26].

It is noteworthy the antimicrobial activity of AMP2041 against the strains derived from the patient with CF. Most patients with CF become chronically infected with wild-type (first infection) *P. aeruginosa* strains early in their life. During the years following the initial colonization, the first infection strains may mutate into mucoid variants [27, 28]. Conversion to the mucoid phenotype is thought to be driven mainly by the unique CF microenvironment [28]. In our case, the *P. aeruginosa* mucoid strain was less sensitive to AMP2041 than the other tested CF strains (Fig. 1b). However, this result was obtained on a single strain and should be further investigated with a wider sample to confirm a higher resistance of the mucoid phenotype compared to the first and chronic infection isolates. The observed lower sensitivity to AMP2041 of the *P. aeruginosa* mucoid strain could be linked to the over production of mucoid exopolysaccharides that hide the negatively charged surface components to which positively charged peptides are attracted.

Mean MBC for dog strains (n = 30, MBC = 6.4 μg/ml—see Fig. 1a) is higher than values previously found for the reference strain ATCC 27853 (4.35 μg/ml) and other dog isolates (n = 6, MBC = 2.44 μg/ml) [8]. Therefore, the increased sample size allowed us to re-evaluate the MBC average value previously obtained.

The bacterial killing assay indicated a CFU reduction >90% within 20 min (Fig. 1c). Therefore, the antimicrobial activity of AMP2041 occurs quickly and the killing kinetic profiles of human and animal clinical isolates,

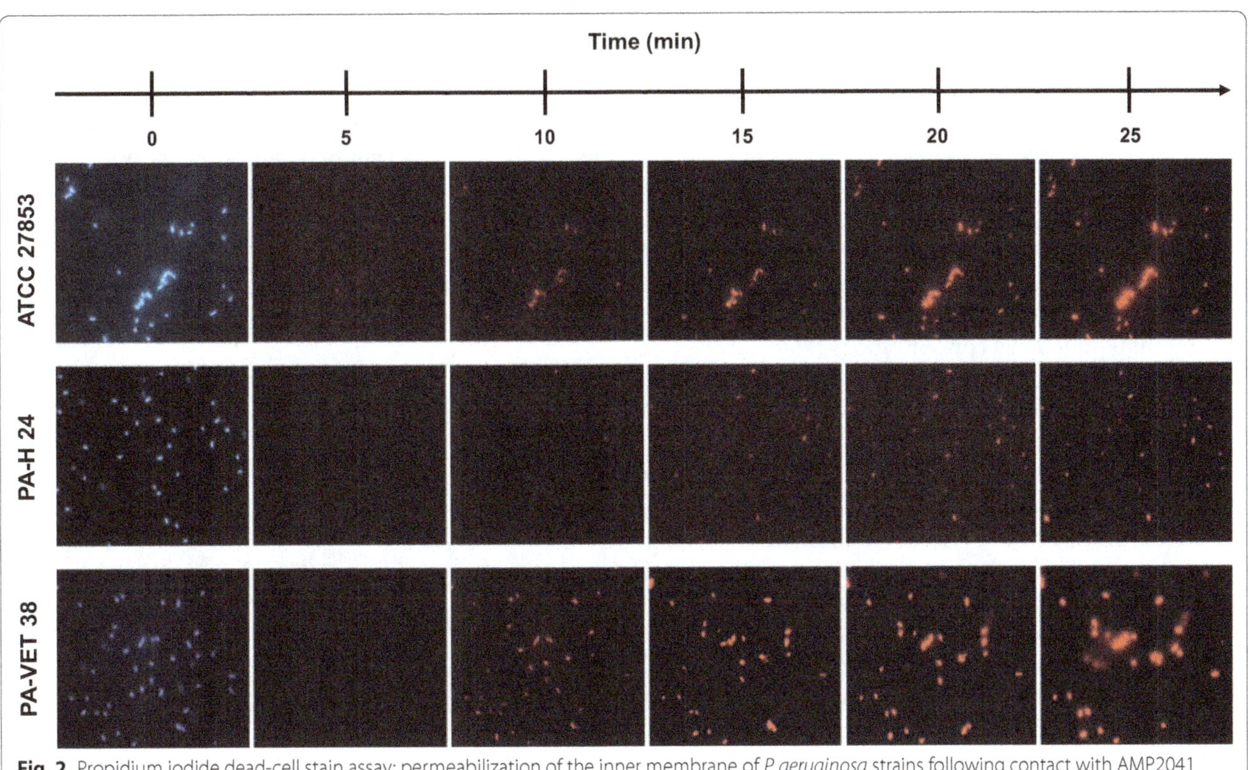

Fig. 2 Propidium iodide dead-cell stain assay: permeabilization of the inner membrane of *P. aeruginosa* strains following contact with AMP2041

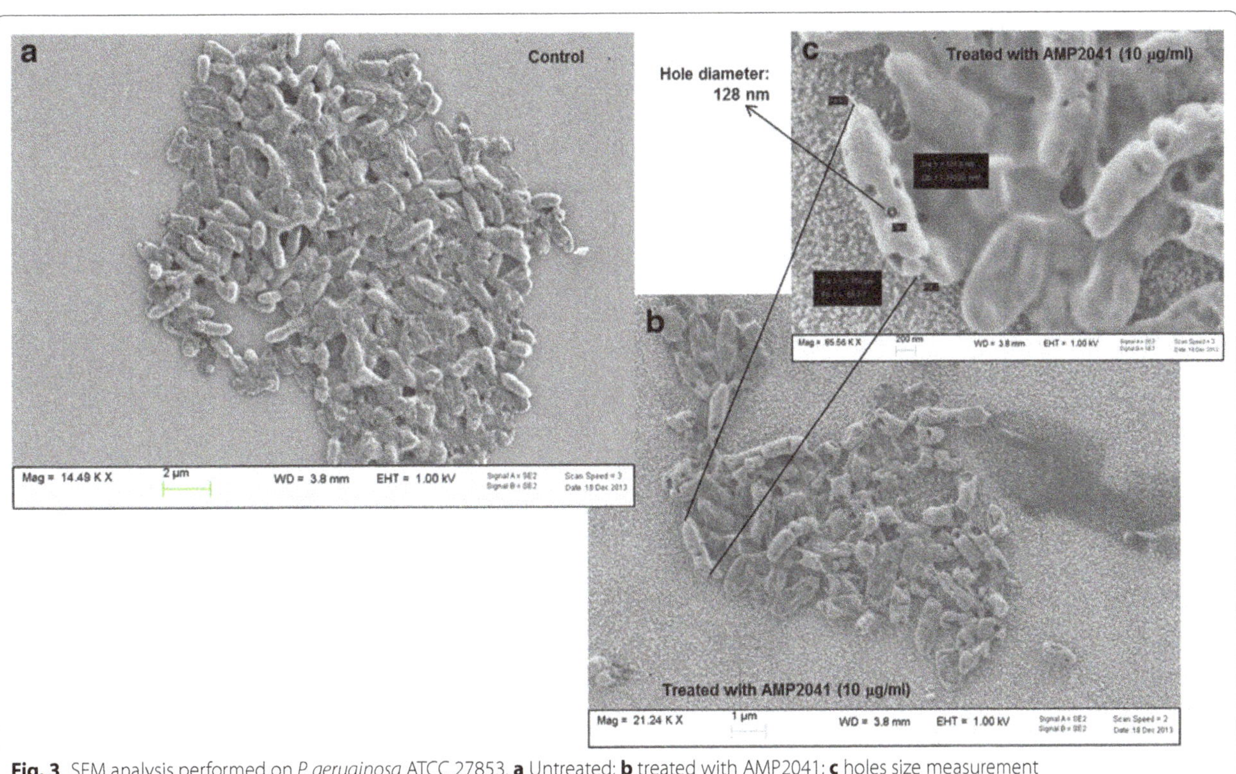

Fig. 3 SEM analysis performed on *P. aeruginosa* ATCC 27853. **a** Untreated; **b** treated with AMP2041; **c** holes size measurement

never investigated before, were similar to that previously reported for *P. aeruginosa* ATCC 27853 [8, 9]. These results were almost unrelated to the sources of strains, suggesting that the mechanism of action was similar for all the examined strains. The killing kinetics are comparable [29] or better [30] than those obtained with other established antimicrobial peptides at their lethal concentration. Saikia et al., instead, showed that two out of four *E. coli* MreB derived peptides completely killed *P. aeruginosa* within 5 min of treatment with the peptides at their minimum lethal concentrations [26]. However, in our case the kinetic of killing of AMP2041 was derived from the testing of many different *P. aeruginosa* strains, while in the other cases only one *P. aeruginosa* strain was tested. Moreover, an interesting fact that emerges from the work of Saikia et al. is that for *P. aeruginosa* there is no direct correlation between the minimum lethal concentration and the rapidity of killing, because the peptide with the best minimum lethal concentration (3 μM) completely killed the bacteria only after 120 min.

The stain-dead assay was performed on the *P. aeruginosa* ATCC 27853 reference strain and on PA-H 24 and PA-VET 38, which were selected for the assay as representative of strains with a high level of antibiotic resistance, being XDR and MDR (see Tables 1, 3), respectively. Results indicated that the inhibitory effect of AMP2041 is linked to an altered permeability of the cellular membrane of *P. aeruginosa* (Fig. 2). This is in accordance with the mechanism of action of cationic antimicrobial peptides which cause cell death through loss of membrane integrity [22]. The timing of the occurrence of red fluorescence was in accordance with time kill results. The membrane damage was evident within 10 min of incubation for the reference strain and the animal isolate PA-VET 38 and within 15 min for the human isolate PA-H 24.

To confirm that the fluorescence increase was due to morphological changes of bacterial membrane, a SEM analysis was performed on the *P. aeruginosa* ATCC 27853 reference strain treated with AMP2041. SEM analysis provided evidence for a direct membrane damage, showing the presence of several holes, dents and bursts throughout cell wall (Fig. 3b, c). Similar membrane changes are also described for other cationic antimicrobial peptides [23, 26, 31]. The microbicidal effect of AMP2041 was also confirmed by the presence of lysed cells.

Conclusions

In conclusion, we assessed the good antimicrobial activity of AMP2041 on *P. aeruginosa* strains of human origin, including those deriving from a CF patient. Moreover, we confirmed the excellent antimicrobial activity of AMP2041 on *P. aeruginosa* strains derived from dog otitis. We also assessed that AMP2041 antimicrobial activity is linked to changes of the *P. aeruginosa* cell wall morphology and the increasing of membrane permeability. This mechanism of action is less prone to induce resistance by the pathogen compared to antimicrobials acting against intracellular targets. However, clinical trials with adequate animal models should be performed to define the therapeutic potential of AMP2041.

Abbreviations

CF: cystic fibrosis; CFU: colony-forming unit; DAPI: 4′,6-diamidino-2-phenylindole; ECDC: European Centre for Disease Prevention and Control; EDTA: ethylenediaminetetraacetic acid; ESKAPE: *Enterococcus faecium* (E) *Staphylococcus aureus* (S) *Klebsiella pneumoniae* (K) *Acinetobacter baumannii* (A) *Pseudomonas aeruginosa* (P) *Enterobacter* Species (E); HPLC: high pressure liquid chromatography; IM: inner membrane; LD: lethal dose; MBC: minimal bactericidal concentration; MDR: multi-drug resistant; PA-H: *Pseudomonas aeruginosa*, human isolate; PA-VET: *Pseudomonas aeruginosa*, animal isolate; PB: phosphate buffer; PDR: pan-drug resistant; PI: propidium iodide; SEM: scanning electron microscopy; XDR: extensively-drug resistant.

Authors' contributions

CSC and ST were involved in all aspects of this study including data collection, analysis and manuscript preparation. AS and DS carried out the laboratory studies. GLA and GG collected and analysed animal strains. EC collected and analysed human strains. All authors read and approved the final manuscript.

Author details

[1] Department of Veterinary Science, University of Parma, Via del Taglio 10, 43126 Parma, Italy. [2] Istituto Zooprofilattico Sperimentale della Lombardia e dell'Emilia Romagna, Via Bianchi 7/9, 25124 Brescia, Italy. [3] Arcispedale S. Maria Nuova, Viale Risorgimento 80, 42123 Reggio Emilia, Italy. [4] Clinica Veterinaria Malpensa, Via Marconi 27, 21017 Samarate, VA, Italy.

Acknowledgements

Not applicable.

Competing interests

CSC is one of the inventors in Italian patent on AMP2041: N. 102012902114114 (MI2012A002263). The patent was purchased by ICF s.r.l., Cremona, Italy. This company had no influence on the study design or the content of this manuscript.

Funding

This study was self-funded.

References

1. Davies JC. *Pseudomonas aeruginosa* in cystic fibrosis: pathogenesis and persistence. Paediatr Respir Rev. 2002;3(2):128–34.
2. Haenni M, Hocquet D, Ponsin C, Cholley P, Guyeux C, Madec J, et al. Population structure and antimicrobial susceptibility of *Pseudomonas aeruginosa* from animal infections in France. BMC Vet Res. 2015;11(9):1–5.
3. Boucher HW, Talbot GH, Bradley JS, Edwards JE, Gilbert D, Rice LB, et al. Bad bugs, no drugs: no ESKAPE! An update from the Infectious Diseases Society of America. Clin Infect Dis. 2009;48(1):1–12.

4. Magiorakos AP, Srinivasan A, Carey RB, Carmeli Y, Falagas ME, Giske CG, et al. Multidrug-resistant, extensively drug-resistant and pandrug-resistant bacteria: an international expert proposal for interim standard definitions for acquired resistance. Clin Microbiol Infect. 2012;18(3):268–81.
5. Mesaros N, Nordmann P, Plesiat P, Roussel-Delvallez M, Van Eldere J, Glupczynski Y, et al. *Pseudomonas aeruginosa*: resistance and therapeutic options at the turn of the new millennium. Clin Microbiol Infect. 2007;13(6):560–78.
6. European commission. Communication from the commission to the European Parliament and the Council. Action plan against the rising threats from antimicrobial resistance. http://ec.europa.eu/dgs/health_food-safety/docs/communication_amr_2011_748_en.pdf. Accessed 24 Feb 2017.
7. Oyston PC, Fox MA, Richards SJ, Clark GC. Novel peptide therapeutics for treatment of infections. J Med Microbiol. 2009;58(8):977–87.
8. Cabassi CS, Taddei S, Cavirani S, Baroni MC, Sansoni P, Romani AA. Broad-spectrum activity of a novel antibiotic peptide against multidrug-resistant veterinary isolates. Vet J. 2013;198(2):534–7.
9. Romani AA, Baroni MC, Taddei S, Ghidini F, Sansoni P, Cavirani S, et al. In vitro activity of novel in silico-developed antimicrobial peptides against a panel of bacterial pathogens. J Pept Sci. 2013;19(9):554–65.
10. European Centre for Disease prevention and Control/European Medicines Agencies (ECDPC/EMA) ECDC/EMEA Joint Technical report. Stockholm: ECDPC/EMA; 2009. The bacterial challenge: time to react. A call to narrow the gap between multidrug-resistant bacteria in the EU and the development of new antibacterial agents.
11. Cabassi CS, Taddei S, Cavirani S, Sala A, Santospirito D, Baroni MC, et al. Antimicrobial activity of 4 novel cyclic peptides against a panel of reference and multi-drug resistant clinical strains of animal origin Pakistan. Vet J. 2015;35(4):522–4.
12. Cerceo EDS, Sherman BM, Amin AN. Multidrug-resistant Gram-negative bacterial infections in the hospital Setting: overview, implications for clinical practice, and emerging treatment options. Microb Drug Resist. 2016;22(5):412–31.
13. Chaparro-Barrios C, Ciancotti-Oliver L, Bautista-Rentero D, Adán-Tomás C, Zanón-Viguer V. A new treatment choice against multi-drug resistant *Pseudomonas aeruginosa*: doripenem. J Bacteriol Parasitol. 2014;5(5):1–4.
14. Tommasi RBD, Walkup GK, Manchester JI, Miller AA. ESKAPEing the labyrinth of antibacterial discovery. Nat Rev Drug Discov. 2015;14(8):529–42.
15. Obritsch MD, Fish DN, MacLaren R, Jung R. Nosocomial infections due to multidrug-resistant *Pseudomonas aeruginosa*: epidemiology and treatment options. Pharmacotherapy. 2005;25(10):1353–64.
16. Liu XBD, Thungrat K, Aly S. Mechanisms accounting for fluoroquinolone multidrug resistance *Escherichia coli* isolated from companion animals. Vet Microbiol. 2012;161(1–2):159–68.
17. Gibson JSMJ, Cobbold RN, Filippich LJ, Trott DJ. Risk factors for multidrug-resistant *Escherichia coli* rectal colonization of dogs on admission to a veterinary hospital. Epidemiol Infect. 2011;139(2):197–205.
18. Scott-Weese J. Antimicrobial resistance in companion animals. Anim Health Res Rev. 2008;9(2):169–76.
19. European Medicines Agency, Committee for Medicinal Products for Veterinary Use. Reflection paper on the risk of antimicrobial resistance transfer from companion animals. http://www.ema.europa.eu/docs/en_GB/document_library/Scientific_guideline/2015/01/WC500181642.pdf. Accessed 24 Feb 2017.
20. Savini V, Passeri C, Mancini G, Iuliani O, Marrollo R, Argentieri AV, et al. Coagulase-positive staphylococci: my pet's two faces. Res Microbiol. 2013;164(5):371–4.
21. Hwang PMVH. Structure–function relationships of antimicrobial peptides. Biochem Cell Biol. 1998;76:235–46.
22. Yeaman MRYN. Mechanisms of antimicrobial peptide action and resistance. Pharmacol Rev. 2003;55(1):27–55.
23. Zhou C, Qi X, Li P, Chen WN, Mouad L, Chang MW, et al. High potency and broad-spectrum antimicrobial peptides synthesized via ring-opening polymerization of alpha-aminoacid-*N*-carboxyanhydrides. Biomacromolecules. 2010;11(1):60–7.
24. Andreu D, Merrifield RB, Steiner H, Boman HG. Solid-phase synthesis of cecropin A and related peptides. Proc Natl Acad Sci U S A. 1983;80(21):6475–9.
25. Agerberth B, Lee JY, Bergman T, Carlquist M, Boman HG, Mutt V, et al. Amino acid sequence of PR-39. Isolation from pig intestine of a new member of the family of proline-arginine-rich antibacterial peptides. Eur J Biochem. 1991;202(3):849–54.
26. Saikia K, Sravani YD, Ramakrishnan V, Chaudhary N. Highly potent antimicrobial peptides from N-terminal membrane-binding region of *E. coli* MreB. Sci Rep. 2017;7:42994.
27. Oliver A, Cantón R, Campo P, Baquero F, Blázquez J. High frequency of hypermutable Pseudomonas aeruginosa in cystic fibrosis lung infection. Science. 2000;288(5469):1251–4.
28. Sousa A, Pereira M. *Pseudomonas aeruginosa* diversification during Infection development in cystic fibrosis lungs—a review. Pathogens. 2014;3(3):680–703.
29. Ge Y, MacDonald DL, Holroyd KJ, Thornsberry C, Wexler H, Zasloff M. In vitro antibacterial properties of pexiganan, an analog of magainin. Antimicrob Agents Chemother. 1999;43(4):782–8.
30. Varkey J, Nagaraj R. Antibacterial activity of human neutrophil defensin HNP-1 analogs without cysteines. Antimicrob Agents Chemother. 2005;49(11):4561–6.
31. Cudic M, Otvos L Jr. Intracellular targets of antibacterial peptides. Curr Drug Targets. 2002;3(2):101–6.

10

Molecular characterization of *Staphylococcus aureus* isolates from various healthcare institutions in Nairobi, Kenya: a cross sectional study

Geoffrey Omuse[1*], Kristien Nel Van Zyl[2], Kim Hoek[2], Shima Abdulgader[3], Samuel Kariuki[4], Andrew Whitelaw[2] and Gunturu Revathi[1]

Abstract

Background: *Staphylococcus aureus* (*S. aureus*) has established itself over the years as a major cause of morbidity and mortality both within the community and in healthcare settings. Methicillin resistant *S. aureus* (MRSA) in particular has been a major cause of nosocomial infections resulting in significant increase in healthcare costs. In Africa, the MRSA prevalence has been shown to vary across different countries. In order to better understand the epidemiology of MRSA in a setting, it is important to define its population structure using molecular tools as different clones have been found to predominate in certain geographical locations.

Methods: We carried out PFGE, MLST, SCC*mec* and *spa* typing of selected *S. aureus* isolates from a private and public referral hospital in Nairobi, Kenya.

Results: A total of 93 *S. aureus* isolates were grouped into 19 PFGE clonal complexes (A–S) and 12 singletons. From these, 55 (32 MRSA and 23 MSSA) representative isolates from each PFGE clonal complex and all singletons were *spa* typed. There were 18 different MRSA *spa* types and 22 MSSA *spa* types. The predominant MRSA *spa* type was t037 comprising 40.6 % (13/32) of all MRSA. In contrast, the MSSA were quite heterogeneous, only 2 out of 23 MSSA shared the same *spa* type. Two new MRSA *spa* types (t13149 and t13150) and 3 new MSSA *spa* types (t13182, t13193 and t13194) were identified. The predominant clonal complex was CC 5 which included multi-locus sequence types 1, 8 and 241.

Conclusion: In contrast to previous studies published from Kenya, there's marked genetic diversity amongst clinical MRSA isolates in Nairobi including the presence of well-known epidemic MRSA clones. Given that these clones are resident within our referral hospitals, adherence to strict infection control measures needs to be ensured to reduce morbidity and mortality associated with hospital acquired MRSA infections.

Keywords: *Staphylococcus aureus*, MRSA, MSSA, Kenya

Background

Staphylococcus aureus (*S. aureus*) has established itself over the years as a major cause of morbidity and mortality globally both within the community and in healthcare settings [1–3]. Its ability to cause disease is aided not only by its impressive repertoire of virulence factors but also its ability to develop resistance to antibiotics used in its treatment epitomized by the emergence of methicillin resistant *S. aureus* (MRSA). Methicillin resistance is conferred by the *mecA* gene that is carried on a staphylococcal cassette chromosome *mec* (SCC*mec*) and codes for a modified penicillin binding protein (PBP2a). This binding protein has reduced affinity to all beta-lactam and

*Correspondence: g_omuse@yahoo.com
[1] Department of Pathology, Aga Khan University Hospital Nairobi, P.O. Box 30270-00100, Nairobi, Kenya
Full list of author information is available at the end of the article

beta-lactam/beta-lactamase inhibitor combination antibiotics [4, 5]. In Africa, the MRSA prevalence has been shown to vary across different countries with a prevalence as low as 7 % reported in Madagascar and as high as 82 % in Egypt [6]. This marked variation could be due to different environmental determinants or simply due to a difference in the genetic diversity of *S. aureus*. In Kenya, there is a marked difference in reported MRSA prevalence in clinical isolates within Nairobi with one recent study reporting a prevalence of 3.7 % while another reported 87.2 % [7, 8]. In order to better understand the epidemiology of MRSA, it is important to define its population structure. Molecular characterization helps in identifying clonal populations which can help in surveillance and investigation of outbreaks.

There is a growing interest in the characterization of MRSA isolates and this stems primarily from its role as a major cause of hospital and community acquired infections [1, 9, 10]. There are various molecular methods used, the more common ones include multi-locus sequence typing (MLST), pulse field gel electrophoresis (PFGE), staphylococcal protein A (*spa*) typing and SCC*mec* typing [11]. Despite *S. aureus* having a very diverse clonal population, MLST studies have shown that a small set of clonal complexes (CC) are associated with most of the MRSA epidemics. These include CC5, CC22, CC30, CC45 and CC80 [6, 12, 13]. A clonal complex can have several sequence types, however the multi-locus sequence types that are regarded as the founders in these clonal complexes are ST5, ST22, ST30, ST45 and ST80 respectively [14]. As regards *spa* types, it has been shown that particular ones are more predominant in certain regions. For example t030 is quite predominant in hospitals in Turkey [15], t042 and t044 are more common in North Africa while t008 is common in the US [16]. Unfortunately, the molecular epidemiology of MRSA in Africa is not very well described. Most of the studies carried out in Africa characterizing MRSA have emanated from a few countries namely Tunisia, Nigeria, South Africa, Algeria and Egypt [6]. There are very few studies from East Africa that have reported on the molecular characterization of *S. aureus* presumably due to lack of readily available technical expertise and laboratory facilities. A study done in Kenya looking at carriage of *S. aureus* by inpatients in a government hospital found that only 6 out of 86 (7 %) *S. aureus* isolates were MRSA and they all belonged to the same clone (MLST ST239; *spa* type t037) [17]. This clone is a globally distributed hybrid of ST8 and ST30 and is known to be responsible for several outbreaks in different continents [18–21]. The only other study from Kenya did not report on *spa* or multi locus sequence types [8].

We set out to characterize selected *S. aureus* isolates from different hospitals in Nairobi, Kenya in order to identify which clonal lineages are present and further shed light on the molecular epidemiology of both MSSA and MRSA in Kenya.

Methods

We obtained archived methicillin susceptible (MSSA) and MRSA isolates from 2 hospitals in Nairobi, Kenya collected between January 2010 and July 2013. The hospitals included a government hospital whose samples we obtained through the Kenya Medical Research Institute (KEMRI) and the Aga Khan University Hospital Nairobi (AKUHN) which is a private referral hospital with a network of satellite clinics and laboratories spread in and around Nairobi as well as different parts of the country. The isolates from the government hospital were part of a previous study done to determine prevalence of MRSA carriage in a paediatric ward and the rest of the isolates were from clinical specimens submitted to the AKUHN laboratory for routine culture and sensitivity. These were convenience isolates that were not collected through a well-structured, formal and documented process. All isolates were stored at −80 °C and grown overnight on sheep blood agar plates at 37 °C.

S. aureus identification

All isolates were confirmed to be *S. aureus* using routine bench identification methods which included growth characteristics on sheep blood agar, gram stain, catalase, coagulase, deoxyribonuclease (DNase) and mannitol fermentation tests. A cefoxitin screen using a 30 µg disc (Oxoid, United Kingdom) was performed to distinguish MSSA from MRSA. Isolates with a diameter $\leq$21 mm were classified as MRSA.

Antibiotic susceptibility

Antibiotic susceptibility was only available for the MRSA isolates obtained from AKUHN. These were performed on Vitek 2 (version 4.01, bioMerieux, Marcy-l'Etoile, France) an automated bacterial identification system that performs antibiotic susceptibility using broth dilution and interpretation based on Clinical Laboratory Standards Institute (CLSI) antimicrobial susceptibility guidelines [22]. Multidrug resistance (MDR) was defined as resistance to three or more drug classes.

DNA derivation

Isolates were grown on blood agar plates (National Health Laboratory Services Media Lab, Cape Town, South Africa) at 37 °C overnight. After incubation, 4–5 large colonies were re-suspended in 200 µL nuclease free water. The samples were incubated at 95 °C for 30 min, followed by −80 °C for 30 min and centrifuged for 10 min at 14,000×*g* when thawed. The supernatant containing

DNA was carefully aspirated without disturbing the pellet of cell debris and stored as DNA aliquots at −20° C until further use.

PFGE

PFGE based on *Sma*I macrorestriction analysis was performed using the CDC laboratory protocol for *S. aureus* [23]. The PFGE was run on a CHEF DR III system (Bio-Rad, California, United States of America) with optimum settings as follows: initial 5 s, switch 30 s, run time 29 h, voltage 6 V/cm and a SeaKem Gold agarose (Lonza, Rockland, USA) gel concentration of 1.4 %. *S. aureus* NCTC 8325 was used as a control in each gel run. Gels were visualized an Alliance 2.7 (UVItec, Cambridge, United Kingdom) gel documentation system after staining with 10 mg/mL ethidium bromide. Analysis of PFGE clusters was performed using the BioNumerics software package (Applied Maths, Sint-Martens-Latem, Belgium), using the Dice coefficient, and visualized as a dendrogram by the unweighted-pair group method, using average linkages with 1 % tolerance and 1 % optimization settings. In order to define a cluster, a cutoff of 80 % similarity was used.

SCC*mec* typing

SCC*mec* typing was performed using multiplex PCR as described by Milheirico et al. [24]. All assays were performed in a GeneAmp 9600 thermocycler (Applied Biosystems). The optimal cycling conditions were the following: 95 °C for 5 min; 35 cycles of 95 °C for 45 s, 57 °C for 45 s, and 72 °C for 1 min; and a final extension at 72 °C for 10 min. Each PCR mixture contained 0.5 µL of the primers listed in Table 1, KAPA2G Robust HotStart ReadyMix PCR (KAPA biosystems) which contains KAPA2G Robust HotStart DNA Polymerase (1 U/25 µL reaction) in a proprietary reaction buffer containing dNTPs (0.2 mM of each dNTP at 1X), $MgCl_2$ (2 mM at 1X), 0.3 µL (3 mM) additional $MgCl_2$, 10.7 µL of PCR grade water and genomic DNA in a final volume of 25 µL. The following *S. aureus* isolates were used as controls: BAA-38, BAA-1681, BAA-39, BAA-1680, BAA-1688 and BAA-42 for SCC*mec* types I–VI respectively. The PCR products were resolved in a 1 % SeaKem Gold Agarose (Lonza, Rockland, USA) gel in 0.5 % Tris–borate-ethylene-diamine-tetra-acetic acid (EDTA) buffer (Bio-Rad, Hercules, CA) at 4 V/cm for 2.5 h and were visualized with ethidium bromide.

spa typing

This was done using the following primers: 1095 F: 5′-AGACGATCCTTCGGTGAGC-3′ and 1517R: 5′-GCTTTTGCAATGTCATTTACTG-3′. PCR reactions consisted of 12.5 uL of KAPA2G Robust HotStart ReadyMix PCR (KAPA biosystems) which contains KAPA2G Robust HotStart DNA Polymerase (1 U per 25 µL reaction) in a proprietary reaction buffer containing dNTPs (0.2 mM of each dNTP at 1X), MgCl2 (2 mM at 1X), 0.5 µM of primers and genomic DNA in a final volume of 25 µL. PCR conditions were 95 °C for 6 min; 30 cycles each of 95 °C for 45 s, 64 °C for 45 s, and 72 °C for 60 s; and a final extension at 72 °C for 6 min. Sequencing was outsourced to inqaba biotec, a biotechnology company based in Pretoria, South Africa. Using the Ridom *spa* server (http://www.spa.server.ridom.de), *spa* sequences were automatically assigned to *spa* types. Sequence types and clonal complexes (*sp*a-CC) were assigned where possible using Based Upon Repeat Patterns (BURP) grouping analysis from the Ridom StaphType software (version 1.4; Ridom GmbH, Würzburg, Germany). For BURP analysis, default parameters were used which allows *spa* types with maximum 4 genetic differences to be grouped into one cluster resulting in a calculated cost between members of a group being less than or equal to 4.

MLST

MLST was done on representative isolates from each PFGE clonal complex and selected singletons according to the protocol published by Enright et al. [25]. The PCRs were carried out as uniplex reactions consisting of 1 µM of the forward and reverse primers, 12.5 µL of 2× KAPA Taq ReadyMix (KAPA Biosystems), 2.5 mM $MgCl_2$, 1 µL of template DNA and nuclease free water up to 25 µL. The PCR conditions were 95 °C for 5 min, followed by 30 cycles of 95 °C for 45 s, 56 °C for 45 s and 72 °C for 1 min. A final elongation step was carried out at 72 °C for 10 min. 5 µL of the PCR product was visualised with gel electrophoresis at 120 V for 1 h. Sequencing was performed on the remainder of the PCR product by Inqaba Biotechnical Industries (Pty) Ltd (Pretoria, South Africa). Sequences were inspected and trimmed in BioEdit Sequence Alignment Editor using reference sequences for each of the seven loci. A consensus sequence was generated from the forward and reverse sequences and used to generate sequence types (STs) on the *S. aureus* MLST database (http://www.saureus.beta.mlst.net/#). Isolates that were not typed by MLST were assigned STs using BURP analysis. Isolates with the same PFGE clonal complex and *spa* type were assigned the same STs. MLST clonal complexes (MLST-CC) were determined using a Java applet found at http://www.eburst.mlst.net that uses the eBURST algorithm. The default setting was used in which STs that share identical alleles at 6 or 7 of MLST loci are put in the same group. Where there was a discrepancy between the CC determined using eBURST and BURP, we considered the MLST-CC as the correct one.

Table 1 Primers used in the updated version of SCC*mec* multiplex PCR

Primer name	Primer sequence (5 33)	Primer specificity (SCC*mec* type, region)	Amplicon size (bp)	Conc. (μM)
CIF2 F2	TTCGAGTTGCTGATGAAGAAGG	I, J1 region	495	0.4
CIF2 R2	ATTTACCACAAGGACTACCAGC			0.4
ccrC F2	GTACTCGTTACAATGTTTGG	V, *ccr* complex	449	0.8
ccrC R2	ATAATGGCTTCATGCTTACC			0.8
RIF5 F10	TTCTTAAGTACACGCTGAATCG	III, J3 region	414	0.4
RIF5 R13	ATGGAGATGAATTACAAGGG			0.4
SCCmec V J1 F	TTCTCCATTCTTGTTCATCC	V, J1 region	377	0.4
SCCmec V J1 R	AGAGACTACTGACTTAAGTGG			0.4
dcs F2	CATCCTATGATAGCTTGGTC	I, II, IV, and VI, J3 region	342	0.8
dcs R1	CTAAATCATAGCCATGACCG			0.8
ccrB2 F2	AGTTTCTCAGAATTCGAACG	II and IV, *ccr* complex	311	0.8
ccrB2 R2	CCGATATAGAAWGGGTTAGC			0.8
kdp F1	AATCATCTGCCATTGGTGATGC	II, J1 region	284	0.2
kdp R1	CGAATGAAGTGAAAGAAAGTGG			0.2
SCCmec III J1 F	CATTTGTGAAACACAGTACG	III, J1 region	243	0.4
SCCmec III J1 R	GTTATTGAGACTCCTAAAGC			0.4
mecI P2	ATCAAGACTTGCATTCAGGC	II and III, *mec* complex	209	0.8
mecI P3	GCGGTTTCAATTCACTTGTC			0.8
mecA P4	TCCAGATTACAACTTCACCAGG	Internal positive control	162	0.8
mecA P7	CCACTTCATATCTTGTAACG			0.8

Results

A total of 93 *S. aureus* isolates underwent PFGE. These were subsequently grouped into 19 PFGE clonal complexes (A–S) and 12 singletons. From these, 55 (32 MRSA and 23 MSSA) representative isolates from each PFGE clonal complex and all singletons were *spa* typed. This comprised 41 isolates from AKUHN and 14 from KEMRI. In total, there were 18 different MRSA *spa* types and 22 different *spa* types amongst the MSSA. The predominant MRSA *spa* type was t037 comprising 40.6 % (13/32) of all MRSA. In contrast, the MSSA were quite heterogeneous, only 2 out of 23 MSSA shared the same *spa* type. Two new MRSA *spa* types (t13149 and t13150) and 3 new MSSA *spa* types (t13182, t13193, t13194) were identified as shown in Table 2. Three *spa* types (t005, t318 and t1476) were found in both MSSA and MRSA. BURP analysis for both MSSA and MRSA revealed 7 spa-clonal complexes and 14 singletons as shown in Fig. 1. The predominant *spa*-CC was *spa*-CC005 which included the new MRSA *spa* type 13149. SCC*mec* type-III [3A] was the predominant type followed by SCC*mec*-IV [2B]. Only one MRSA isolate was non-typeable using the SCC*mec* protocol published by Milheirico et al. [24]

MLST STs were determined and extrapolated for 31 isolates. A total of seven different MRSA and MSSA MLST-CC were identified with the predominant one being MLST-CC 5. This clonal complex comprised STs 1, 5, 8 and 241 as shown in Table 2. An isolate belonging to ST241 (t2029) that was detected in a pus sample from AKUHN hospital was found to harbor SCC*mec* type IV [2B].

Out of the 16 MRSA from AKUHN, 13 were MDR including the two new *spa* types. Resistance was commonly seen to clindamycin, erythromycin and trimethoprim/sulfamethoxazole (TMP/SMX). A number of isolates had intermediate resistance to levofloxacin. However, two isolates were only resistant to beta lactams but susceptible to all other antibiotics including TMP/SMX as shown in Table 3. None of the MRSA was resistant to vancomycin, linezolid, mupirocin, teicoplanin or tigecycline.

Discussion

This study reveals a markedly heterogeneous population of *S. aureus* isolates as well as the presence of well described MRSA clonal complexes 5, 22 and 30 that are responsible for several outbreaks worldwide [13, 26]. CC5 has been identified as the major clonal complex causing HA-MRSA in Africa with MRSA ST239/ST241-III [3A] having been identified in several African countries [6]. The main clonal complex in our study was CC5 that included ST 241, a single locus variant of ST 239 also known as the "Brazilian/Hungarian clone". ST 239 and ST 239 like isolates are well-known epidemic clones responsible for several healthcare associated MRSA outbreaks globally. They have been found to be a cause of hospital

Table 2 Molecular characterization of methicillin susceptible and resistant *Staphylococcus aureus*

Isolate No.	Hospital	Sample	ID	*spa* type	*spa*-CC	SCC*mec* type	MLST/*spa* ST	MLST CC	PFGE CC	PFGE pulsotype
36	AKUHN	Pus swab	MSSA	t645	sng		1841[a]	121	A	A2
84	AKUHN	Pus swab	MSSA	t314	sng		121[a]	121	B	B2
78	AKUHN	Pus swab	MSSA	t355	sng		152[a]	152	C	C1
48	AKUHN	Pus swab	MSSA	t355	sng		152[b]	152	C	C4
91	AKUHN	Nasal swab	MRSA	t005	5	IV	22[a]	22	D	D2
28	AKUHN	Nasal swab	MRSA	t005	5	IV	22[b]	22	D	D3
83	AKUHN	Sputum	MRSA	t005	5	IV	22[b]	22	D	D3
89	AKUHN	Pus swab	MRSA	t13149[d]	5	IV	ND[c]		D	D1
22	KEMRI	Nasal swab	MRSA	t022	5	IV	22[a]	22	E	E2
75	AKUHN	Blood	MRSA	t9622	sng	IV	ND[c]		E	E1
15	AKUHN	Pus swab	MSSA	t005	5		22[a]	22	F	F6
12	AKUHN	Pus swab	MSSA	t223	5		22[a]	22	G	G2
71	AKUHN	Pus swab	MSSA	t122	sng		30[a]	30	H	H1
88	AKUHN	Tracheal aspirate	MSSA	t318	sng		30[a]	30	I	I5
16	AKUHN	Pus swab	MSSA	t021	21		30[a]	30	I	I7
23	AKUHN	Sputum	MRSA	t1339	3202/186	UT	88[a]	88	J	J2
49	KEMRI	Nasal swab	MRSA	t3202	3202/186	UT	ND[c]		J	J1
19	AKUHN	Axillary swab	MSSA	t3841	sng		672[a]	672	K	K2
6	AKUHN	Nasal swab	MRSA	t091	NF3	V	789[a]	7	L	L2
69	AKUHN	Pus swab	MSSA	t2505	NF3		789[a]	7	L	L1
14	AKUHN	Tracheal aspirate	MSSA	t002	sng		5[a]	5	M	M3
79	AKUHN	Pus swab	MRSA	t13150[d]	sng	II	5[a]	5	M	M2
52	AKUHN	Blood	MSSA	t2473	sng		72[a]	72	N	N3
92	AKUHN	Blood	MSSA	t13193[d]	5		22[a]	22	O	O1
87	AKUHN	Blood	MSSA	t127	sng		1[a]	5	P	P3
81	AKUHN	Ear swab	MRSA	t1476	NF2	V	8[a]	5	Q	Q1
45	AKUHN	Pus swab	MSSA	t1476	NF2		8[a]	5	Q	Q2
31	AKUHN	Pus swab	MSSA	t064	sng		8[a]	5	R	R4
33	KEMRI	Nasal swab	MRSA	t104	NF1	IV	8[a]	5	R	R2
7	KEMRI	Nasal swab	MRSA	t689	NF1	I	ND[c]		R	R1
25	AKUHN	Blood	MRSA	t852	5	IV	ND[c]		R	R5
4	AKUHN	Sputum	MRSA	t037	NF4	III	241[a]	5	S	S1
2	KEMRI	Nasal swab	MRSA	t037	NF4	III	241[b]	5	S	S10
3	KEMRI	Nasal swab	MRSA	t037	NF4	III	241[b]	5	S	S10
1	AKUHN	Blood	MRSA	t037	NF4	III	241[b]	5	S	S11
47	KEMRI	Nasal swab	MRSA	t037	NF4	III	241[b]	5	S	S2
38	KEMRI	Nasal swab	MRSA	t037	NF4	III	241[b]	5	S	S3
34	KEMRI	Nasal swab	MRSA	t037	NF4	III	241[b]	5	S	S4
20	KEMRI	Nasal swab	MRSA	t037	NF4	III	241[b]	5	S	S5
18	KEMRI	Nasal swab	MRSA	t037	NF4	III	241[b]	5	S	S6
37	KEMRI	Nasal swab	MRSA	t037	NF4	III	241[b]	5	S	S7
27	KEMRI	Nasal swab	MRSA	t037	NF4	III	241[b]	5	S	S9
29	AKUHN	Pus swab	MRSA	t2029	NF4	IV	241[a]	5	S	S8
13	AKUHN	Pus swab	MRSA	t037	NF4	III	239/240/241[c]			Sng12
11	AKUHN	Pus swab	MRSA	t037	NF4	III	239/240/241[c]			Sng6
17	AKUHN	Pus swab	MSSA	t13182[d]	sng		ND[c]			Sng 3
44	AKUHN	Urine	MSSA	t13194[d]	sng		ND[c]			Sng7
73	AKUHN	Pus swab	MSSA	t1839	345		ND[c]			Sng5
58	AKUHN	Blood	MSSA	t186	3202/186		88[c]			Sng4

Table 2 continued

Isolate No.	Hospital	Sample	ID	*spa* type	*spa*-CC	SCC*mec* type	MLST/*spa* ST	MLST CC	PFGE CC	PFGE pulsotype
70	AKUHN	Blood	MSSA	t224	345		97[c]			Sng8
21	AKUHN	Pus swab	MRSA	t293	sng	IV	ND[c]			Sng 2
43	KEMRI	NASAL SWAB	MRSA	t318	sng	IV	30[c]			Sng 1
35	AKUHN	Pus swab	MRSA	t345	345	V	ND[c]			Sng10
40	AKUHN	Urine	MRSA	t648	NF2	IV	ND[c]			Sng11
85	AKUHN	Vulval swab	MSSA	t131	345		ND[c]			Sng9

sng singleton, *NF* no founder, *UT* untypeable, *ND* not defined on the Ridom database Accessed on 07/10/2015

[a] MLST ST

[b] MLST ST extrapolated based on similar *spa* type and pulsotype

[c] *spa* ST

[d] New *spa* type

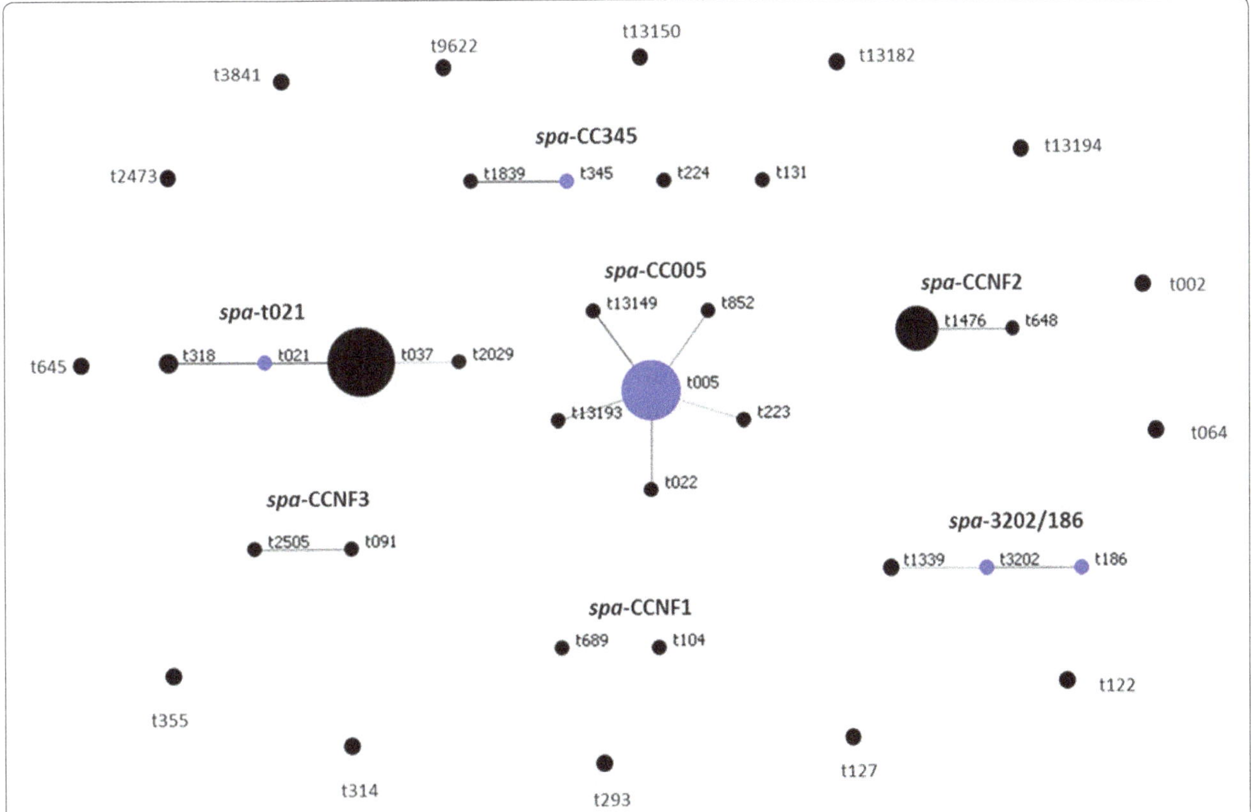

Fig. 1 Based upon repeat pattern clustering analysis for all identified *S. aureus* isolates: the clustering analysis resulted in seven *spa*-clonal complexes and 14 singletons. The *blue circle* represents the group founder and the circle size is proportional to the frequency of the *spa* type

acquired infections in other African countries including Algeria, Ghana, Morocco, South Africa and Nigeria [6]. A study done by Aiken et al. [17] in a public hospital that is approximately 40 km from Nairobi identified t037-ST239 as the predominant clone carried by inpatients in a surgical ward. Most of the nasal swabs in our study were obtained from children in a paediatric ward situated in a public referral hospital. The high proportion of t037-ST241 among our MRSA isolates is not necessarily reflective of the true prevalence of this *spa* type in Nairobi due to a selection bias in the manner in which the isolates were collected. Nevertheless, it is quite concerning that a clone known to be associated with MRSA epidemics is resident within hospitals in Nairobi indicating an urgent need for proper infection control interventions and regular surveillance.

Table 3 Molecular characterization and antibiotic susceptibility of MRSA isolates from AKUHN

Isolate No.	Sample	*spa* type	SCC*mec* type	Antibiogram		
				R	S	I
21	Pus swab	t293	IV [2B]	TOB, CLI, ERY, LEV	LNZ, TEI, VAN, TET, TIG, MUP, RIF, SXT, MOX	
23	Sputum	t1339	UT	SXT	TOB, MOX, ERY, CLI, VAN, TET, TIG, MUP, RIF, LEV	
79	Pus swab	t13150[a]	II [2A]	ERY, CLI, LEV, MOX, TOB	TET, SXT, VAN, MUP, RIF, TIG, TEI, LNZ	
40	Urine	t648	IV [2B]	–	ERY, CLI, TET, SXT, VAN, MUP, MOX, RIF, TIG, TOB, TEI, LNZ, LEV	
25	Blood	t852	IV [2B]	CLI#, ERY	LNZ, MUP, MOX, RIF, SXT, TET, TEI, TIG, TOB, VAN	LEV
35	Pus swab	t345	V [5C]	RIF, SXT, TET, TOB	CLI, ERY, LNZ, MUP, MOX, TEI, TIG, VAN	LEV
13	Pus swab	t037	III [3A]	CLI, ERY, SXT, TOB	LNZ, MUP, MOX, RIF, TET, TEI, TIG, VAN	LEV
11	Pus swab	t037	III [3A]	CLI#, SXT, TET, TOB	ERY, LNZ, MUP, MOX, RIF, TEI, TIG, VAN	LEV
89	Pus swab	t13149[a]	IV [2B]	TOB, SXT, ERY	CLI, LNZ, TEI, VAN, TET, TIG, MUP, RIF, LEV, MOX	
75	Blood	t9622	IV [2B]	–	ERY, CLI, TET, SXT, VAN, MUP, MOX, RIF, TIG, TOB, TEI, LNZ	LEV
83	Sputum	t005	IV [2B]	TOB, ERY, CLI#	MOX, LNZ, TEI, VAN, TET, TIG, MUP, RIF, SXT	LEV
28	Nasal swab	t005	IV [2B]	ERY, CLI#, TOB, LEV	TET, SXT, VAN, LNZ, TEI, MUP, MOX, RIF, TIG	
81	Ear swab	t1476	V [5C]	ERY, CLI#, TET, SXT, LEV	VAN, MUP, MOX, RIF, TIG, TEI, LNZ	TOB
6	Nasal swab	t091	V [5C]	SXT, TET, TOB	CLI, ERY, LNZ, MUP, MOX, RIF, TEI, TIG, VAN	LEV
29	Pus swab	t2029	IV [2B]	CLI, ERY, RIF, SXT, TET, TOB	LNZ, MUP, MOX, TEI, TIG, VAN	LEV
1	Blood	t037	III [3A]	ERY, CLI#, TET, SXT, RIF, TOB, LEV	VAN, MUP, MOX, TIG, TEI, LNZ	

R resistant, *S* susceptible, *I* intermediate, *ERY* erythromycin, *CLI* clindamycin, *CLI#* inducible clindamycin resistance, *TET* tetracycline, *SXT* trimethoprim/sulfamethoxazole, *VAN* vancomycin, *GENT* gentamicin, *MUP* mupirocin, *MOX* moxifloxacin, *RIF* rifampicin, *TIG* tigecycline, *TOB* tobramycin, *TEI* teicoplanin, *LNZ* linezolid, *LEV* levofloxacin

[a] New spa type

Unlike the study by Aiken et al. [17] that only found one MRSA clone, we identified 18 distinct *spa* types amongst the MRSA isolates belonging to very diverse sequence types, including 2 MRSA *spa* types (t13149 and t13150) that have not previously been described. The *spa* type t13150 was found to belong to ST5-II [2A] which has also been found in Nigeria and Senegal [27, 28]. We identified MRSA belonging to ST22 which in Africa has only previously been found in Algeria, Tunisia and South Africa. This clone has been widely associated with hospital epidemics especially in new born units [29]. The "West Australia MRSA-2 clone" (WA-MRSA-2), ST88-IV [2B] which has been reported in Cameroon and Madagascar was not found and the European MRSA clone ST80-IV that has been found in North African countries was not present in our collection. None of the MRSA in this study belonged to *spa* type t008, the prevalent *spa* type associated with the USA300 pulsotype that has been identified as the major cause of community acquired skin and soft tissue infections in North America [30, 31]. Although the isolates included in our study were few, they represent a fairly diverse collection from both a public and private referral hospital and we can therefore conclude that USA300 is not common in Nairobi.

The 23 MSSA belonged to 22 different *spa* types highlighting their marked genetic diversity in contrast to the MRSA. There were 3 *spa* types (t005, t318 and t1476) that were found in both MSSA and MRSA suggesting the possibility of local acquisition of an SCC*mec* element. One of the MSSA *spa* types belongs to t002 which is associated with the MRSA pulsotype USA100 [16]. The *spa* type t064 was also found which is associated with one of the major MRSA clones (ST612- SCC*mec* IV [2B] found in South Africa [32]. ST241 has frequently been associated with SCC*mec* III [3A], however, one isolate belonging to ST241 harbored SCCmec IV [2B] (this SCC*mec* element was more common in AKUHN hospital). This particular clone was previously observed in a large university clinic in Nigeria [33]. SCC*mec* types IV and V are small in size and can be transmitted both in the community and healthcare settings. Potentially, this could result in the emergence of well-known epidemic MRSA clones like the predominant European CA-MRSA clone ST80-IV [2B] whose for bearer is thought to be a PVL-positive MSSA from sub-Saharan Africa that acquired the SCC*mec* IV [2B] [34]. The MSSA strain t021-ST30 has also been associated with a known PVL positive CA-MRSA clone [35].

The multi-drug resistant patterns for the MRSA in this study are in keeping with what has been described in other countries in Africa [17, 32, 36, 37]. Most of the MRSA were resistant to macrolide–lincosamide, tetracycline and sulphonamide group of antibiotics which is fairly common amongst MRSA especially those that are healthcare associated. However two of the isolates showed resistance to only beta lactam antibiotics suggesting that they may be community acquired (based on their molecular structure) given that they belonged to SCC*mec* type IV which has been associated with CA-MRSA.

The major limitation of this study is that the isolates characterized were not collected in a structured and consistent manner and as such the proportions reported do not necessarily represent a true picture of the relative distributions of different clones in Nairobi due to a selection bias. The over representation of nasal swab specimens from a paediatric population from one hospital may have exaggerated the prevalence of t037-ST 241. We also did not carry out MLST and *spa* typing on all isolates due to financial constraints. However, we did ensure that a representative isolate from each PFGE clonal complex was included in the isolates that were further characterized using MLST and *spa* typing.

Conclusion

To the best of our knowledge, this is the largest study from Kenya that has carried out PFGE, MLST, *spa* and SCC*mec* typing on a diverse collection of MRSA isolates. This study highlights the marked genetic diversity of MSSA and MRSA isolates in Nairobi including the presence of well-known epidemic MRSA clones and new MRSA *spa* types. Given the evolution of *S. aureus* over the years, there is need for continuous surveillance in order to keep track of emerging clones. The existence of epidemic MRSA clones further justifies the need to strengthen infection control measures within our hospitals so as to avoid nosocomial *S. aureus* infections.

Abbreviations

AKUHN: Aga Khan University Hospital Nairobi; BURP: based upon repeat pattern; CC: clonal complex; CLSI: Clinical Laboratory Standards Institute; DNA: deoxyribonucleic acid; dNTP: deoxynucleotide triphosphate; EDTA: ethylene-diamine-tetraacetic acid; KEMRI: Kenya Medical Research Institute; MDR: multidrug resistance; MLST: multi-locus sequence Type; MSSA: methicillin susceptible *Staphylococcus aureus*; MRSA: methicillin resistant *Staphylococcus aureus*; ND: not defined; NF: no founder; PBP2a: penicillin binding protein 2a; PCR: polymerase chain reaction; *S. aureus*: *Staphylococcus aureus*; SCC*mec*: Staphylococcal cassette chromosome *mec*; ST: sequence type; UT: untypeable.

Authors' contributions

GO conceptualized the study, collected isolates, carried out molecular analysis and drafted the manuscript. KNVZ and KH assisted in molecular analysis of samples and drafting of the manuscript. SA helped in carrying out BURP and eBURST analysis, drafting and critiquing the manuscript. SK, AW and GV assisted in designing the study, getting samples, interpreting of results and drafting the manuscript. All authors read and approved the final manuscript.

Author details

[1] Department of Pathology, Aga Khan University Hospital Nairobi, P.O. Box 30270-00100, Nairobi, Kenya. [2] Division of Medical Microbiology, Department of Pathology, Stellenbosch University, P. O. Box 19063, Western Cape, South Africa. [3] Division of Medical Microbiology, Department of Pathology, Faculty of Health Sciences, University of Cape Town, South Africa, P.O. Box 7925, Cape Town, South Africa. [4] Center of Microbiology Research, Kenya Medical Research Institute, P.O. Box 54840-00200, Nairobi, Kenya.

Acknowledgements

We acknowledge the use of the *S. aureus* MLST database which is located at Imperial College London and is funded by the Wellcome Trust.

Competing interests

The authors declare that they have no competing interests.

Funding

All the molecular work was done in the Microbiology section, Department of Pathology, Tygerberg Hospital, Cape Town, South Africa. This was facilitated through a technology transfer grant awarded to Prof Andrew Whitelaw by Stellenbosch University.

References

1. Diekema DJ, Pfaller MA, Schmitz FJ, Smayevsky J, Bell J, Jones RN, Beach M. Survey of infections due to Staphylococcus species: frequency of occurrence and antimicrobial susceptibility of isolates collected in the United States, Canada, Latin America, Europe, and the Western Pacific region for the SENTRY Antimicrobial Surveillanc. Clin Infect Dis. 2001;32(Suppl 2):S114–32.
2. Chambers HF. The changing epidemiology of *Staphylococcus aureus*? Emerg Infect Dis. 2001;7:178–82.
3. Grundmann H, Aires-de-Sousa M, Boyce J, Tiemersma E. Emergence and resurgence of meticillin-resistant *Staphylococcus aureus* as a public-health threat. Lancet. 2006;368:874–85.
4. Seybold U, Kourbatova EV, Johnson JG, Halvosa SJ, Wang YF, King MD, Ray SM, Blumberg HM. Emergence of community-associated methicillin-resistant *Staphylococcus aureus* USA300 genotype as a major cause of health care-associated blood stream infections. Clin Infect Dis. 2006;42:647–56.
5. Chambers HF. Methicillin resistance in staphylococci: molecular and biochemical basis and clinical implications. Clin Microbiol Rev. 1997;10:781–91.
6. Abdulgader SM, Shittu AO, Nicol MP, Kaba M. Molecular epidemiology of methicillin-resistant *Staphylococcus aureus* in Africa: a systematic review. Front Microbiol. 2015;6:348.
7. Omuse G, Kabera B, Revathi G. Low prevalence of methicillin resistant *Staphylococcus aureus* as determined by an automated identification system in two private hospitals in Nairobi, Kenya: a cross sectional study. BMC Infect Dis. 2014;14:669.
8. Maina EK, Kiiyukia C, Wamae CN, Waiyaki PG, Kariuki S. Characterization of methicillin-resistant *Staphylococcus aureus* from skin and soft tissue infections in patients in Nairobi, Kenya. Int J Infect Dis. 2012;17:e115–9.
9. Zinn CS, Westh H, Rosdahl VT. An international multicenter study of antimicrobial resistance and typing of hospital *Staphylococcus aureus* isolates from 21 laboratories in 19 countries or states. Microb Drug Resist. 2004;10:160–8.
10. Cookson BD. Methicillin-resistant *Staphylococcus aureus* in the community: new battlefronts, or are the battles lost? Infect Control Hosp Epidemiol. 2000;21:398–403.

11. Falagas ME, Karageorgopoulos DE, Leptidis J, Korbila IP. MRSA in Africa: filling the global map of antimicrobial resistance. PLoS ONE. 2013;8:e68024.
12. Chatterjee SS, Otto M. Improved understanding of factors driving methicillin-resistant *Staphylococcus aureus* epidemic waves. Clin Epidemiol. 2013;5:205–17.
13. Stefani S, Chung DR, Lindsay JA, Friedrich AW, Kearns AM, Westh H, Mackenzie FM. Meticillin-resistant *Staphylococcus aureus* (MRSA): global epidemiology and harmonisation of typing methods. Int J Antimicrob Agents. 2012;39:273–82.
14. Enright MC, Robinson DA, Randle G, Feil EJ, Grundmann H, Spratt BG. The evolutionary history of methicillin-resistant *Staphylococcus aureus* (MRSA). Proc Natl Acad Sci USA. 2002;99:7687–92.
15. Bozdoğan B, Yıldız O, Oryaşın E, Kırdar S, Gülcü B, Aktepe O, Arslan U, Bayramoğlu G, Coban AY, Coşkuner SA, Güdücüoğlu H, Karabiber N, Oncü S, Tatman Otkun M, Ozkütük N, Ozyurt M, Sener AG. t030 is the most common spa type among methicillin-resistant *Staphylococcus aureus* strains isolated from Turkish hospitals. Mikrobiyol Bul. 2013;47:571–81.
16. David MZ, Taylor A, Lynfield R, Boxrud DJ, Short G, Zychowski D, Boyle-Vavra S, Daum RS. Comparing pulsed-field gel electrophoresis with multilocus sequence typing, spa typing, Staphylococcal Cassette Chromosome mec (SCC mec) typing, and PCR for Panton–Valentine Leukocidin, arcA, and opp3 in methicillin-resistant *Staphylococcus aureus* Isola. J Clin Microbiol. 2013;51:814–9.
17. Aiken AM, Mutuku IM, Sabat AJ, Akkerboom V, Mwangi J, Scott JAG, Morpeth SC, Friedrich AW, Grundmann H. Carriage of *Staphylococcus aureus* in Thika level 5 Hospital, Kenya: a cross-sectional study. Antimicrob Resist Infect Control. 2014;3:22.
18. Robinson DA, Enright MC. Evolution of *Staphylococcus aureus* by large chromosomal replacements. J Bacteriol. 2004;186:1060–4.
19. de Aires de Sousa M, Sanches IS, Ferro ML, Vaz MJ, Saraiva Z, Tendeiro T, Serra J, de Lencastre H. Intercontinental spread of a multidrug-resistant methicillin-resistant *Staphylococcus aureus* clone. J Clin Microbiol. 1998;36:2590–6.
20. Xu BL, Zhang G, Ye HF, Feil EJ, Chen GR, Zhou XM, Zhan XM, Chen SM, Pan WB. Predominance of the Hungarian clone (ST 239-III) among hospital-acquired meticillin-resistant *Staphylococcus aureus* isolates recovered throughout mainland China. J Hosp Infect. 2009;71:245–55.
21. Edgeworth JD, Yadegarfar G, Pathak S, Batra R, Cockfield JD, Wyncoll D, Beale R, Lindsay JA. An outbreak in an intensive care unit of a strain of methicillin-resistant *Staphylococcus aureus* sequence type 239 associated with an increased rate of vascular access device-related bacteremia. Clin Infect Dis. 2007;44:493–501.
22. Wayne P. Performance standards for antimicrobial susceptibility testing; twentieth informational supplement. M100-S20. Clin Lab Stand Inst. 2010:29.
23. CDC. Oxacillin—resistant *Staphylococcus aureus* on PulseNet (OPN): Laboratory Protocol for Molecular Typing of *S. aureus* by Pulsed—field gel electrophoresis (pfge) growing cultures : plug preparation . Natl Mol Subtyping Netw foodborne Dis Surveill. 2013:1–24.
24. Milheirico C, Oliveira DC, de Lencastre H. Update to the multiplex PCR strategy for assignment of mec element types in *Staphylococcus aureus*. Antimicrob Agents Chemother. 2007;51:4537.
25. Enright MC, Day NP, Davies CE, Peacock SJ, Spratt BG. Multilocus sequence typing for characterization of methicillin-resistant and methicillin-susceptible clones of *Staphylococcus aureus*. J Clin Microbiol. 2000;38:1008–15.
26. Deurenberg RH, Stobberingh EE. The evolution of *Staphylococcus aureus*. Infect Genet Evol. 2008;8:747–63.
27. Breurec S, Fall C, Pouillot R, Boisier P, Brisse S, Diene-Sarr F, Djibo S, Etienne J, Fonkoua MC, Perrier-Gros-Claude JD, Ramarokoto CE, Randrianirina F, Thiberge JM, Zriouil SB, Garin B, Laurent F. Epidemiology of methicillin-susceptible *Staphylococcus aureus* lineages in five major African towns: high prevalence of Panton–Valentine leukocidin genes. Clin Microbiol Infect. 2011;17:633–9.
28. Raji A, Ojemhen O, Umejiburu U, Ogunleye A, Blanc DS, Basset P. High genetic diversity of *Staphylococcus aureus* in a tertiary care hospital in Southwest Nigeria. Diagn Microbiol Infect Dis. 2013;77:367–9.
29. Pinto AN, Seth R, Zhou F, Tallon J, Dempsey K, Tracy M, Gilbert GL, O'Sullivan MVN. Emergence and control of an outbreak of infections due to Panton–Valentine leukocidin positive, ST22 methicillin-resistant *Staphylococcus aureus* in a neonatal intensive care unit. Clin Microbiol Infect. 2013;19:620–7.
30. Al-Rawahi GN, Reynolds S, Porter SD, Forrester L, Kishi L, Chong T, Bowie WR, Doyle PW. Community-associated CMRSA-10 (USA-300) is the predominant strain among methicillin-resistant *Staphylococcus aureus* strains causing skin and soft tissue infections in patients presenting to the emergency department of a Canadian tertiary care hospital. J Emerg Med. 2010;38:6–11.
31. Ray GT, Suaya JA, Baxter R. Incidence, microbiology, and patient characteristics of skin and soft-tissue infections in a U.S. population: a retrospective population-based study. BMC Infect Dis. 2013;13:252.
32. Shittu A, Nübel U, Udo E, Lin J, Gaogakwe S. Characterization of meticillin-resistant *Staphylococcus aureus* isolates from hospitals in KwaZulu-Natal province, Republic of South Africa. J Med Microbiol. 2009;58(Pt 9):1219–26.
33. Ghebremedhin B, Olugbosi MO, Raji AM, Layer F, Bakare RA, Konig B, Konig W. Emergence of a community-associated methicillin-resistant *Staphylococcus aureus* strain with a unique resistance profile in Southwest Nigeria. J Clin Microbiol. 2009;47:2975–80.
34. Stegger M, Wirth T, Andersen PS, Skov RL, De Grassi A, Simões PM, Tristan A, Petersen A, Aziz M, Kiil K, Cirković I, Udo EE, del Campo R, Vuopio-Varkila J, Ahmad N, Tokajian S, Peters G, Schaumburg F, Olsson-Liljequist B, Givskov M, Driebe EE, Vigh HE, Shittu A, Ramdani-Bougessa N, Rasigade J-P, Price LB, Vandenesch F, Larsen AR, Laurent F. Origin and evolution of European community-acquired methicillin-resistant Staphylococcus aureus. MBio. 2014;5:e01044.
35. Monecke S, Coombs G, Shore AC, Coleman DC, Akpaka P, Borg M, Chow H, Ip M, Jatzwauk L, Jonas D, Kadlec K, Kearns A, Laurent F, O'Brien FG, Pearson J, Ruppelt A, Schwarz S, Scicluna E, Slickers P, Tan HL, Weber S, Ehricht R. A field guide to pandemic, epidemic and sporadic clones of methicillin-resistant *Staphylococcus aureus*. PLoS One. 2011;6:e17936.
36. Egyir B, Guardabassi L, Sørum M, Nielsen SS, Kolekang A, Frimpong E, Addo KK, Newman MJ, Larsen AR. Molecular Epidemiology and antimicrobial susceptibility of clinical *Staphylococcus aureus* from Healthcare Institutions in Ghana. PLoS ONE. 2014;9:e89716.
37. Marais E, Aithma N, Perovic O, Oosthuysen WF, Musenge E, Dusé AG. Antimicrobial susceptibility of methicillin-resistant *Staphylococcus aureus* isolates from South Africa. S Afr Med J. 2009;99:170–3.

11

Performance evaluation of a rapid whole-blood immunoassay for the detection of IgG antibodies against *Helicobacter pylori* in daily clinical practice

Dietmar Enko[1*], Gabriele Halwachs-Baumann[1], Robert Stolba[1], Ortrun Rössler[2] and Gernot Kriegshäuser[1]

Abstract

Background: A growing number of rapid *Helicobacter pylori* antibody tests are commercially available now, however, some of these tests are often used without sufficient evaluation. The aim of this study was to evaluate the performance of a commercially available rapid whole-blood immunoassay (gabControl® *H. pylori*; gabmed GmbH, Köln, Germany), for the qualitative detection of IgG antibodies against *H. pylori* with the ^{13}C-urea breath test (^{13}C-UBT) serving as a reference method.

Methods: A total of 108 consecutive outpatients, who were referred for ^{13}C-UBT by general practitioners and specialists, were also tested for *H. pylori* infection by the gabControl® *H. pylori* immunoassay. The clinical performance of this rapid whole-blood test was evaluated by determining the sensitivity, specificity, positive predictive value (PPV), and negative predictive value (NPV) compared to the ^{13}C-UBT. The agreement between the two tests was calculated using Cohen's Kappa (κ) with 95 % confidence intervals (CI).

Results: The agreement between the gabControl® *H. pylori* assay and the ^{13}C-UBT was 0.62 [95 % confidence intervals (CIs) 0.47–0.76; $P < 0.001$]. With the ^{13}C-UBT serving as the non-invasive gold standard method of *H. pylori* diagnosis, the gabControl® *H. pylori* assay demonstrated a sensitivity and specificity of 91.4 and 76.7 %, respectively, with a PPV of 65.3 % and a NPV of 94.9 %. Seventeen (15.7 %) individuals with a positive *H. pylori* anamnesis showed a negative ^{13}C-UBT and were typed positive by the gabControl® *H. pylori* assay. Of these, 13 (76.5 %) and 3 individuals (17.6 %) had completed one and two eradication therapies, respectively.

Conclusions: The gabControl® *H. pylori* immunoassay is a rapid and easy to use first line screening tool for *H. pylori* IgG antibody detection in daily clinical practice. However, this assay should not be used for confirmation of the successful *H. pylori* eradication after antibiotic treatment.

Keywords: *Helicobacter pylori*, Immunoassay, Laboratory diagnosis

Background

Helicobacter pylori infection is still a common condition worldwide. In North Europe and North America, about one-third of adults are infected, whereas in South-East Europe, South America, and in Asia, the *H. pylori* prevalence is reported to be higher than 50 % [1].

Since the *H. pylori* infection was recognized as a causative agent of chronic active gastritis and a risk factor for ulcer disease, gastric cancer and the mucosa-associated lymphoid tissue (MALT) lymphoma, numerous invasive and non-invasive methods for the accurate detection of this bacterium have been developed. Invasive techniques include biopsy-based histological methods, culture of the bacterium, the rapid urease test, and molecular tests (e.g. real-time PCR). Non-invasive methods encompass the ^{13}C-urea breath test (^{13}C-UBT), the stool antigen test,

*Correspondence: dietmar.enko@gespag.at
[1] Institute of Clinical Chemistry and Laboratory Medicine, General Hospital Steyr, Sierningerstraße 170, 4400 Steyr, Austria
Full list of author information is available at the end of the article

and the *H. pylori* antibody detection by serological tests [2–4].

The ^{13}C-UBT is considered the non-invasive gold standard method of *H. pylori* diagnosis [5–7]. It is a simple and safe test, which is easily repeated and provides excellent accuracy for the initial diagnosis of *H. pylori* infection, as well as the confirmation of its eradication after treatment [7, 8]. In the presence of the *H. pylori* produced enzyme urease, the ingested labeled urea (^{13}C-urea) is metabolized into labeled carbon dioxide ($^{13}CO_2$) and ammonia (NH_3). The produced $^{13}CO_2$ diffuses into the blood vessels and is eliminated via the lungs. The expired air is collected in order to measure the activity of labeled carbon so as to detect individuals with *H. pylori* infection [5, 9, 10].

Since individuals infected with *H. pylori* develop a local and systematic immune response [11, 12], specific *H. pylori* antibodies can be detected by rapid serological assays. These tests are easy to perform, inexpensive, and enable immediate patient testing for *H. pylori* antibodies in general practice surgeries [13]. A previous study, which evaluated a rapid whole-blood test, demonstrated, that there was no difference in diagnostic accuracy between capillary (fingerstick) and venous blood (venipuncture) collection [14]. A growing number of rapid *H. pylori* antibody tests are commercially available now, however, some of these tests are often used without sufficient evaluation.

The aim of this study was to evaluate the performance of a commercially available rapid whole blood immunoassay (gabControl® *H. pylori*; gabmed GmbH, Köln, Germany), for the qualitative detection of IgG antibodies against *H. pylori* with the ^{13}C-UBT serving as a reference method.

Methods

Patients

In total, 108 patients, who were consecutively referred for ^{13}C-UBT by general practitioners and specialists to our outpatient clinic, were also tested for *H. pylori* infection by the gabControl® *H. pylori* immunoassay (gabmed GmbH, Köln, Germany). The study period was from January to December 2015. The inclusion criteria were a minimum age of >15 years, an overnight fasting state and a non-smoking period >12 h before the ^{13}C-UBT. Patients with antibiotic-based therapy at least 4 weeks before and/or proton pump inhibitor (PPI) therapy at least 2 weeks before the ^{13}C-UBT were excluded from the study. An anamnesis was carried out about the history of *H. pylori* infections, completed eradication therapies, and intake of medication. Written informed consent was provided from all the patients. The ethical approval for this study was obtained from the Ethical Committee of Upper Austria, Linz, Austria. The study was carried out in accordance with the latest version of the Declaration of Helsinki.

^{13}C-UBT

Isotope ratio mass spectrometry was employed using the IRIS®-^{13}C-Infrared Isotope Analyzer System (Wagner Analysen Technik GmbH, Bremen, Germany). The ^{13}C-UBT was performed according to the manufacturer's instructions. Briefly: after a 12 h fasting period, breath samples were obtained before (baseline) and 30 min after the test drink intake (75 mg ^{13}C-urea from the capsule dissolved in 200 mL fruit juice) early in the morning (8:00–10.00 a. m.). ^{13}C/^{12}C-isotope ratio differences between the value at 30 min and the baseline value were determined and expressed in delta over baseline (DOB, ‰). A sample was considered positive if the 30 min value was above a 4 ‰ cut-off level [15]. Eating, drinking and/or smoking were not allowed until the ^{13}C-UBT was completed.

GabControl® *H. pylori*

This commercially available test is a qualitative membrane based immunoassay for the qualitative detection of *H. pylori* IgG antibodies in whole-blood, serum or plasma. The test was performed in accordance with the manufacturer's instructions. Approximately 50 µL of fingerstick whole-blood was sampled in a glass capillary tube and transferred to the specimen well (S) on the test device (Fig. 1a–c). One drop (approximately 40 µL) of dilution buffer containing *H. pylori* antigen-coated particles was added and allowed to migrate along a lateral-flow membrane thereby interacting with anti-human IgG antibodies immobilized as parallel lines. The test results were read after 10 min: a red control (C) line signal together with a red test (T) line signal (intense or faint) indicated the presence of *H. pylori* IgG antibody (Fig. 1a, b); showing a single red C line signal only, the assay was interpreted as negative (Fig. 1c). Assay read-out was performed independently by two physicians (i.e. four eyes principle), which were both blinded to the respective ^{13}C-UBT result.

Statistical analysis

The agreement between the ^{13}C-UBT and the gabControl® *H. pylori* assay was calculated using Cohen's Kappa (κ) with 95 % confidence intervals (CIs) [16]. Sensitivity, specificity, positive predictive value (PPV) and negative predictive value (NPV) of the gabControl® *H. pylori* assay were calculated compared to the ^{13}C-UBT. No adjustment for type I error was made. Therefore the concerning P values are only descriptive. Analyse-it® software version 2.30 (Analyse-it Software, Ltd, Leeds, United Kingdom) was used for statistical analysis.

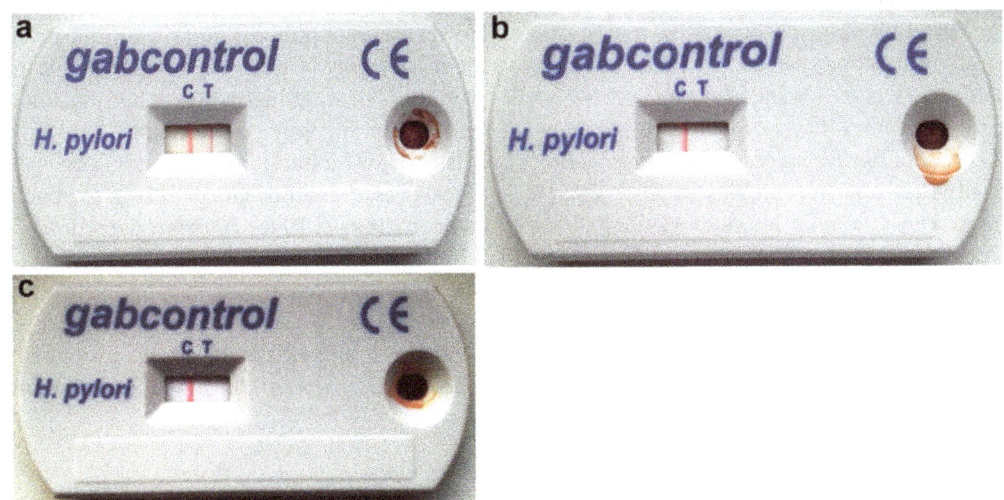

Fig. 1 Typical reactivity patters obtained for the gabControl® *H. pylori* immunoassay: **a** thirty-four (31.5 %) individuals showed an intense T line signal, **b** 15 (13.9 %) individuals were observed with faint to faintest T line signals, **c** 59 (54.6 %) patients demonstrated a C line signal only. *C* control line; *T* test line

Results

Study population characteristics

Of 108 consecutively enrolled patients, 36 (33.3 %) were male and 72 (66.7 %) were female. The median age was 44.0 (range: 15–88) years. The main demographic and clinical characteristics of the study population are provided in Table 1. Fifty-eight (53.7 %) individuals had a positive history of previous *H. pylori* infections.

Performance of the gabControl® *H. pylori* assay

The gabControl® *H. pylori* assay was found positive and negative in 49/108 (45.4 %) and 59/108 (54.6 %) patients, respectively (Table 2). Of those patients with a positive result, fifteen (30.6 %) individuals showed faint red colored changes in the test line region (T) only (Fig. 1b).

The agreement between the gabControl® *H. pylori* assay and the ^{13}C-UBT was 0.62 (95 % CI 0.47–0.76; P < 0.001). With the ^{13}C-UBT serving as the non-invasive gold standard method of *H. pylori* diagnosis [5–7], the gabControl® *H. pylori* assay demonstrated a sensitivity and specificity of 91.4 and 76.7 %, respectively, with a PPV of 65.3 % and a NPV of 94.9 % (Table 2).

Thirty-five (32.4 %) individuals had a positive ^{13}C-UBT. Twenty-seven (77.1 %) of these patients had a positive *H. pylori* anamnesis, whereas in 8 patients (22.9 %) *H. pylori* infection was detected for the first time. Seventeen (15.7 %) individuals with a positive *H. pylori* anamnesis showed a negative ^{13}C-UBT and were typed positive by the gabControl® *H. pylori* assay. Of these, 13 (76.5 %) and 3 individuals (17.6 %) had completed one and two eradication therapies, respectively. One patient (5.9 %), however, did not undergo any kind of antibiotic treatment.

Table 1 Basic characteristics of the study population

	Study population
Patients	n = 108
Gender	
Male	n = 36 (33.3 %)
Female	n = 72 (66.7 %)
Median age (years)	44 (range: 15–88)
History of previous H. pylori infections	
Negative history	n = 50 (46.3 %)
Positive history	n = 58 (53.7 %)
Completed eradication therapies (one or more)	n = 54 (50 %)

Discussion

This study aimed to compare the performance of the gabControl® *H. pylori* rapid immunoassay with the ^{13}C-UBT in 108 patients, who were referred by general practitioners and specialists to our outpatient clinic. As the ^{13}C-UBT

Table 2 GabControl® *H. pylori* versus ^{13}C-UBT

	n = 108	
	GabControl® *H. pylori* [a] +	GabControl® *H. pylori* [a] −
^{13}C-UBT +	32 (29.6 %)	3 (2.8 %)
^{13}C-UBT −	17 (15.7 %)	56 (51.9 %)

[a] The gabControl® *H. pylori* immunoassay showed a sensitivity of 91.4 % and a specificity of 76.7 % with the ^{13}C-UBT serving as a reference method

was considered the non-invasive gold standard method of *H. pylori* diagnosis [5–7], the gabControl® *H. pylori* assay demonstrated a sensitivity and specificity of 91.4 and 76.7 %, respectively, with a PPV of 65.3 % and a NPV of 94.9 %.

Several previous studies have evaluated other rapid whole blood test kits for *H. pylori* antibody detection, reporting sensitivities and specificities of 80.3–89.5 % and 78.0–93.5 %, and PPVs and NPVs of 83–92.9 % and 57.4–93.5 %, respectively [13, 17–19].

Herein, seventeen patients (15.7 %), who had a negative ^{13}C-UBT result were found positive for *H. pylori* antibody by the gabControl® *H. pylori* testing. Of these, 16 (94.1 %) individuals had a positive *H. pylori* anamnesis with one or two completed eradication therapies most likely responsible for the relatively low specificity of 76.7 % observed for the gabControl® *H. pylori* assay as well as the substantial agreement of 0.62 (95 % CI 0.47–0.76; $P < 0.001$) between the two methodologies investigated here. Patients with previous eradication therapy might recently have overcome their infection and the ^{13}C-UBT, as an indicator of current active infection, might be negative [20, 21]. Furthermore, it is known that it may take more than 1 year for *H. pylori* antibody to disappear after successful eradication [22]. Moreover, post-treatment circulating *H. pylori* antibodies are considered to remain positive for a significant period or perhaps indefinitely in some patients [3, 4, 20].

The intake of proton pump inhibitors (PPIs) may be another possible explanation of discrepant test results between the ^{13}C-UBT and the gabControl® *H. pylori* assay. While PPI intake at least 2 weeks before the ^{13}C-UBT was an exclusion criterion of this study, the authors cannot guarantee, that all individuals strictly followed this instruction. Individuals with PPI intake within 2 weeks before the ^{13}C-UBT may have false-negative breath test results, whereas *H. pylori* antibodies are serologically detectable [23–25].

Previous studies, which were performed in various populations with different geographical and socio-economic status, demonstrated, that the prevalence of antibodies against *H. pylori* increases with age [26–28]. A cross-sectional population study in Germany comprising 1797 individuals showed a *H. pylori* antibody prevalence of 48 % [29]. These seroprevalence data are in agreement with our study that found IgG antibodies against *H. pylori* in 49/108 (45.4 %) individuals.

In clinical practice, it should be considered, that a positive IgG serology does not necessarily indicate an ongoing infection [30]. As a consequence the ^{13}C-UBT may not be replaced through rapid whole-blood IgG antibody screening tests for confirmation of the successful *H. pylori* eradication after antibiotic treatment.

Using finger-stick blood samples the gabControl® *H. pylori* assay is rapid and easy to perform as centrifugation is no necessary and results are available within 10 min. However, low antibody titers resulting in faintest signal intensities may lead to false negative read-outs as interpretation becomes highly subjective and should therefore be based on the four eyes principle.

The major limitation of this study is the lack of invasive biopsy-based methods (e.g. histology, bacterial culture and real-time PCR) for *H. pylori* detection.

In conclusion, the gabControl® *H. pylori* immunoassay is a rapid and easy to use first-line screening tool for *H. pylori* IgG antibody detection in daily clinical practice. However, it should not be used for confirmation of the successful *H. pylori* eradication after antibiotic treatment.

Abbreviations

H: Helicobacter; MALT: Mucosa-associated lymphoid tissue; ^{13}C-UBT: ^{13}C-urea breath test; CO_2: Carbon dioxide; NH_3: Ammonia; DOB: Delta over baseline; κ: Kappa; PPV: Positive predictive value; NPV: Negative predictive value; PPI: proton pump inhibitor.

Authors' contributions

All authors contributed to the design of the study. DE and GK collected the data. DE analyzed the data and wrote the first draft of the manuscript. GK revised the paper critically. All authors read and approved the final manuscript.

Author details

[1] Institute of Clinical Chemistry and Laboratory Medicine, General Hospital Steyr, Sierningerstraße 170, 4400 Steyr, Austria. [2] Institute of Pathology, General Hospital Steyr, Sierningerstraße 170, 4400 Steyr, Austria.

Competing interests

The authors declare that they have no competing interests.

References

1. Eusebi LH, Zagari RM, Bazzoli F. Epidemiology of *Helicobacter pylori* infection. Helicobacter. 2014;19(Suppl 1):1–5.
2. Mentis A, Lehours P, Mégraud F. Epidemiology and diagnosis of *Helicobacter pylori* infection. Helicobacter. 2015;20(Suppl 1):1–7.
3. Cutler AF, Prasad VM. Long-term follow-up of *Helicobacter pylori* serology after successful eradication. Am J Gastroenterol. 1996;91(1):85–8.
4. Sharma TK, Young EL, Miller S, Cutler AF. Evaluation of a rapid, new method for detecting serum IgG antibodies to *Helicobacter pylori*. Clin Chem. 1997;43(5):832–6.
5. Patel SK, Pratap CB, Jain AK, Gulati AK, Nath G. Diagnosis of *Helicobacter pylori*: what should be the gold standard? World J Gastroenterol. 2014;20(36):12847–59.
6. Parente F, Bianchi Porro G. The (13)C-urea breath test for non-invasive diagnosis of *Helicobacter pylori* infection: which procedure and which measuring equipment? Eur J Gastroenterol Hepatol. 2001;13(7):803–6.
7. Savarino V, Vigneri S, Celle G. The 13C urea breath test in the diagnosis of *Helicobacter pylori* infection. Gut. 1999;45(Suppl 1):I18–22.
8. Lopes AI, Vale FF, Oleastro M. *Helicobacter pylori* infection—recent developments in diagnosis. World J Gastroenterol. 2014;20(28):9299–313.
9. Epple HJ, Kirstein FW, Bojarski C, Frege J, Fromm M, Riecken EO, Schulzke JD. 13C-urea breath test in *Helicobacter pylori* diagnosis and eradication. Correlation to histology, origin of "false" results, and influence of food intake. Scand J Gastroenterol. 1997;32(4):308–14.
10. Kawakami E, Machado RS, Reber M, Patrício FR. 13 C-urea breath test with infrared spectroscopy for diagnosing *Helicobacter pylori* infection in children and adolescents. J Pediatr Gastroenterol Nutr. 2002;35(1):39–43.

11. Blanchard TG, Nedrud JG, Czinn SJ. Local and systematic antibody responses in humans with *Helicobacter pylori* infection. Can J Gastroenterol. 1999;13(7):591–4.
12. Rathbone BJ, Wyatt JI, Worsley BW, Shires SE, Trejdosiewicz LK, Heatley RV, Losowsky MS. Systemic and local antibody responses to gastric *Campylobacter pyloridis* in non-ulcer dyspepsia. Gut. 1986;27(6):642–7.
13. Hackelsberger A, Schultze V, Peitz U, Günther T, Nilius M, Diete U, Schumacher M, Roessner A, Malfertheiner P. Performance of a rapid whole blood test for *Helicobacter pylori* in primary care: a German multicenter study. Helicobacter. 1998;3(3):179–83.
14. Chen TS, Chang FY, Lee SD. No difference of accuracy between capillary and venous blood in rapid whole blood test for diagnosis of *Helicobacter pylori* infection. Dig Dis Sci. 2002;47(11):2519–22.
15. Burucoa C, Delchier JC, Courillon-Mallet A, de Korwin JD, Mégraud F, Zerbib F, Raymond J, Fauchère JL. Comparative evaluation of 29 commercial *Helicobacter pylori* serological kits. Helicobacter. 2013;18(3):169–79.
16. Viera AJ, Garrett JM. Understanding interobserver agreement: the kappa statistic. Fam Med. 2005;37(5):360–3.
17. Jones R, Phillips I, Felix G, Tait C. An evaluation of near-patient testing for *Helicobacter pylori* in general practice. Aliment Pharmacol Ther. 1997;11(1):101–5.
18. Harrison JR, Bevan J, Furth EE, Metz DC. AccuStat whole blood fingerstick test for *Helicobacter pylori* infection: a reliable screening method. J Clin Gastroenterol. 1998;27(1):50–3.
19. Laine L, Knigge K, Faigel D, Margaret N, Marquis SP, Vartan G, Fennerty MB. Fingerstick *Helicobacter pylori* antibody test: better than laboratory serological testing? Am J Gastroenterol. 1999;94(12):3464–7.
20. Newell DG, Hawtin PR, Stacey AR, MacDougall MH, Ruddle AC. Estimation of prevalence of *Helicobacter pylori* infection in an asymptomatic elderly population comparing [14C] urea breath test and serology. J Clin Pathol. 1991;44(5):385–7.
21. Domínguez-Muñoz JE, Leodolter A, Sauerbruch T, Malfertheiner P. A citric acid solution is an optimal test drink in the 13C-urea breath test for the diagnosis of *Helicobacter pylori* infection. Gut. 1997;40(4):459–62.
22. Kim SG, Jung HK, Lee HL, Jang JY, Lee H, Kim CG, Shin WG, Shin ES, Lee YC, Korean College of Helicobacter and Upper Gastrointestinal Research. Guidelines for the diagnosis and treatment of *Helicobacter pylori* infection in Korea, 2013 revised edition. J Gastroenterol Hepatol. 2014;29(7):1371–86.
23. Laine L, Estrada R, Trujillo M, Knigge K, Fennerty MB. Effect of proton-pump inhibitor therapy on diagnostic testing for *Helicobacter pylori*. Ann Intern Med. 1998;129(7):547–50.
24. Graham DY, Opekun AR, Hammoud F, Yamaoka Y, Reddy R, Osato MS, El-Zimaity HM. Studies regarding the mechanism of false negative urea breath tests with proton pump inhibitors. Am J Gastroenterol. 2003;98(5):1005–9.
25. Mana F, Van Laer W, Bossuyt A, Urbain D. The early effect of proton pump inhibitor therapy on the accuracy of the 13C-urea breath test. Dig Liver Dis. 2005;37(1):28–32.
26. Jones DM, Eldridge J, Fox AJ, Sethi P, Whorwell PJ. Antibody to the gastric campylobacter-like organism ("*Campylobacter pyloridis*")—clinical correlations and distribution in the normal population. J Med Microbiol. 1986;22(1):57–62.
27. Mégraud F, Brassens-Rabbé MP, Denis F, Belbouri A, Hoa DQ. Seroepidemiology of *Campylobacter pylori* infection in various populations. J Clin Microbiol. 1989;27(8):1870–3.
28. Veldhuyzen van Zanten SJ, Pollak PT, Best LM, Bezanson GS, Marrie T. Increasing prevalence of Helicobacter pylori infection with age: continuous risk of infection in adults rather than cohort effect. J Infect Dis. 1994;169(2):434–7.
29. Michel A, Pawlita M, Boeing H, Gissmann L, Waterboer T. *Helicobacter pylori* antibody patterns in Germany: a cross-sectional population study. Gut Pathog. 2014;6:10. doi:10.1186/1757-4749-6-10.
30. Zagari RM, Romano M, Ojetti V, Stockbrugger R, Gullini S, Annibale B, Farinati F, Ierardi E, Maconi G, Rugge M, Calabrese C, Di Mario F, Luzza F, Pretolani S, Savio A, Gasbarrini G, Caselli M. Guidelines for the management of *Helicobacter pylori* infection in Italy: The III Working Group Consensus Report 2015. Dig Liver Dis. 2015;47(11):903–12.

12

Antibiotic resistance and biofilm production among the strains of *Staphylococcus aureus* isolated from pus/wound swab samples in a tertiary care hospital in Nepal

Ankit Belbase[1], Narayan Dutt Pant[2*], Krishus Nepal[1], Bibhusan Neupane[1], Rikesh Baidhya[1], Reena Baidya[3] and Binod Lekhak[4]

Abstract

Background: The increasing drug resistance along with inducible clindamycin resistance, methicillin resistance and biofilm production among the strains of *Staphylococcus aureus* are present as the serious problems to the successful treatment of the infections caused by *S. aureus*. So, the main objectives of this study were to determine the antimicrobial susceptibility patterns along with the rates of inducible clindamycin resistance, methicillin resistance and biofilm production among the strains of *S. aureus* isolated from pus/wound swab samples.

Methods: A total of 830 non-repeated pus/wound swab samples were processed using standard microbiological techniques. The colonies grown were identified on the basis of colony morphology, Gram's stain and biochemical tests. Antimicrobial susceptibility testing was performed by Kirby–Bauer disc diffusion technique. Detection of inducible clindamycin resistance was performed by D test, while detection of methicillin resistant *S. aureus* (MRSA) was performed by determination of minimum inhibitory concentration of oxacillin by agar dilution method. Similarly, detection of biofilm formation was performed by microtiter plate method. Strains showing resistance to three or more than three different classes of antibiotics were considered multidrug resistant.

Results: Total 76 samples showed the growth of *S. aureus*, among which 36 (47.4%) contained MRSA and 17 (22.4%) samples were found to have *S. aureus* showing inducible clindamycin resistance. Among the *S. aureus* isolated from outpatients, 41.9% were MRSA. Highest rates of susceptibility of *S. aureus* were seen toward linezolid (100%) and vancomycin (100%). Similarly, *S. aureus* isolated from 35 (46.1%) samples were found to be biofilm producers. Higher rate of inducible clindamycin resistance was seen among MRSA in comparison to methicillin susceptible *S. aureus* (MSSA). Similarly, higher rates of multidrug resistance and methicillin resistance were found among biofilm producing strains in comparison to biofilm non producing strains.

Conclusions: The rate of isolation of MRSA from community acquired infections was found to be high in Nepal. Increased rate of inducible clindamycin resistance as compared to previous studies in Nepal was noted. So for the proper management of the infections caused by *S. aureus*, D test for the detection of inducible clindamycin resistance should be included in the routine laboratory diagnosis. Further, detection of biofilm production should also be included in the routine tests. Linezolid and vancomycin can be used for the preliminary treatment of the serious infections caused by *S. aureus*.

Keywords: *S. aureus*, Inducible clindamycin resistance, Biofilm, MRSA, Linezolid, Vancomycin

*Correspondence: ndpant1987@gmail.com
[2] Department of Microbiology, Grande International Hospital, Dhapasi, Kathmandu, Nepal
Full list of author information is available at the end of the article

Background

The increasing rates of drug resistance among *S. aureus* to commonly used antibiotics and emergence of methicillin resistant strains for which limited treatment options exist have created a great problem to the management of the infections caused by *S. aureus* [1]. The accurate local antibiotic susceptibility data along with knowledge about the local prevalence of methicillin resistance may be helpful for starting proper preliminary treatment of the infections caused by *S. aureus* [1]. The increased prevalence of drug resistance mainly methicillin resistance among the strains of *S. aureus* has impelled the usage of macrolide–lincosamide–streptogramin B (MLS_B) antibiotics mainly clindamycin for the treatment of the infections caused by *S. aureus* [2]. However, there are reports of increasing resistance to MLS_B therapy particularly to clindamycin due to haphazard use of these antibiotics [2]. The inducible clindamycin resistance is responsible for treatment failure of the infections caused by *S. aureus* treated with clindamycin, as it can not be detected in the routine laboratory tests if the erythromycin and clindamycin are not kept adjacent to each other while performing antimicrobial susceptibility testing [2–4]. D test is one of the easiest methods that can be employed to detect the strains of *S. aureus* showing inducible clindamycin resistance.

Similarly, another problem with the treatment of infections caused by *S. aureus* is biofilm formation. Biofilm formation is a defense mechanism of *S. aureus* [5]. Bacteria protected by biofilms are resistant to host defense mechanisms and show resistance to standard antibiotic therapy [5].

So, in this study we determined the drug susceptibility patterns of the strains of *S. aureus* isolated from pus/wound swab samples. Further, we also studied the prevalence of inducible clindamycin resistance and methicillin resistance along with rate of biofilm production.

Methods

A cross sectional descriptive study was conducted among the patients attending B & B hospital, Lalitpur, Nepal from March 2015 to September 2015. A total of 830 pus/wound swab samples (400 from inpatients and 430 from out patients) received were processed using standard microbiological techniques [6]. The colonies grown were identified on the basis of colony morphology, Gram's stain, and biochemical tests [7]. Yellow colored colonies on mannitol salt agar, which were Gram positive cocci, catalase positive, slide and tube coagulase positive, hydrolysed gelatin, showed beta-hemolysis on blood agar, methyl red positive, Voges–Proskauer positive, nitrate reduction positive, fermentative, urease positive, DNase producing, lactose, mannitol, maltose, mannose, sucrose and trehalose fermenting, alkaline phosphatase positive were confirmed as *S. aureus*. Antimicrobial susceptibility testing was performed by Kirby Bauer disc diffusion technique following clinical and laboratory standards institute (CLSI) guidelines [8]. The concentration of suspension of the test organism was made equivalent to 0.5 McFarland standards. And lawn culture was performed on Mueller–Hinton agar plate. Then the antibiotic discs were placed over the lawn culture and the plate was incubated aerobically at 35 °C for 24 h. Finally the plate was observed for zone of inhibition and interpreted according to CLSI guidelines. The antibiotic discs used were penicillin-G (10 units), cefoxitin (30 µg), ciprofloxacin (5 µg), clindamycin (2 µg), chloramphenicol (30 µg), erythromycin (15 µg), gentamicin (10 µg), tetracycline (30 µg), cotrimoxazole (25 µg), vancomycin (30 µg) and linezolid (30 µg). Strains showing resistance to three or more than three different classes of antibiotics were considered multidrug resistant [9].

Detection of methicillin resistant *S. aureus*

The strains of methicillin resistant *S. aureus* were detected by determination of minimum inhibitory concentration of oxacillin by agar dilution method [8, 10]. Different concentrations of oxacillin ranging from 0.0625 to 32 µg/ml were prepared. One milliliter of each of these concentrations was added to 19 ml of Mueller–Hinton agar cooled to around 50 °C and allowed to solidify in sterilized petri plates. Then the concentration of the broth containing test organism was adjusted to 0.5 McFarland standards. Prior to inoculation, further (1:10) dilution of the broth containing test organism was performed. The plates were then inoculated with the test organisms and were incubated aerobically at 35 °C for 24 h, which were then examined for bacterial growth and interpreted according to CLSI guidelines.

Screening of inducible clindamycin resistance in *S. aureus*

The inducible clindamycin resistance was detected by D test [8]. Erythromycin (15 µg) disc and clindamycin (2 µg) disc were placed 15–26 mm edge to edge apart in Mueller–Hinton agar plate inoculated with the test isolate. The plates were incubated aerobically at 35 °C for 16–18 h. Flattening of the zone of inhibition of clindamycin adjacent to the erythromycin disc was regarded as D test positive.

Screening of biofilm production among the strains of *S. aureus*

The detection of biofilm production among the strains of *S. aureus* was performed by microtiter plate method [11]. The *S. aureus* was grown in 96 welled microtiter plate containing trypticase soya broth with 2% glucose, at 35 °C for 48 h. The optical density value of the bacteria that coat the wall of the wells was determined with the help of enzyme linked immunosorbent assay reader after staining with crystal violet. The organisms were identified as biofilm producer or biofilm non producer on the basis of the observed optical density values.

For quality control S. *aureus* ATCC 25923 was used.

Data analysis

For data analysis SPSS version 21.0 was used. Chi square test was applied and *p* value <0.05 was considered statistically significant.

Results

Among total 830 pus/wound swab samples processed, 364 (43.9%) were culture positive. Out of which, *S. aureus* was isolated from 76 (20.9%) samples. Among the 76 *S. aureus* isolated, 45 (59.2%) were MDR, 36 (47.4%) were MRSA, 17 (22.4%) were D test positive and 35 (46.1%) were biofilm producers.

Out of 76 *S. aureus* isolated, 43 (56.6%) were isolated from outpatients, whereas 33 (43.4%) were isolated from inpatients. Among the *S. aureus* isolated from outpatients, 41.9% were MRSA, while among the *S. aureus* isolated from inpatients 54.5% were MRSA.

Antimicrobial susceptibility patterns of *S. aureus* isolated

Among all the *S. aureus,* highest rates of susceptibility were seen toward linezolid (100%) and vancomycin (100%) followed by tetracycline (98.7%) and chloramphenicol (94.7%) (Table 1).

Inducible clindamycin resistance among strains of *S. aureus*

Among 76 *S. aureus,* inducible macrolide–lincosamide–streptogramin B (MLS_B) resistance, constitutive MLS_B resistance and macrolide–streptogramin B (MS_B) resistance were seen in 17 (22.4%), 8 (10.5%) and 17 (22.4%) *S. aureus* respectively. Inducible MLS_B resistance was higher among MRSA in comparison to MSSA ($p < 0.05$) (Table 2).

Table 1 Antimicrobial susceptibility patterns of *S. aureus* isolates

Antibiotics	MRSA (n = 36)	MSSA (n = 40)	Total (n = 76)
Penicillin	0 (0%)	2 (5%)	2 (2.6%)
Cefoxitin	0 (0%)	40 (100%)	40 (52.6%)
Ciprofloxacin	8 (22.2%)	13 (32.5%)	21 (27.6%)
Cotrimoxazole	10 (27.8%)	18 (45%)	28 (36.8%)
Gentamicin	22 (61.2%)	30 (75%)	52 (68.4%)
Chloramphenicol	35 (97.2%)	37 (92.5%)	72 (94.7%)
Erythromycin	10 (27.8%)	24 (60%)	34 (44.7%)
Clindamycin	32 (88.9%)	36 (90%)	68 (89.5%)
Tetracycline	35 (97.2%)	40 (100%)	75 (98.7%)
Vancomycin	36 (100%)	40 (100%)	76 (100%)
Linezolid	36 (100%)	40 (100%)	76 (100%)

Biofilm production among *S. aureus*

Thirty five (46.1%) *S. aureus* were found to be biofilm producers. Out of which, 23 (65.7%) were MRSA and 24 (68.6%) were MDR. Among 41 (53.9%) biofilm non producers, 13 (31.7%) were MRSA and 21 (51.2%) were MDR.

Discussion

Similar rates of MRSA as in our study were reported by Shrestha et al. (44.9%) [12] and Ansari et al. (43.1%) [13]. In our study, higher percent of MRSA isolates were isolated from admitted patients. The colonized health care workers in the hospitals are the main sources of MRSA in hospitalized patients causing higher rates of infections among them [14]. However, the rate of isolation of MRSA among the out patients was also very high (41.9%). This high rate of community acquired MRSA infections indicates a frightening situation. The main source for the community acquired MRSA infections may be the colonized health care workers who transfer the MRSA to their household, spreading it to the community [14]. Further, the admitted patients who got colonized during hospital stay may also act as the alternative sources for the community acquired MRSA infections.

In our study, the rate of inducible clindamycin resistance was found to be 22.4%, which was very high in comparison to the rates reported in previous studies by Ansari et al. (12.4%) [13] and Adhikari et al. (10%) [15] in Nepal. Such difference could be due to the difference in resistance patterns of *S. aureus* in different patient groups, hospitals, time periods and geographical locations [12]. This showed the increasing prevalence of inducible clindamycin resistance among the clinical isolates of *S. aureus* in Nepal. We reported higher rate of inducible clindamycin resistance among the strains of MRSA in comparison to the strains of MSSA, which was in accordance to the result reported by Shrestha et al. [12]. Clindamycin is considered as one of the drugs of choice for treatment of the infection caused by MRSA [13]. But due to increasing rates of inducible clindamycin resistance among strains of *S. aureus* mainly MRSA, there is high chance of treatment failure if clindamycin is used for the treatment of the infections caused by strains showing inducible clindamycin resistance [1]. So, a simple test like D test for detection of inducible clindamycin resistance is crucial to guide the treatment of the infections caused by *S. aureus* and is recommended to include in the routine laboratory tests.

As in a study by Ansari et al. (94.7%) [13], high rate of resistance to penicillin (97.4%) was reported in

Table 2 Inducible clindamycin resistance among strains of *S. aureus*

Resistant and susceptible phenotypes	Erythromycin	Clindamycin	D test	Total *S. aureus* (n = 76)	MRSA (n = 36)	MSSA (n = 40)
Inducible MLS_B	R	S	+	17 (22.4%)	15 (41.7%)	2 (5%)
Constitutive MLS_B	R	R	–	8 (10.5%)	4 (11.1%)	4 (10%)
MS_B	R	S	–	17 (22.4%)	7 (19.4%)	10 (25%)
Susceptible	S	S	–	34 (44.7%)	10 (27.8%)	24 (60%)

MLS_B macrolide–lincosamide–streptogramin B, *MS_B* macrolide–streptogramin B

our study. This is because only a small numbers of strains of *S. aureus* do not produce beta-lactamases [13]. We reported similar rate of resistance to ciprofloxacin (72.4%) as reported by Ansari et al. (63.7%) [13]. However, lower rate of resistance was reported toward gentamicin (31.6%) in comparison to the rate reported by Ansari et al. (60.4%) [13]. Further, higher rate of resistance to erythromycin (55.3%) was noted in contrast to 32.7% in a study by Ansari et al. [13]. In addition, resistance to cotrimoxazole was 63.2% in comparison to 81.7% noted in a previous study by Ansari et al. [13]. As previous studies in Nepal, no resistance was seen toward vancomycin and linezolid [13]. But among the commonly used antibiotics, the highest rate of susceptibility of *S. aureus* including MRSA, was found toward tetracycline followed by chloramphenicol suggesting the possibility of using these drugs for preliminary treatment of the infections caused by *S. aureus* in our settings. In the developing countries like Nepal, the low cost of these drugs will be an extra benefit.

In our study, higher rates of multidrug resistance and methicillin resistance were found among biofilm producing strains in comparison to biofilm non producing strains. These findings were in favor of the results reported by Ghasemian et al. [16]. Due to protective nature of the biofilm, the bacteria growing in it are intrinsically resistant to many antibiotics [17]. The antibiotic resistance among the strains of the bacteria residing in biofilm may increase up to 1000 times [17]. The main reasons for this may be difficulty in penetration of biofilm by antibiotics, slow growth rate of the bacteria and presence of antibiotic degradation mechanisms [17]. Further, biofilm formation gives platform for horizontal gene transfer among bacteria, causing the spread of drug resistance markers and other virulence factors [18].

In this study, due to lack of resources we could not use molecular methods to confirm our results but there are molecular methods like coagulase (coa) gene detection by polymerase chain reaction for identification of *S. aureus* [19] and detection of mecA gene for identification of methicillin resistant *S. aureus* [15].

Conclusions

In our study, high rates of drug resistance among the strains of *S. aureus* to commonly used drugs were observed. The rate of isolation of MRSA from community acquired infections was found to be high in Nepal. Inducible clindamycin resistance is presenting as serious problem to the management of infections caused by *S. aureus*, as its prevalence is increasing in Nepal. So, D test for the detection of inducible clindamycin resistance should be included in the routine laboratory diagnosis to guide the treatment. Further, keeping in mind the high rate of biofilm production among the strains of *S. aureus* and high rate of drug resistance among the biofilm producing strains, detection of biofilm formation should also be included in the routine tests. On the basis of the antimicrobial susceptibility testing report of our study, among the commonly used drugs tetracycline and chloramphenicol can be used for the preliminary treatment of the infections caused by *S. aureus* including MRSA in our settings. However, we recommend to use linezolid and vancomycin for the preliminary treatment of the serious infections caused by *S. aureus*.

Abbreviations

MRSA: methicillin resistant *S. aureus*; MDR: multidrug resistant; MSSA: methicillin susceptible *S. aureus*; MLS_B: macrolide–lincosamide–streptogramin B; ATCC: American Type Culture Collection; SPSS: statistical package for the social sciences; MS_B: macrolide–streptogramin B.

Authors' contributions

NDP and AB designed and conceived the study, carried out the research works, analyzed data, and prepared the final manuscript. KN, BN and RB carried out the research works and analyzed the data. RS and BL monitored the study. All authors read and approved the final manuscript.

Author details

[1] Department of Microbiology, GoldenGate International College, Battisputali, Kathmandu, Nepal. [2] Department of Microbiology, Grande International Hospital, Dhapasi, Kathmandu, Nepal. [3] Department of Pathology, B&B Hospital, Gwarko, Lalitpur, Nepal. [4] Central Department of Microbiology, Tribhuvan University, Kirtipur, Nepal.

Acknowledgements
The authors would like to thank, Golden Gate International College, Kathmandu, Nepal and B and B Teaching Hospital, Lalitpur, Nepal for providing the opportunity to conduct this research. The authors would also like to thank all the patients and the technical staffs for their help during the study.

Competing interests
The authors declare that they have no competing interests.

Ethics statement
Ethical approval for this study was obtained from Institutional Review committee of B&B Hospital, Lalitpur, Nepal. Informed consent was taken from all the patients or patient's guardians.

References

1. Prabhu K, Rao S, Rao V. Inducible clindamycin resistance in *Staphylococcus aureus* isolated from clinical samples. J Lab Physicians. 2011;3(1):25–7.
2. Deotale V, Mendiratta DK, Raut U, Narang P. Inducible clindamycin resistance in *Staphylococcus aureus* isolated from clinical samples. Indian J Med Microbiol. 2010;28:124–6.
3. Lim HS, Lee H, Roh KH, Yum JH, Yong D, Lee K, et al. Prevalence of inducible clindamycin resistance in staphylococcal isolates at Korean Tertiary Care Hospital. Yonsei Med J. 2006;47:480–4.
4. Steward CD, Raney PM, Morrell AK, Williams PP, McDougal LK, Jevitt L, et al. Testing for induction of clindamycin resistance in erythromycin resistant isolates of *Staphylococcus aureus*. J Clin Microbiol. 2005;43:1716–21.
5. Croes S, Deurenberg RH, Boumans ML, Beisser PS, Neef C, Stobberingh EE. *Staphylococcus aureus* Biofilm formation at the physiologic glucose concentration depends on the *S. aureus* Lineage. BMC Microbiol. 2009;9:229.
6. Cheesbrough M. District laboratory practice in tropical countries, part II. 2nd ed. New York: Cambridge University Press; 2006.
7. Holt JG, Krieg NR, Sneath PHA, Staley JT, Williams ST. Bergey's manual of determinative bacteriology. Baltimore: Williamsons and Wilkins; 1994.
8. Clinical and Laboratory Standards Institute. CLSI Document M100-S25. Performance standards for antimicrobial susceptibility testing: twenty fifth informational supplement edition. Wayne: CLSI; 2015.
9. Magiorakos AP, Srinivasan A, Carey RB, Carmeli Y, Falagas ME, Giske CG, et al. Multidrug-resistant, extensively drug-resistant and pandrug-resistant bacteria: an international expert proposal for interim standard definitions for acquired resistance. Clin Microbiol Infect. 2012;18:268–81.
10. Andrews JM. Determination of minimum inhibitory concentrations. J Antimicrob Chemother. 2001;1:5–16.
11. Los R, Sawicki R, Juda M, Stankevic M, Rybojad P, Sawicki M, et al. A comparative analysis of phenotypic and genotypic methods for the determination of the biofilm-forming abilities of *Staphylococcus epidermidis*. FEMS Microbiol Lett. 2010;310(2):97–103.
12. Shrestha B, Pokhrel BM, Mohapatra TM. Phenotypic characterization of nosocomial isolates of *Staphylococcus aureus* with reference to MRSA. J Infect Dev Ctries. 2009;3(7):554–60.
13. Ansari S, Nepal HP, Gautam R, Rayamajhi N, Shrestha S, Upadhyay G, et al. Threat of drug resistant *Staphylococcus aureus* to health in Nepal. BMC Infect Dis. 2014;14:157.
14. Pant ND, Sharma M. Carriage of methicillin resistant *Staphylococcus aureus* and awareness of infection control among health care workers working in Intensive Care Unit of a Hospital in Nepal. Braz J Infect Dis. 2016;20(2):218–9.
15. Adhikari R, Pant ND, Neupane S, Neupane M, Bhattarai R, Bhatta S, et al. Detection of methicillin resistant *Staphylococcus aureus* and determination of minimum inhibitory concentration of vancomycin for *Staphylococcus aureus* isolated from pus/wound swab samples of the patients attending a Tertiary Care Hospital in Kathmandu Nepal. Can J Infect Dis Med Microbiol. 2017;2017:2191532.
16. Ghasemian A, Peerayeh SN, Bakhshi B, Mirzaee M. Several virulence factors of multidrug resistant *Staphylococcus aureus* isolates from hospitalized patients in Tehran. Int J Enteric Pathog. 2015;3(2):e25196.
17. Neupane S, Pant ND, Khatiwada S, Chaudhary R, Banjara MR. Correlation between biofilm formation and resistance toward different commonly used antibiotics along with extended spectrum beta lactamase production in Uropathogenic *Escherichia coli* isolated from the patients suspected of urinary tract infections visiting Shree Birendra Hospital, Chhauni, Kathmandu Nepal. Antimicrob Resist Infect Control. 2016;5:5.
18. Soto SM. Importance of biofilms in urinary tract infections: new therapeutic approaches. Adv Biol. 2014;2014:543974.
19. Tiwari HK, Sapkota D, Sen MR. Evaluation of different tests for detection of *Staphylococcus aureus* using Coagulase (coa) gene PCR as the gold standard. Nepal Med Coll J. 2008;10(2):129–31.

13

Hematologic manifestations of babesiosis

Tamer Akel[1*] and Neville Mobarakai[2]

Abstract

Background: Babesiosis, a zoonotic parasitic infection transmitted by the Ixodes tick, has become an emerging health problem in humans that is attracting attention worldwide. Most cases of human babesiosis are reported in the United States and Europe. The disease is caused by the protozoa of the genus Babesia, which invade human erythrocytes and lyse them causing a febrile hemolytic anemia. The infection is usually asymptomatic or self-limited in the immunocompetent host, or follows a persistent, relapsing, and/or life threatening course with multi-organ failure, mainly in the splenectomized or immunosuppressed patients. Hematologic manifestations of the disease are common. They can range from mild anemia, to severe pancytopenia, splenic rupture, disseminated intravascular coagulopathy (DIC), or even hemophagocytic lymphohistiocytosis (HLH).

Case presentation: A 70 year old immunocompetent female patient living in New York City presented with a persistent fever, night sweats, and fatigue of 5 days duration. Full evaluation showed a febrile hemolytic anemia along with neutropenia and thrombocytopenia. Blood smear revealed intraerythrocytic Babesia, which was confirmed by PCR. Bone marrow biopsy was remarkable for dyserythropoiesis, suggesting possible HLH, supported by other blood workup meeting HLH-2004 trial criteria.

Conclusion: Human babesiosis is an increasing healthcare problem in the United States that is being diagnosed more often nowadays. We presented a case of HLH triggered by Babesia *microti* that was treated successfully. Also, we presented the hematologic manifestations of this disease along with their pathophysiologies.

Background

Human babesiosis, an emerging zoonosis caused by the hemoparasites of the genus Babesia, the second most common blood-borne parasites of mammals after trypanosomes [2]. Infection of the human host is being diagnosed more often, probably due to increasing number of travelers, immunocompromised individuals, blood transfusions, and better diagnostic methods. The first case of human babesiosis was reported in a Yugoslavian farmer in 1956 [3]. More than 100 Babesia species infect a wide variety of domestic and wild animals, but only few infect humans [4]. The main species of Babesia that are thought to cause the majority of human babesiosis are *Babesia microti*, *Babesia divergens* and *Babesia venatorum* [2, 4].

*Correspondence: tamer.akel.88@gmail.com
[1] Department of Internal Medicine, Staten Island University Hospital, 475 Seaview Avenue, Staten Island, NY 10305, USA
Full list of author information is available at the end of the article

In the northeastern part of the US, babesiosis is usually caused by the rodent species *B. microti*, which is transmitted by the tick, *Ixodes scapularis*, the same tick vector responsible for the transmission of anaplasmosis and Lyme disease; and thus co-infection with *Anaplasma phagocytophilum* and *Borrelia burgdorferi* should always be considered and tested for [5]. A study of 1000 patients who are seropositive for *B. burgdorferi* found that 10% of them had antibodies to *B. microti* [6]. In Europe, human babesiosis is mainly caused by the cattle species *B. divergens* which is also transmitted by the Ixodes tick (*Ixodes ricinus* being the most important) [2]. The incubation period for babesiosis is somewhere between 5 and 30 days [7]. Moreover, the disease has been increasingly acquired over the past decade by blood transfusions; the incubation period in such cases has been reported to be as long as 63 days, and in one case, up to 6 months [7, 8]. The incidence of transfusion-transmitted Babesia has been reported to be about 1.1 cases per million packed

RBCs across the United States [9]. More specifically, in endemic areas like Rhode Island, the incidence once approached 1 case per 9000 units of blood transfused [10].

The presentation of the disease is variable, ranging from subclinical, self limited asymptomatic infection to a life threatening one depending on the immune system of the host. Symptoms are usually non-specific and constitutional; initially start as fatigue, generalized weakness, and malaise, followed by abdominal pain, nausea, vomiting, photophobia, and anorexia. Hematuria and jaundice can also be observed depending on the degree of hemolysis. In a review of 139 patients hospitalized with babesiosis in New York, the most common symptoms were: fever (91%), fatigue, malaise, and weakness (91%), shaking chills (77%), and diaphoresis (69%) [11]. Physical examination is usually remarkable for fever, tachycardia or bradycardia, hepatosplenomegaly might be present, and lymphadenopathy is usually absent. The disease is more severe in splenectomized and immunosuppressed patients, and may require multiple blood transfusions or even exchange transfusion. In addition, these patients might relapse and the parasite might persist despite treatment [2].

Babesia parasites can be visualized on blood smears using the Giemsa-Wright stain. They are intraerythrocytic ring forms that resemble plasmodium, the causative agent of malaria. There are a couple of distinguishing features that can hint towards one organism over the other on light microscopy [12]. In Babesia, the parasite can form tetrads or maltese cross, although rare with *B. microti* but pathognomonic of babesiosis. In addition, Babesia does not generate hemozoin (malaria pigment) in the affected RBCs. Nevertheless, hemozoin is also not found during the early trophozoites of plasmodia. Additionally, Babesia has extracellular merozoites [12]. Furthermore, the blood smear might not show the parasites when the degree of RBCs infection is minimal i.e. <0.01%. Light microscopy has excellent sensitivity for Babesia detection, and should only be performed by an experienced microscopist, especially when thick blood smears are done, as the organisms might appear as simple chromatin dots that could be mistaken for a stain precipitate or iron inclusion bodies [13]. In the immunocompetent host, parasitemia can be hard to detect on a peripheral blood smear given that it rarely exceeds 5%, in comparison to the asplenic patient where parasitemia may amount up to 85% [7, 14]. Other diagnostic tests can be used such as real-time quantitative PCR or conventional PCR. The detection limit of PCR is usually 50 parasites per ml, while that of light microscopy is approximately 0.001% parasitemia, which is around 5000 infected erythrocytes per mL [7, 15]. Since babesiosis typically presents with a parasitemia of >0.1%, the assay is exceedingly sensitive for the detection of most clinical specimens [1]. Antibody testing can also be used, since sero-conversion is always required for complete clearance of the parasites [16]. Nearly all infected patients will have detectable antibodies in an acute phase serum sample; this might not be the case in immunocompromised patients, however [13]. Immunofluorescence assays are used to detect titers for *B. microti* in specific. Titers from 1:32 to 1:160 were reported to be both diagnostic and specific, with 88–96% sensitivity, 90–100% specificity [17].

Case presentation

A 70-year-old female patient, who recently immigrated to New York City, United States of America presented to the emergency department in mid-September 2015 for episodic high grade fever associated with confusion, chills, night sweats, fatigue, nausea, headache and palpitations for 5 days. She had moved from South Korea to the United States in June 2015. Prior to presentation, she was prescribed a course of amoxicillin–clavulonic acid for three days for a possible upper respiratory tract infection. Her past medical history is remarkable only for hypertension controlled with hydrochlorothiazide. The patient denied any recent travel history, contact with pets or tick bites and stated that she lives in New York City, and occasionally visits the city's gardens next to her house. Her social history is only remarkable for smoking half a pack of cigarettes daily; she denied any alcohol or drug use. She had never been hospitalized. In the emergency department she was hypotensive, tachycardic, and febrile with a temperature of 39.3 °C, a pulse of 102 bpm and a blood pressure of 92/58 mmHg. She was awake, alert but not oriented. Physical examination was unremarkable except for disorientation which resolved after becoming normothermic. Her blood pressure responded to 1L of normal saline.

Blood tests showed abnormal cell counts with neutropenia (1.23×10^9/L; ANC <1.5×10^9/L), lymphopenia (0.57×10^9/L; ALC <1×10^9/L), anemia (Hemoglobin of 6.8 g/dL; Hb <12 g/dL), thrombocytopenia (45×10^9/L), and MCV of 85 fL. Serum chemistries were all normal. Liver function tests were only remarkable for a mild elevation in total bilirubin (1.7 mg/dL) with an indirect bilirubin of 1.35 mg/dL. Other blood tests showed elevated C-reactive protein (11.6 mg/dL), LDH of 476 IU/L, ferritin of 1316 ng/mL, reticulocyte production index of 0.7% and an undetectable haptoglobin. A blood smear was ordered on the third day of hospitalization for the evaluation of hemolysis which was only remarkable for schistocytes without any detectable parasites.

She was started on broad spectrum antibiotics for a working diagnosis of sepsis. Blood cultures were sent with no bacterial growth reported few days later. Imaging studies done along with a lumbar puncture were all unremarkable. Febrile hemolytic anemia was our working diagnosis with an infectious etiology being highest on our differential. Testing for HIV, EBV, CMV, Lyme disease, West Nile virus, parvovirus B19, *Anaplasma phagocytophilum* and *Babesia microti* were all sent out, but took at least four days to get reported. Meanwhile, an immunological workup done was also unremarkable. Direct coombs test was negative.

She was actively hemolyzing with persistently daily high grade fevers despite antibiotics. The patient was given steroids for possible coombs negative autoimmune hemolysis without any response. During her 10 day hospital stay she required multiple RBCs' transfusions to keep the hemoglobin above 7 mg/dL. Bone marrow biopsy was performed on the fourth day of hospitalization which showed dyserythropoeisis. She continued to be pancytopenic; repeat blood smear on the seventh day showed intraerythrocytic Babesia in 4% of the RBCs. Infectious serology testing on blood using IFA sent initially was remarkable for positive IgM antibodies against *B. microti* with a titer of 1:256 along with a positive real-time PCR for the 18S rRNA gene [1]. Atovaquone 750 mg every 12 h orally and Clindamycin 600 mg every 8 h were started and the patient responded well. After 10 days of hospitalization, the patient was discharged, and followed up with an outside physician who reported that she was doing well. Repeated CBC showed resolution of the hemolytic anemia. A follow up peripheral blood smear was clear of hemoparasites.

Discussion

Human babesiosis is increasingly seen more often among the immunocompetent host, especially in the aging population. Age related decline in cellular immunity might help explain the severity of babesiosis in patients older than 50 years of age [4]. This can be reflected by a mouse model which showed age-associated loss of immunity against *B. microti* [18]. The patient we presented was an elderly woman without any other known risk factors. However, she followed a moderate-to-severe course of the disease and became transfusion-dependant on a daily basis for one week.

Clinical manifestations of severe babesiosis can have multiple complications; these include acute respiratory failure, non-cardiogenic edema, congestive heart failure, renal failure, DIC, splenic infarction or even HLH. Complications can occur early or late in the course of the disease. One review of 34 cases of babesiosis who were hospitalized in Long Island confirmed that acute respiratory failure is the most common complication (happened in 7 out of 34 cases), followed by DIC (happened in 6 out of 34 cases) [19].

An extremely rare, yet can be a fatal complication of babesiosis is HLH. HLH is likely an under-diagnosed disease that can result in multi-organ failure and death [20]. It is a condition characterized by excessive inflammation, hypercytokinemia, abnormal immune activation and tissue destruction. This results from a lack of normal down-regulation of activated macrophages and lymphocytes [21]. The dysregulation is due to the inability of natural killer cells and cytotoxic lymphocytes to eliminate the activated macrophages. This dysregulation along with the excessive secretion of cytokines cause tissue damage. HLH is classified into a primary form and a secondary form. The primary form typically manifests in young adults with genetic abnormalities of the cytotoxic function of natural killer cells and T cells. The secondary form of the disease occurs in older people who usually have an underlying condition, such as infection, malignancy or an autoimmune disorder without any identifiable genetic defect. Infectious diseases associated with HLH include epstein-barr virus, cytomegalovirus, human herpes virus-8, herpes simplex virus, varicella-zoster virus, H1N1 influenza virus, measles virus, parechovirus, parvovirus, and HIV. Leishmaniasis has also been reported to precipitate HLH, although more reported in the pediatric population.

The diagnostic criteria have been derived from the HLH-2004 trial [22]. Five out of the 8 criteria listed in Table 1 need to be met to diagnose HLH [22, 23].

It should also be noted that these diagnostic criteria were used in clinical trials, and thus may not identify every single case of HLH. In the literature, there are only 4 cases reported since 1986 with HLH secondary to babesiosis. The first reported case was in a patient with cryptosporidium infection [25]. The second case was

Table 1 Diagnostic criteria for HLH used in the HLH-2004 trial

Five of the eight criteria listed below should be fulfilled
Fever ≥38.5 °C
Splenomegaly
Cytopenias (affecting at least 2 of 3 lineages in the peripheral blood)
Hemoglobin <9 g/dL (in infants <4 weeks: hemoglobin <10 g/dL)
Platelets <100 × 10^3/mL
Neutrophils <1 × 10^3/mL
Hypertriglyceridemia (fasting, >265 mg/dL) and/or hypofibrinogenemia (<150 mg/dL)
Hemophagocytosis in bone marrow, spleen, lymph nodes, or liver[a]
Ferritin >500 ng/mL
Elevated sCD25 (α-chain of sIL-2 receptor)
Low or absent NK-cell activity

[a] Findings in up to two-thirds of initial bone marrow aspirates may be nondiagnostic; an additional bone marrow finding includes dyserythropoiesis, which has been observed in the absence of hemophagocytic histiocytes [24]

in an asplenic renal transplant patient on immunosuppressive therapy [26, 27]. Another case report suggested a possible HLH in a man with amyopathic dermatomyositis and ILD who is on rituximab therapy [28]. The last case report was a possible HLH in an immunocompetent patient who presented with severe pancytopenia and hemophagocytosis on bone marrow biopsy [29]. In our case, the patient had pancytopenia, fever, dyserythropoiesis, hypofibrinogenemia, and a high ferritin level meeting the criteria defined by HLH-2004 trial. Hence, we hypothesize that he had HLH triggered by Babesia. When HLH is triggered by acute infection, and the patient is stable, the appropriate therapy is removal of the stimulus that is activating the immune system. This strategy may allow patients to avoid HLH specific therapy which is potentially toxic and should be reserved for patients who are severely ill. However, in our case, we highlight the role of prednisone given initially, as it is difficult to conclude whether it had a role on the disease itself. Corticosteroids are part of the initial therapy for HLH, since it has a role in controlling the over-activation of the immune system. Conversely, since the precipitating etiology in our case was infectious, it is difficult to tell whether steroids had a role in exacerbating the disease, or whether it was beneficial in preventing progression to severe HLH. In Table 2, we compare our case to other reported cases of babesiosis in the literature using the HLH criteria.

Hematologic manifestations of Babesia are common in the human host. Thrombocytopenia is one of its major features. It is usually caused by hypersplenism which results in increased platelet sequestration and destruction by splenic macrophages [30]. In severe babesiosis, thrombocytopenia could be secondary to DIC. Immune mediated destruction of platelets has also been reported along with autoimmune hemolytic anemia [31]. Shatzel et al. reported two cases of Evans syndrome, the first one had a history of Hodgkin's lymphoma in remission, along with a history of autoimmune hemolytic anemia 12 years prior to presentation which was treated with splenectomy; he presented again with severe AIHA and thrombocytopenia, but this time after getting infected with Babesia [31]. The second patient had a history of Evans Syndrome treated with splenectomy, but relapsed three weeks post-splenectomy after a babesial infection [31]. Many other case reports described AIHA in patients with babesiosis; this leads us to conclude that there might be an element of immune deregulation precipitated by Babesia [19, 31–34].

Anemia (defined her as hemoglobin ≤10 g/dL) is another well documented hematologic abnormality in babesiosis. Its presence is associated with further complications [19]. Anemia happens after the egress of the parasite from RBCs causing lysis. Hemolysis alone does not really explain the severity of the anemia, since it is more pronounced than the level of parasitemia usually. Otsuka et al. found that cultures of parasitized RBCs of dogs with *Babesia gibsoni* had a significantly higher production of superoxide, which indicates that lipid peroxidation was greater in the infected cells and thus clarifying the role of oxidative damage in host erythrocytes; this could also be the case in human RBCs [35, 36]. There could also be an element of autoimmune hemolysis triggered by Babesia as described previously.

Table 2 Reported cases of HLH and babesiosis (*Babesia microti*) with our case

Author, year (Ref.)	Auerbach et al. [25]	Gupta et al. [27] Slovut et al. [26]	Poisnel et al. [29]	Mecchella et al. [28]	Our case
Underlying disease	Cryptosporidium	Renal transplant	None	Amyopathic DM and ILD	None
Medication	None	Prednisone, azathioprine	None	Rituximab/MMF/prednisone	Prednisone
Parasitemia %	7	13	3	<1	4
Cytopenia (as per HLH-2004)	No	Yes	Yes	Yes	Yes
Ferritin, ng/mL	Not reported	Not reported	5953	1665	1316
Fibrinogen, mg/dL	Not reported	Not reported	Not reported	Not reported	98
Bone marrow biopsy	Hemophagocytic histiocytes	Hemophagocytic histiocytes	Hemophagocytic histiocytes	Not done	Dyserythropoiesis
LDH, units/L	485	3510	620	586	476
Haptoglobin mg/dL	Not reported	<3	Undetectable	<10	<3
Splenomegaly	Yes	Asplenic		Not reported	No
Fever	Yes	Yes	Yes, value not reported	Yes, but low grade	Yes
Coombs test	Not reported	Positive	Not reported	Negative	Negative

In addition, the reticulocyte count is usually high to compensate for hemolysis, however, it can also be low as in our patient suggesting a bone marrow complication like HLH. If the patient has severe anemia, partial or complete red cell exchange transfusion is recommended as per the guidelines of the IDSA in the context of high levels of parasitemia (≥10%); or if the patient has any signs of end organ damage [13].

White blood cell involvement can also happen. Lymphopenia is a common finding among patients with babesiosis, one report described 17 patients with documented babesiosis; among them 13 where identified as lymphopenic [37]. Neutropenia on the other hand is not listed as a common hematologic finding associated with babesiosis [4]. On this contrary some clinicians may view neutropenia as inconsistent with babesiosis leading them to search for another cause [38]. One report assessed the frequency of neutropenia among 51 adult patients who were diagnosed with babesiosis between 2010 and 2013, 18 of them had neutropenia defined as an absolute neutrophil count ≤1800 neutrophils/μL [38]. Mechanisms of WBCs involvement is yet to be clarified whether it's a result of direct damage to the hematopoietic precursor cells, increased neutrophil adherence, splenic sequestration or a combination of all. In fact a high WBC count i.e. more than 5×10^9/L is a strong predictor of severe babesiosis [11].

The spleen is a vital organ in clearing erythrocytes infected with Babesia, and its absence is a major risk factor for severe infection. The role of the spleen can be illustrated by the mechanism of sequestration, since the parasitized erythrocytes lack the deformability needed to transit the splenic sinusoids and are therefore sequestered within the spleen by resident macrophages [39]. Complications involving this organ can happen, more specifically splenic infarction or rupture. In reviewing the literature we found 11 cases with this complication. Table 3 summarizes these cases.

Accordingly, we conclude that babesiosis can cause splenic rupture, just like malaria which is a well documented cause of this pathology. Mechanisms for malarial splenic rupture may also apply to babesiosis. During infection, pro-inflammatory cytokines are released, specifically TNF, IL-1, IL-6 and IFN-g leading to increased expression of adhesion molecules on the surface of the vascular endothelium. This in turn results in cytoadherence of the infected erythrocytes to the vascular endothelium causing erythrocyte sequestration and obstruction of the vascular flow [48]. In addition, hyperplasia of the reticuloendothelial system may lead to sub-capsular hemorrhage, and eventual splenic capsule breakdown with rupture into the peritoneum [46]. Conversely, one report examined tissue sections from a splenectomized patient who died from multi-organ failure resulting from severe babesiosis. None of the parasitized erythrocytes examined were close enough to the vascular walls to suggest any degree of sequesteration [49]. Animal models confirmed sequestration of infected erythrocytes (with *B. gibsoni* and Babesia *WA-1*) over the capillary endothelial cells [50, 51]. This has to be clarified by more histological sections in the human host. It is reasonable to conclude from published cases of splenic rupture that this is a complication of the immunocompetent individual. Since all cases had some degree of splenomegaly, it is possible to hypothesize that the development of subclinical splenomegaly due to splenic erythrophagocytosis may render the spleen more susceptible to spontaneous rupture with minor trauma [39, 42].

Conclusion

The incidence of human babesiosis is increasing in the United States, mainly in endemic regions like the Northeastern part. The present case illustrates the importance of considering blood-borne infections in patients presenting with febrile hemolytic anemia. We conclude that human babesiosis is a well documented cause of

Table 3 Reported cases of splenic rupture due to babesiosis

Author, year (Ref.)	Splenomegaly	Immunity status	Urgent splenectomy
Siderits et al. [39]	Had splenomegaly	Immunocompetent	Yes
Florescu et al. [40]	2 cases both had splenomegaly	2 cases both are immunocompetent	No
Kuwayama and Briones [41]	Subclinical splenomegaly	Immunocompetent	Yes
Froberg et al. [42]	Had splenomegaly	Immunocompetent	Yes
Reis et al. [43]	Not reported	Immunocompetent	Treated by splenic artery embolization
El Khoury et al. [44]	2 cases both had splenomegaly	2 cases both are immunocompetent	No
Tobler Jr. et al. [45]	Had splenomegaly	Immunocompetent	No
Seible et al. [46]	Not reported	Immunocompetent	No
Farber et al. [47]	Subclinical splenomegaly	Immunocompetent	Yes

pancytopenia, hemolysis, splenic rupture and should be considered as a potentially treatable cause of HLH.

Abbreviations

AIHA: autoimmune hemolytic anemia; ALC: absolute lymphocyte count; ANC: absolute neutrophile count; CBC: complete blood count; CMV: cytomegalovirus; DIC: disseminated intravascular coagulopathy; EBV: epstein barr virus; Hb: hemoglobin; HIV: human immunodefieicny virus; HLH: hemophagocytic lymphohistiocytosis; IDSA: Infectious Diseases Society of America; IFA: immunofluorescence assay; IL: interleukin; ILD: interstitial lung disease; LDH: lactate dehydrogenase; MCV: mean corpuscular volume; NK: natural Killer; PCR: polymerase chain reaction; RBC: red blood cells; WBC: white blood cells.

Author details

[1] Department of Internal Medicine, Staten Island University Hospital, 475 Seaview Avenue, Staten Island, NY 10305, USA. [2] Department of Infectious Diseases, Staten Island University Hospital, 475 Seaview Avenue, Staten Island, NY 10305, USA.

Acknowledgements

The authors gratefully acknowledge Mrs. Katrina Tohme for her technical and linguistic support.

Competing interests

The authors declare that they have no competing interests.

References

1. Teal AE, Habura A, Ennis J, Keithly JS, Madison-Antenucci S. A new real-time PCR assay for improved detection of the parasite *Babesia microti*. J Clin Microbiol. 2012;50(3):903–8.
2. Hildebrandt A, Gray JS, Hunfeld KP. Human babesiosis in Europe: what clinicians need to know. Infection. 2013;41(6):1057–72.
3. Skrabalo Z, Deanovic Z. Piroplasmosis in man; report of a case. Doc Med Geogr Trop. 1957;9(1):11–6.
4. Vannier E, Krause PJ. Human babesiosis. N Engl J Med. 2012;366(25):2397–407.
5. Weiss LM. Babesiosis in humans: a treatment review. Expert Opin Pharmacother. 2002;3(8):1109–15.
6. Krause PJ, Telford SR, Spielman A, Sikand V, Ryan R, Christianson D, Burke G, Brassard P, Pollack R, Peck J, Persing DH. Concurrent Lyme disease and babesiosis. Evidence for increased severity and duration of illness. JAMA. 1996;275(21):1657–60.
7. Rozej-Bielicka W, Stypulkowska-Misiurewicz H, Golab E. Human babesiosis. Przegl Epidemiol. 2015;69(3):489–94.
8. Herwaldt BL, Linden JV, Bosserman E, Young C, Olkowska D, Wilson M. Transfusion-associated babesiosis in the United States: a description of cases. Ann Intern Med. 2011;155(8):509–19.
9. Tonnetti L, Eder AF, Dy B, Kennedy J, Pisciotto P, Benjamin RJ, Leiby DA. Transfusion complicationS: transfusion–transmitted Babesia microti identified through hemovigilance. Transfusion. 2009;49(12):2557–63.
10. Asad S, Mermel L, Sweeney J. Transfusion transmitted babesiosis in Rhode Island, Transfusion. Oxford: Blackwell Publishing; 2008. p. 32A–3A.
11. White DJ, Talarico J, Chang HG, Birkhead GS, Heimberger T, Morse DL. Human babesiosis in New York State: review of 139 hospitalized cases and analysis of prognostic factors. Arch Intern Med. 1998;158(19):2149–54.
12. Bonoan JT, Johnson DH, Cunha BA. Life-threatening babesiosis in an asplenic patient treated with exchange transfusion, azithromycin, and atovaquone. Heart Lung. 1998;27(6):424–8.
13. Wormser GP, Dattwyler RJ, Shapiro ED, Halperin JJ, Steere AC, Klempner MS, Krause PJ, Bakken JS, Strle F, Stanek G, Bockenstedt L, Fish D, Dumler JS, Nadelman RB. The clinical assessment, treatment, and prevention of lyme disease, human granulocytic anaplasmosis, and babesiosis: clinical practice guidelines by the Infectious Diseases Society of America. Clin Infect Dis. 2006;43(9):1089–134.
14. Martinot M, Zadeh MM, Hansmann Y, Grawey I, Christmann D, Aguillon S, Jouglin M, Chauvin A, De Briel D. Babesiosis in immunocompetent patients, Europe. Emerg Infect Dis. 2011;17(1):114–6.
15. Beugnet F, Moreau Y. Babesiosis. Rev Sci Tech. 2015;34(2):627–39.
16. Ruebush TK, Chisholm ES, Sulzer AJ, Healy GR. Development and persistence of antibody in persons infected with *Babesia microti*. Am J Trop Med Hyg. 1981;30(1):291–2.
17. Krause PJ, Telford SR, Ryan R, Conrad PA, Wilson M, Thomford JW, Spielman A. Diagnosis of babesiosis: evaluation of a serologic test for the detection of *Babesia microti* antibody. J Infect Dis. 1994;169(4):923–6.
18. Vannier E, Borggraefe I, Telford SR, Menon S, Brauns T, Spielman A, Gelfand JA, Wortis HH. Age-associated decline in resistance to *Babesia microti* is genetically determined. J Infect Dis. 2004;189(9):1721–8.
19. Hatcher JC, Greenberg PD, Antique J, Jimenez-Lucho VE. Severe babesiosis in Long Island: review of 34 cases and their complications. Clin Infect Dis. 2001;32(8):1117–25.
20. Rosado FG, Kim AS. Hemophagocytic lymphohistiocytosis: an update on diagnosis and pathogenesis. Am J Clin Pathol. 2013;139(6):713–27.
21. Filipovich A, McClain K, Grom A. Histiocytic disorders: recent insights into pathophysiology and practical guidelines. Biol Blood Marrow Transplant. 2010;16(1 Suppl):S82–9.
22. Henter JI, Horne A, Arico M, Egeler RM, Filipovich AH, Imashuku S, Ladisch S, McClain K, Webb D, Winiarski J, Janka G. HLH-2004: diagnostic and therapeutic guidelines for hemophagocytic lymphohistiocytosis. Pediatr Blood Cancer. 2007;48(2):124–31.
23. Jordan MB, Allen CE, Weitzman S, Filipovich AH, McClain KL. How I treat hemophagocytic lymphohistiocytosis. In: Blood, vol 118. Washington, DC; 2011. p 4041–52.
24. Schwartz RA, Coppes M. Lymphohistiocytosis (Hemophagocytic Lymphohistiocytosis). 2011.
25. Auerbach M, Haubenstock A, Soloman G. Systemic babesiosis. Another cause of the hemophagocytic syndrome. Am J Med. 1986;80(2):301–3.
26. Slovut DP, Benedetti E, Matas AJ. Babesiosis and hemophagocytic syndrome in an asplenic renal transplant recipient. Transplantation. 1996;62(4):537–9.
27. Gupta P, Hurley RW, Helseth PH, Goodman JL, Hammerschmidt DE. Pancytopenia due to hemophagocytic syndrome as the presenting manifestation of babesiosis. Am J Hematol. 1995;50(1):60–2.
28. Mecchella JN, Rigby WF, Zbehlik AJ. Pancytopenia and cough in a man with amyopathic dermatomyositis. Arthritis Care Res (Hoboken). 2014;66(10):1587–90.
29. Poisnel E, Ebbo M, Berda-Haddad Y, Faucher B, Bernit E, Carcy B, Piarroux R, Harle JR, Schleinitz N. *Babesia microti*: an unusual travel-related disease. BMC Infect Dis. 2013;13:99.
30. Pantanowitz L. Mechanisms of thrombocytopenia in tick-borne diseases. Internet J Infect Dis. 2003:2(2).
31. Shatzel JJ, Donohoe K, Chu NQ, Garratty G, Mody K, Bengtson EM, Dunbar NM. Profound autoimmune hemolysis and Evans syndrome in two asplenic patients with babesiosis. Transfusion. 2015;55(3):661–5.
32. Evenson DA, Perry E, Kloster B, Hurley R, Stroncek DF. Therapeutic apheresis for babesiosis. J Clin Apher. 1998;13(1):32–6.
33. Wolf CF, Resnick G, Marsh WL, Benach J, Habicht G. Autoimmunity to red blood cells in babesiosis. Transfusion. 1982;22(6):538–9.
34. Herman JH, Ayache S, Olkowska D. Autoimmunity in transfusion babesiosis: a spectrum of clinical presentations. J Clin Apher. 2010;25(6):358–61.
35. Otsuka Y, Yamasaki M, Yamato O, Maede Y. Increased generation of superoxide in erythrocytes infected with Babesia gibsoni. J Vet Med Sci. 2001;63(10):1077–81.
36. Otsuka Y, Yamasaki M, Yamato O, Maede Y. The effect of macrophages on the erythrocyte oxidative damage and the pathogenesis of anemia in *Babesia gibsoni*-infected dogs with low parasitemia. J Vet Med Sci. 2002;64(3):221–6.
37. Kim N, Rosenbaum GS, Cunha BA. Relative bradycardia and lymphopenia in patients with babesiosis. Clin Infect Dis. 1998;26(5):1218–9.
38. Wormser GP, Villafuerte P, Nolan SM, Wang G, Lerner RG, Saetre KL, Maria MH, Branda JA. Neutropenia in congenital and adult Babesiosis. Am J Clin Pathol. 2015;144(1):94–6.
39. Siderits R, Mikhail N, Ricart C, Abello-Poblete MV, Wilcox C, Godyn JJ. Babesiosis, Significance of spleen function illustrated by postsplenectomy course in 3 cases. Infect Dis Clin Pract. 2008;16(3):182–6.

40. Florescu D, Sordillo PP, Glyptis A, Zlatanic E, Smith B, Polsky B, Sordillo E. Splenic infarction in human babesiosis: two cases and discussion. Clin Infect Dis. 2008;46(1):e8–11.
41. Kuwayama DP, Briones RJ. Spontaneous splenic rupture caused by Babesia microti infection. Clin Infect Dis. 2008;46(9):e92–5.
42. Froberg MK, Dannen D, Bernier N, Shieh WJ, Guarner J, Zaki S. Case report: spontaneous splenic rupture during acute parasitemia of Babesia microti. Ann Clin Lab Sci. 2008;38(4):390–2.
43. Reis SP, Maddineni S, Rozenblit G, Allen D. Spontaneous splenic rupture secondary to Babesia microti infection: treatment with splenic artery embolization. In J Vasc Interv Radiol, United States. 2011;22:732–4.
44. El Khoury MY, Gandhi R, Dandache P, Lombardo G, Wormser GP. Non-surgical management of spontaneous splenic rupture due to *Babesia microti* infection. Ticks Tick Borne Dis. 2011;2(4):235–8.
45. Tobler WD Jr, Cotton D, Lepore T, Agarwal S, Mahoney EJ. Case Report: successful non-operative management of spontaneous splenic rupture in a patient with babesiosis. World J Emerg Surg. 2011;6:4.
46. Seible DM, Khatana SA, Solomon MP, Parr JB. Hoof beats may mean zebras: atraumatic splenic rupture. Am J Med. 2013;126(9):778–80.
47. Farber FR, Muehlenbachs A, Robey TE. Atraumatic splenic rupture from Babesia: a disease of the otherwise healthy patient. Ticks Tick Borne Dis. 2015;6(5):649–52.
48. Krause PJ, Daily J, Telford SR, Vannier E, Lantos P, Spielman A. Shared features in the pathobiology of babesiosis and malaria. Trends Parasitol. 2007;23(12):605–10.
49. Clark IA, Budd AC, Hsue G, Haymore BR, Joyce AJ, Thorner R, Krause PJ. Absence of erythrocyte sequestration in a case of babesiosis in a splenectomized human patient. Malar J. 2006;5:69.
50. O'Connor RM, Long JA, Allred DR. Cytoadherence of Babesia bovis-infected erythrocytes to bovine brain capillary endothelial cells provides an in vitro model for sequestration. Infect Immun. 1999;67(8):3921–8.
51. Dao AH, Eberhard ML. Pathology of acute fatal babesiosis in hamsters experimentally infected with the WA-1 strain of Babesia. Lab Invest. 1996;74(5):853–9.

14

A combination of silver nanoparticles and visible blue light enhances the antibacterial efficacy of ineffective antibiotics against methicillin-resistant *Staphylococcus aureus* (MRSA)

Fatma Elzahraa Akram[1], Tarek El-Tayeb[2], Khaled Abou-Aisha[1] and Mohamed El-Azizi[1*]

Abstract

Background: Silver nanoparticles (AgNPs) are potential antimicrobials agents, which can be considered as an alternative to antibiotics for the treatment of infections caused by multi-drug resistant bacteria. The antimicrobial effects of double and triple combinations of AgNPs, visible blue light, and the conventional antibiotics amoxicillin, azithromycin, clarithromycin, linezolid, and vancomycin, against ten clinical isolates of methicillin-resistant *Staphylococcus aureus* (MRSA) were investigated.

Methods: The antimicrobial activity of AgNPs, applied in combination with blue light, against selected isolates of MRSA was investigated at 1/2–1/128 of its minimal inhibitory concentration (MIC) in 24-well plates. The wells were exposed to blue light source at 460 nm and 250 mW for 1 h using a photon emitting diode. Samples were taken at different time intervals, and viable bacterial counts were determined. The double combinations of AgNPs and each of the antibiotics were assessed by the checkerboard method. The killing assay was used to test possible synergistic effects when blue light was further combined to AgNPs and each antibiotic at a time against selected isolates of MRSA.

Results: The bactericidal activity of AgNPs, at sub-MIC, and blue light was significantly ($p < 0.001$) enhanced when both agents were applied in combination compared to each agent alone. Similarly, synergistic interactions were observed when AgNPs were combined with amoxicillin, azithromycin, clarithromycin or linezolid in 30–40 % of the double combinations with no observed antagonistic interaction against the tested isolates. Combination of the AgNPs with vancomycin did not result in enhanced killing against all isolates tested. The antimicrobial activity against MRSA isolates was significantly enhanced in triple combinations of AgNPs, blue light and antibiotic, compared to treatments involving one or two agents. The bactericidal activities were highest when azithromycin or clarithromycin was included in the triple therapy compared to the other antibiotics tested.

Conclusions: A new strategy can be used to combat serious infections caused by MRSA by combining AgNPs, blue light, and antibiotics. This triple therapy may include antibiotics, which have been proven to be ineffective against MRSA. The suggested approach would be useful to face the fast-growing drug-resistance with the slow development of new antimicrobial agents, and to preserve last resort antibiotics such as vancomycin.

*Correspondence: mohamed.el-azizi@guc.edu.eg

[1] Department of Microbiology, Immunology, and Biotechnology, German University in Cairo, GUC, New Cairo City, Cairo, Egypt

Full list of author information is available at the end of the article

Keywords: Nonconventional antimicrobials, Double and triple combinations, Multidrug-resistance, Checkerboard assay, Linezolid, Vancomycin, Azithromycin, Clarithromycin

Background

Treatment of infections caused by *Staphylococcus aureus* has become more difficult because of the emergence of multidrug-resistant isolates [1, 2]. Methicillin-resistant *S. aureus* (MRSA) presents problems for patients and healthcare facility-staff whose immune system is compromised, or who have open access to their bodies via wounds, catheters or drips. The infection spectrum ranges from superficial skin infections to more serious diseases such as bronchopneumonia [3].

Failure of antibiotics to manage infections caused by multidrug-resistant (MDR) pathogens, especially MRSA, has triggered much research effort for finding alternative antimicrobial approaches with higher efficiency and less resistance developed by the microorganisms. Silver has long been known to exhibit antimicrobial activity against wide range of microorganisms and has demonstrated considerable effectiveness in bactericidal applications [4] and silver nanoparticles (AgNPs) have been reconsidered as a potential alternative to conventional antimicrobial agents [5].

It has been estimated that 320 tons of nanosilver are used annually [6] with 30 % of all currently registered nano-products contain nanosilver [7]. The use of AgNPs alone or in combination with other antimicrobial agents has been suggested as a potential alternative for traditional treatment of infections caused by MDR pathogens [5]. AgNPs were found to exhibit antibacterial activity against MRSA in vitro when tested alone or in combination with other antimicrobial agents [8–10].

Metal nanostructures attract a lot of attention due to their unique properties. AgNPs is a potential biocide that has been reported to be less toxic compared to Silver ions [11]. AgNPs can be incorporated into antimicrobial applications such as bandages, surface coatings, medical equipment, food packaging, functional clothes and cosmetics [12].

Blue light is recently attracting increasing attention as a novel phototherapy-based antimicrobial agent that has significant antimicrobial activity against a broad range of bacterial and fungal pathogens with less chance to resistance development compared to antibiotics [13, 14]. Further, blue light has been shown to be highly effective against MRSA and other common nosocomial bacterial pathogens [15, 16].

The present investigation aims to evaluate the effectiveness of triple combination of AgNPs, blue light and the conventional antibiotics vancomycin, linezolid, amoxicillin, azithromycin, and clarithromycin against clinical isolates of MRSA. To the best of our knowledge, this is the first study, which utilizes this triple combination against pathogenic bacteria.

Methods

Chemicals

Unless otherwise indicated all chemicals were purchased from Sigma-Aldrich, USA.

Antibiotics

Amoxicillin (AMX), oxacillin (OXA), vancomycin (VAN) were purchased from Sigma Chemical Co., ST. Louis, Missouri, USA. Linezolid (LNZ) was provided by Pharmacia & Upjohn, Kalamazoo, MI, USA. Azithromycin (AZM) was provided by Pfizer, USA. Clarithromycin (CLR) was provided by Abbott Laboratories, USA.

Microorganisms

Ten clinical MRSA isolates were collected from The National Cancer Institute and from Abbasseya Hospital in Cairo, Egypt. The collected isolates were identified using conventional microbiological techniques.

According to genotyping results, the isolates were sub-classified into 14 different pulsed field patterns, 11 *spa*-types and 8 *multiple locus sequence typing* (MLST) sequence types. The pulsed field type A was the predominant pulsed field type, which corresponded to *spa*-type t-037 and MLST sequence type ST-239, and belonged to clonal complex 8 (CC8) according to eBURST analysis (Table 1) (Unpublished data, Master Thesis, Moussa et al. 2010).

Oxacillin susceptibility

The isolates were inoculated onto Mueller–Hinton agar (Lab M, UK) plates supplemented with 4 % NaCl and 6 μg/mL oxacillin, followed by incubation at 37 °C for 24 h. Isolates that showed more than one colony were considered as MRSA [17].

Preparation of the AgNPs

The AgNPs used for the purpose of this research are silver magnetite nanoparticles. To prepare the AgNPs, 0.127 g silver nitrate were dissolved in 75 mL of distilled water then 10 mL of an aqueous solution containing 0.08 g trisodium citrate and 0.2 g polyvinylpyrrolidone (PVP) were added. Ten milliliter of 0.1 M sodium borohydride were dissolved and added to the mixture. The

Table 1 Characteristics of the MRSA clinical isolates used in this study

Isolate designation	Spa-repeats	MLST	Clonal complex (eBURST)	*SCCmec*
C51	t-186	ST-88	CC88	IIIa
C6	t-5711	ST-22	CC22	IVa
C43	t-037	ST-239	CC8	III
N11	t-363	ST-239	CC8	III
N5	t-037	ST-239	CC8	III
N8	t-037	ST-239	CC8	III
C34	t-037	ST-239	CC8	III
C19	t-037	ST-239	CC8	III
C12	t-037	ST-239	CC8	III
C41	t-1234	ST-97	CC97	III

solution turned dark brown indicating the conversion of silver nitrate to silver nanoparticles. The nanoparticles were characterized spectrophotometrically, where a surface plasmon resonance peak appeared between 390 and 410 nm [18]. The particles size was also characterized by Malvern Zetasizer Nano ZS (United Kingdom) and by Tecnai G20, Super twin, double tilt (FEI) ultra-high resolution Transmission Electron Microscope, which showed a uniform distribution of the nanoparticles, with an average size of 15–20 nm.

Susceptibility of the isolates to AgNPs and the antibiotics

MIC of the AgNPs was determined by the broth microdilution method using cation-adjusted Mueller–Hinton broth (MHB) based on the guidelines of the Clinical Laboratory Standard Institute (CLSI) [19]. The minimum bactericidal concentration (MBC) was determined by streaking 10 μL samples from bacterial cultures supplemented with AgNPs or the antibiotics at their MICs and higher concentrations, onto the surfaces of Muller Hinton agar plates. After a 24 h incubation period, the number of colony forming units per mL (CFU/mL) was determined and the MBC, defined as the concentration that kills 99.9 % of bacteria, was recorded.

Double combination of AgNPs with blue light against MRSA

AgNPs were tested at 1/2, 1/4, 1/8, 1/16, 1/32, 1/64 and 1/128 of its MIC in 24-wells plates. Briefly, bacterial suspensions were pipetted into the wells, which contained the AgNPs at the tested concentrations in MHB to give an initial inoculum size of 1×10^5 CFU/mL and a final volume of 2 mL/well. The wells were exposed to visible blue light source at 460 nm and 250 mW for 1 h using Photon Emitting Diode (Photon Scientific, Egypt). Samples were taken after 0, 2, 4, 6, 8 and 10 h of inoculation, where viable bacterial counts were determined. Briefly, 10 μL aliquots were withdrawn and spread onto nutrient agar plates before being incubated at 37 °C for 24 h. The same procedure was repeated with nanoparticles-free and light-free wells. The experiment was performed in triplicates and the results were compared to drug-free samples.

Double combination of AgNPs with the antibiotics against MRSA

The efficiency of double combination of AgNPs and amoxicillin, vancomycin, linezolid, azithromycin, or clarithromycin against the ten clinical isolates of MRSA was assessed by the checkerboard method. The combination response was evaluated by calculation of the Fraction Inhibitory Index ($\sum$ FIC) as follow:

$$\sum \text{FIC} = \frac{MIC\ of\ drug\ A,\ in\ combination}{MIC\ of\ drugA,\ tested\ along} + \frac{MIC\ of\ drug\ B,\ in\ combination}{MIC\ of\ drug\ B,\ tested\ along}$$

The interaction is defined as synergistic if the FIC index is 0.5 or less; indifferent, if the FIC index is >0.5 and <4; and antagonistic if the FIC index is >4 [20].

Triple combination of AgNPs, blue light, and the antibiotics against MRSA

The purpose of this experiment was to test the effectiveness of AgNPs in combination with blue light and each of the following antibiotics at a time: amoxicillin, vancomycin, linezolid, azithromycin, or clarithromycin, against selected isolates of MRSA. Two isolates from the combination of AgNPs and each of the tested antibiotics were chosen on the basis of the synergistic response in the checkerboard assay.

The experiments were carried out in 24 multi-well plates where eight wells were designated as: drug- and light-free, blue light exposure, AgNPs alone, the antibiotic alone, blue light and AgNPs, blue light and the antibiotic, AgNPs and the antibiotic, and finally, the triple combination blue light, AgNPs and the antibiotic. The 24 multi-well plates were used because the diameter of their wells fits the tip of the Photon Emitting Diode, where the diode was placed at a distance of 5 mm over the surface of the bacterial culture in the well to ensure optimal exposure to the light and reduce light scattering. Only the wells in the four corners of one plate were used in parallel treatments to avoid the scattered light from adjacent wells, if any; all other wells were left empty.

The AgNPs and the antibiotics were tested at concentrations that resulted in the best combination in checkerboard assay against the selected isolates. Bacterial suspensions were pipetted into the wells, which contained the AgNPs alone or in combination with the antibiotics at the test concentrations in MHB to give an initial inoculum size of 1×10^5 CFU/mL and a final volume of 2 mL/well. The wells designated for light treatment were exposed to the light source emitting blue light at a wavelength of 460 nm for 1 h. The plates were then incubated at 37 °C for 24 h after which viable cell counts were determined. The experiment was performed in triplicate, and the results obtained were compared to the drug- and blue light-free wells.

Effects of triple combination of AgNPs, blue light, and azithromycin on MRSA isolate using transmission electron microscopy (TEM)

Ten milliliter of MHB medium were inoculated with 1×10^5 CFU/mL of MRSA isolate (N8) in 15 mL conical centrifuge tubes (Falcon, USA). The suspensions were then incubated at 37 °C for 4 h till the bacteria reached the logarithmic phase. The suspensions were then centrifuged at 2800×*g* for 10 min and the cell pellets were re-suspended in 10 mL of the fresh drug-free MHB, or containing 0.25 μg/mL (1/16 MIC) of AgNPs, or 0.25 μg/mL of azithromycin or both agents. Two milliliter aliquots of the suspension were transferred to 24 multi-wells plates. The plates were incubated at room temperature during which the blue light wells were exposed to the light at 460 nm for 1 h. One milliliter samples were then taken and prepared for TEM as previously described [21]. Briefly, the samples were centrifuged, and the bacterial pellets were fixed in 1 mL of 3 % glutaraldehyde for 2 h and then centrifuged and washed with 7.2 % phosphate buffer. A secondary fixative, osmium tetraoxide, was then added to the pellets, incubated for 1 h before being washed with phosphate buffer saline. The samples were then subjected to a series of dehydration steps using different concentrations of ethanol, starting with ethanol 50–95 %. During each step, the samples were left for 10 min and then put in absolute ethanol for 20 min. The samples were then embedded in resin blocks that were subsequently cut into semi- then ultra-thin thickness and finally stained with uranyl acetate and lead citrate before being examined by TEM JEOL (JEM-1400). The results were compared to drug- and light-free control experiments.

Statistical analysis

The statistical analysis of the data was done using GraphPad Prism (version 5.0) software. One-way- and two-way analysis of variance (ANOVA) were used to test the significance among the different treatment groups, and 5 % error was accepted in the statistics. Error bars in the graphical presentation of data express the standard deviation of the means between samples.

Results

Susceptibility of the isolates to AgNPs and the antibiotics

The MIC of AgNPs was found to be 4 μg/mL with MBC range of 8–16 μg/mL, and MBC_{90} (The minimum bactericidal concentration of the antibiotic required to kill 99.9 % of bacteria in 90 % of the isolates) was 8 μg/mL (Table 2). Vancomycin is the only antibiotic, which showed activity against the tested isolates with MIC_{90} (the minimum inhibitory concentration of the antibiotic required to inhibit the growth of 90 % of the isolates) and MBC_{90} values of 2 and 8 μg/mL, respectively (Table 2). The isolates were resistant to linezolid with MIC_{90} of 32 μg/mL, and to amoxicillin, azithromycin and clarithromycin with MIC_{90} >64 μg/mL.

Combination of AgNPs with blue light against MRSA

The antimicrobial activity of AgNPs in combination with blue light against one of the MRSA isolates was investigated. The AgNPs were tested at 1/2, 1/4, 1/8, 1/16, 1/32, 1/64 and 1/128 of its MIC in 24-wells plates. The antimicrobial activity of these combinations against the tested isolate was significantly higher ($p < 0.001$) than each agent alone. All bacteria were killed after 8 h of exposure to the combined therapy at all tested concentrations. Figure 1 shows the results for the combinations tested at 1/2, 1/4, 1/8, and 1/16 of the MIC of AgNPs (data for lower concentrations are not shown).

Combination of AgNPs with the antibiotics against MRSA

The efficiency of the double combination of the AgNPs and each of amoxicillin, vancomycin, linezolid, azithromycin, or clarithromycin, against the ten clinical MRSA isolates was assessed using the checkerboard method. The

Table 2 Susceptibility of the tested isolates to AgNPs and the antibiotics

Antimicrobial agents	Concentration (μg/mL)[a]	
	MIC_{90}	MBC_{90}
AgNPs	4	8
Amoxicillin	>64	>64
Azithromycin	>64	>64
Clarithromycin	>64	>64
Linezolid	32	>64
Vancomycin	2	8

[a] MIC_{90}: The minimum inhibitory concentration of the antibiotic required to inhibit the growth of 90 % of the isolates. MBC_{90}: The minimum bactericidal concentration of the antibiotic required to kill 99.9 % of bacteria in 90 % of the isolates

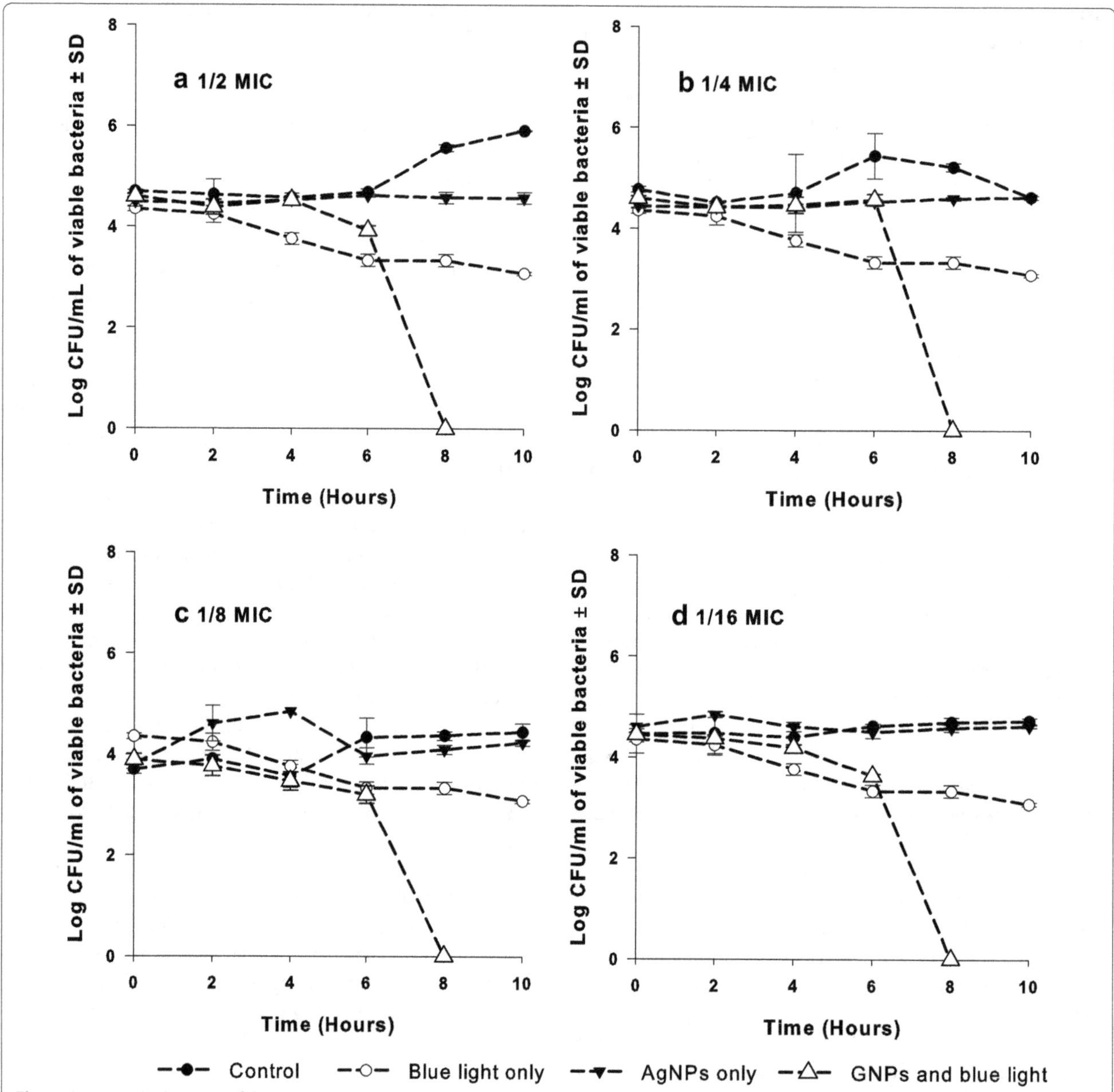

Fig. 1 Antimicrobial activity of the AgNPs at different concentrations in combination with blue light against MRSA isolates. Cell suspensions were exposed to either the silver compound alone at sub-MICs (**a** 1/2, **b** 1/4, **c** 1/8, and **d** 1/16 MIC), or blue light alone at 460 nm and 250 mW for 1 h, or combination of both agents. Viable colony count was recorded as mean ± SD of three independent experiments. *AgNPs* silver nanoparticles, *CFU* colony forming unit, *MIC* minimum inhibitory concentration, *SD* standard deviation

combination of AgNPs with amoxicillin resulted in synergistic activity against four isolates whereas indifference response was observed in six isolates. Similar results were observed when the AgNPs were combined with azithromycin, clarithromycin or linezolid, where synergism was observed against 4, 3 and 3 isolates, respectively, whereas indifferent interaction prevailed for the remaining isolates. On the other hand, combination of AgNPs with vancomycin was indifferent for all tested isolates (Fig. 2).

Triple combination of AgNPs, blue light, and the antibiotics against MRSA isolates

The effectiveness of the AgNPs in combination with blue light and amoxicillin, linezolid, azithromycin, or clarithromycin, was tested against selected isolates of MRSA. Two isolates from each combination of AgNPs and antibiotic were selected based on the synergistic results of the checkerboard assay. Vancomycin was excluded because its combination with the AgNPs was indifferent against all isolates.

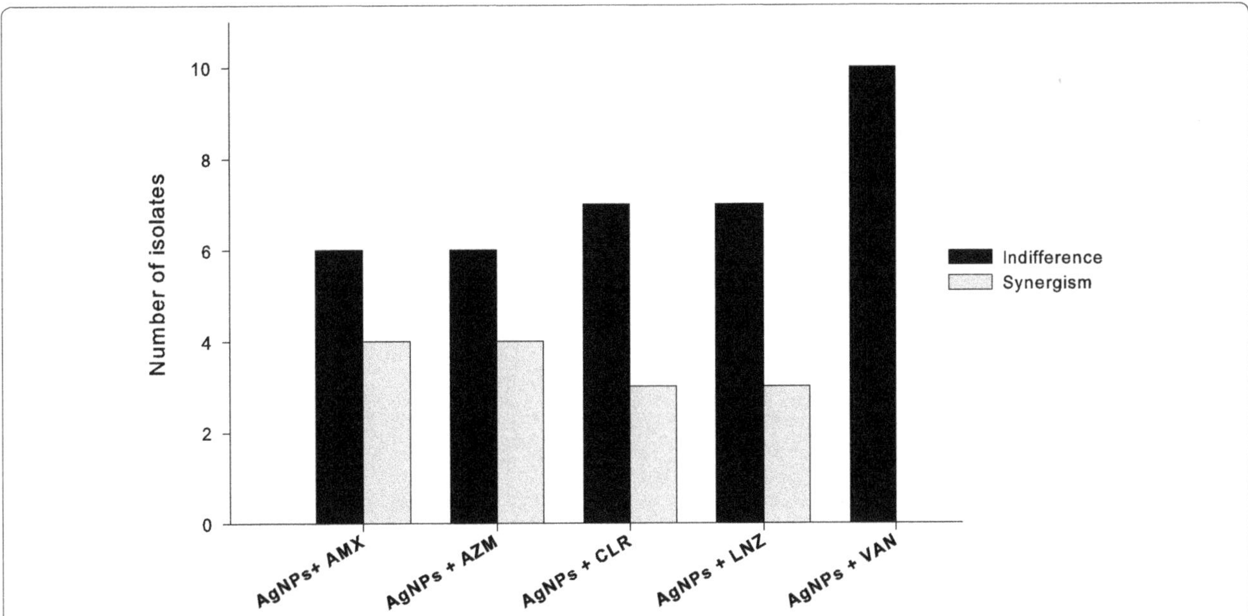

Fig. 2 Double combination of AgNPs with the amoxicillin, vancomycin, linezolid, azithromycin or clarithromycin against ten MRSA isolates. The combination was assessed by the checkerboard method and the response was evaluated by calculation of the fraction inhibitory index (FIC) as follow: synergistic if the FIC index is 0.5 or less, indifference if the FIC index more than 0.5 and less than four, and antagonistic if the FIC index more than four. *AgNPs* silver nanoparticles, *AMX* amoxicillin, *AZM* azithromycin, *CLR* clarithromycin, *LNZ* linezolid, *VAN* vancomycin

The AgNPs and the antibiotics were tested at the concentrations, which gave the best results in checkerboard assay. Isolates N8 and C41 were used to assess the triple combination of AgNPs at 1/16 MIC, the blue light, and azithromycin at 0.25 and 2 µg/mL, respectively. The triple combination resulted in significantly higher ($p < 0.001$) killing effect of isolate C41 with $\log_{10}$ CFU/mL reductions of 8.4, 3.2, compared to the drug-free samples and to the double combinations of the antibiotic with the AgNPs (Fig. 3a). The triple combinations against isolate N8 resulted in killing of all bacteria compared to all other treatments, which showed lower activity with $\log_{10}$ CFU/mL reduction range of 1.0–2.0 (Fig. 3b).

Triple combinations that included clarithromycin were tested against isolates C51 and C41, at 1/8 and 1/512 of the MIC, respectively, of the AgNPs and 0.25 µg/mL of the antibiotic. The bactericidal activity of the three-agent combination was significantly higher ($p < 0.001$) than that attained with other treatment combinations with $\log_{10}$ CFU/mL reduction of 13.02 and 5.84 compared to the control of the two isolates, respectively (Fig. 4a, b).

The antimicrobial efficacy of linezolid at 0.25 and 8 µg/mL was evaluated against isolate C19 and N5, respectively, when combined with the silver compound at its 1/2 MIC and blue light. Synergistic interaction was observed when the AgNPs were combined with either the antibiotic or the blue light or with both of them, where the bacteria were completely killed following treatment with all combinations (Fig. 5a, b). The same effect was observed when amoxicillin at 1 and 0.25 µg/mL was combined with blue light and AgNPs at 1/32 and 1/256 of its MIC against isolates C12 and N8, respectively (data not shown).

TEM examination of MRSA isolate (N8) after treatment with the AgNPs, blue light, and azithromycin alone or in triple combination

The antimicrobial efficiency of the AgNPs at 1/16 MIC, blue light for 1 h and azithromycin at 0.25 µg/mL against isolate N8 was visualized by TEM when each of them was used alone or in triple combination (Fig. 6a–e). Bacteria treated with AgNPs alone showed accumulation of the silver particles inside the cells concomitant with signs of membrane damage and lysis (Fig. 6b). Cell lysis was also observed when the bacteria were treated with either blue light or azithromycin alone (Fig. 6c, d). On the other hand, bacterial cell lysis was more pronounced following treatment with the three agents in combination, where the cells were severely affected (Fig. 6e).

Discussion

Antibiotic resistance by isolates of *S. aureus* has become a global alarming problem that limits the availability of effective antimicrobial agents [22]. Antibiotic-misuse, the failure of some patients to comply with their treatment regimen, and the high capability of bacteria to

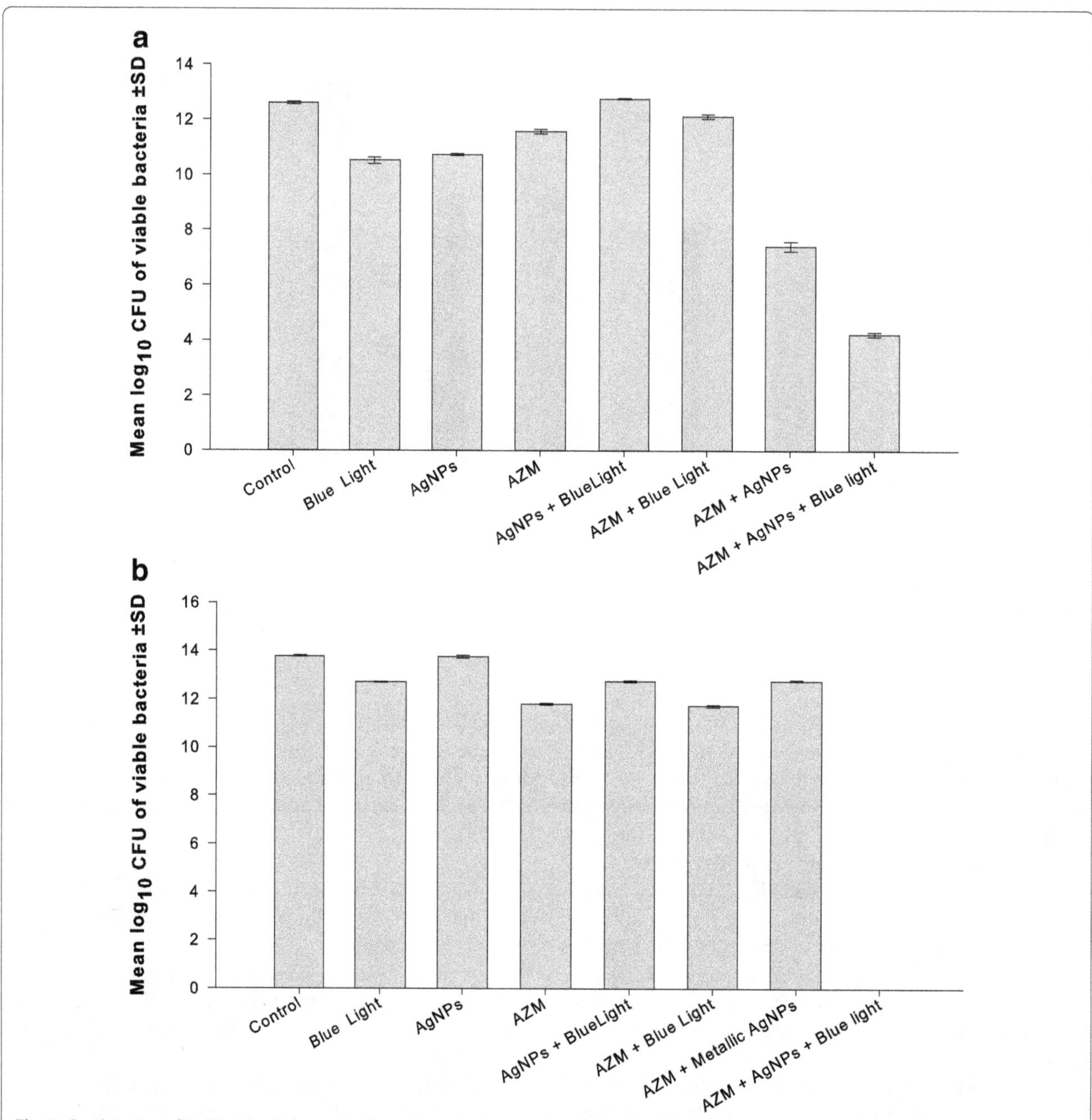

Fig. 3 Combination of AgNPs, blue light, and azithromycin against two isolates of MRSA. The triple combination of AgNPs with the blue light and azithromycin against two isolates of MRSA was assessed. The isolates were selected on the basis of synergistic response in checkerboard assay. Based on the best result of the combination in the checkerboard assay, the concentrations of the two agents were used as follow: **a** Isolate C41: AgNPs at 1/16 of the MIC, and azithromycin at 2 μg/mL. **b** Isolate N8: AgNPs at 1/16 of the MIC, and azithromycin at 0.25 μg/mL. *AgNPs* silver nanoparticles, *CFU* colony forming unit, *AZM* azithromycin, *SD* standard deviation

mutate, are among the major factors contributing to the emergence of bacterial resistance. Antibiotic resistance leads to the failure of treatment of life-threatening bacterial infections and increases costs due to longer stay in healthcare settings [23, 24]. The use of non-conventional therapy to which bacteria are improbably to develop resistance, would be the best alternative. AgNPs are potential antimicrobials agents, which can be considered as an alternative to antibiotics for the treatment of infections caused by MDR bacteria [5]. AgNPs have been shown to possess strong and broad-spectrum antimicrobial activity due to a combined effect between their physical properties and the released free silver ions [25].

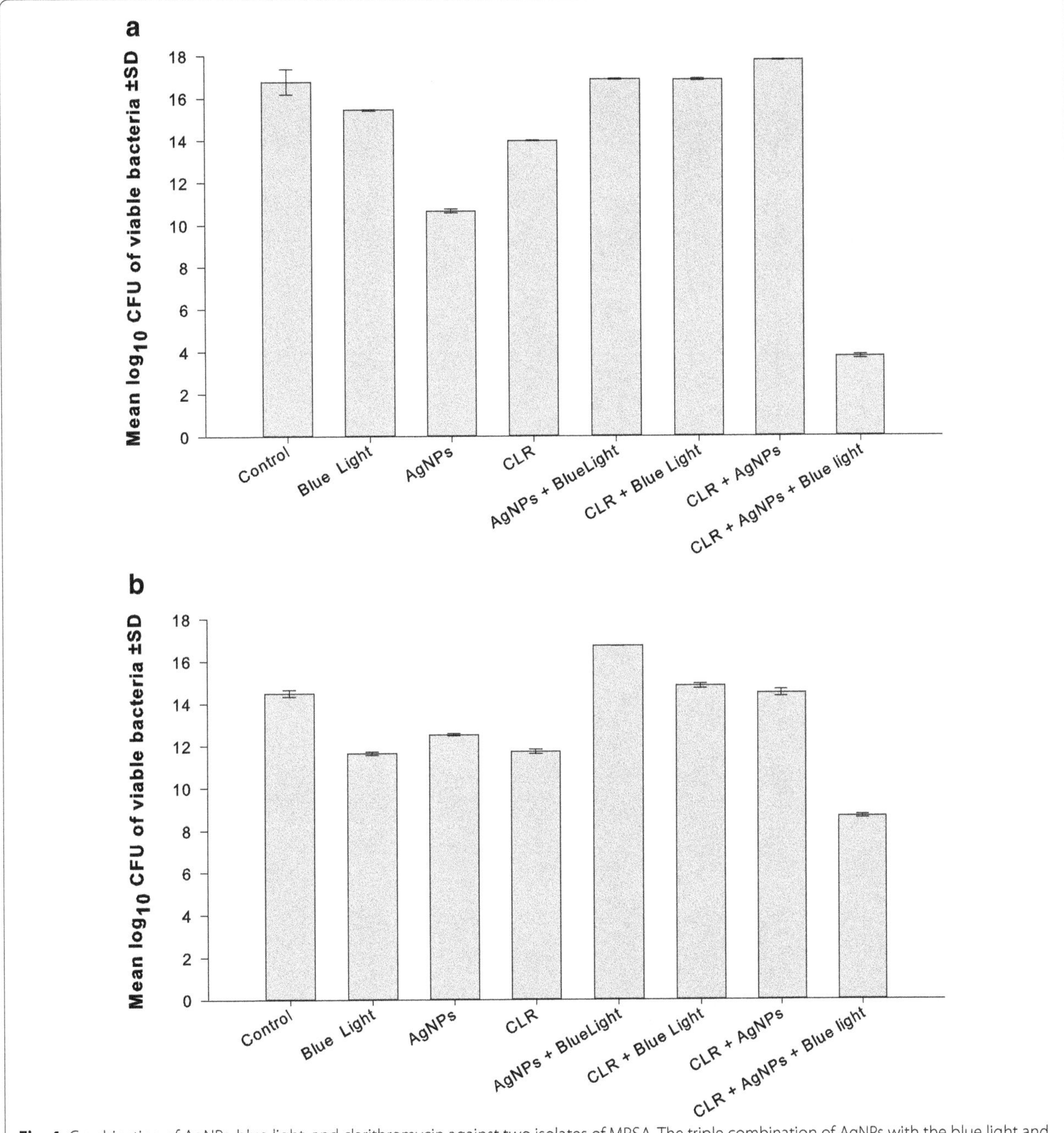

Fig. 4 Combination of AgNPs, blue light, and clarithromycin against two isolates of MRSA. The triple combination of AgNPs with the blue light and clarithromycin against two isolates of MRSA was assessed. The isolates were selected on the basis of synergistic response in checkerboard assay. Based on the best result of the combination in the checkerboard assay, the concentrations of the two agents were used as follow: **a** Isolate C51: AgNPs at 1/8 of the MIC, and azithromycin at 0.25 μg/mL. **b** Isolate C41: AgNPs at 1/512 of the MIC, and azithromycin at 0.25 μg/mL. *AgNPs* silver nanoparticles, *CFU* colony forming unit, *CLR* clarithromycin, *SD* standard deviation

Methicillin-resistant *S. aureus* was used as a model in our study to assess the efficiency of combination of AgNPs, blue light, and anti-staphylococcal antibiotics. The isolates had been collected from different hospital units to guarantee the most possible representation of the Egyptian genotype population of *S. aureus*. We have previously found that members of CC8 are the prevailing MRSA clone in Egypt (Unpublished data, Master Thesis, Moussa et al. 2010). Infections caused by *S. aureus* are among the most frequent causes of both

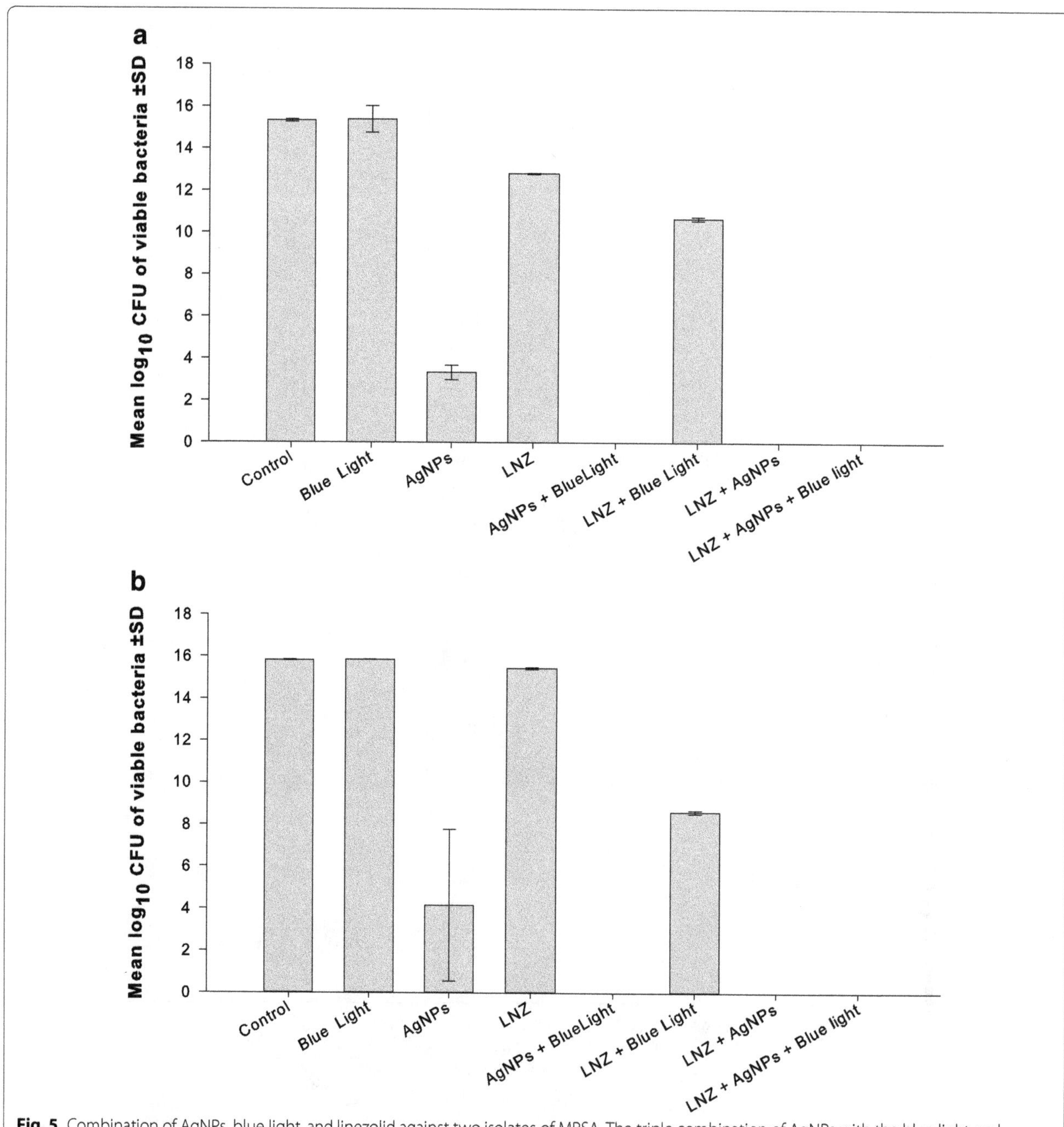

Fig. 5 Combination of AgNPs, blue light, and linezolid against two isolates of MRSA. The triple combination of AgNPs with the blue light and linezolid against two isolates of MRSA was assessed. The isolates were selected on the basis of synergistic response in checkerboard assay. Based on the best result of the combination in the checkerboard assay, the concentrations of the two agents were used as follow: **a** Isolate C19: AgNPs at 1/2 of the MIC, and azithromycin at 0.25 µg/mL. **b** Isolate N5: AgNPs at 1/2 of the MIC, and azithromycin at 8 µg/mL. *AgNPs* silver nanoparticles, *CFU* colony forming unit, *LNZ* linezolid, *SD* standard deviation

healthcare-associated and community-onset infections [26]. MRSA and coagulase-negative staphylococci are among the leading causes of nosocomial blood stream infections in the USA [27]. Staphylococci cause biofilm-associated infections by forming biofilms on damaged tissues, and indwelling vascular catheters [28–32].

Five antibiotics were selected from different conventional classes including beta-lactam (amoxicillin), macrolides (azithromycin and clarithromycin), oxazolidinones (linezolid), and glycopeptides (vancomycin). Based on the European Committee on Antimicrobial Susceptibility Testing (EUCAST) MIC breakpoint guideline

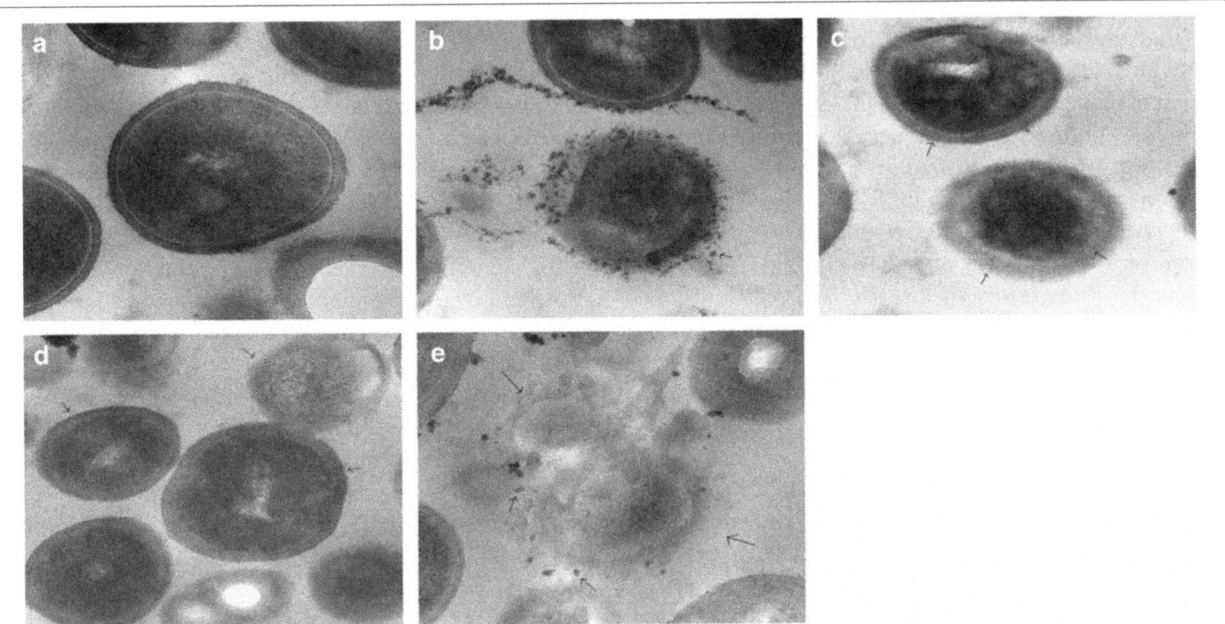

Fig. 6 Visualization of the effect of combination of AgNPs, blue light, and azithromycin on MRSA isolate N8 using transmission electron microscope (TEM). The antimicrobial efficacy of the AgNPs at 1/16 MIC, blue light and azithromycin at 0.25 μg/mL alone and in triple combination against isolate N8 was visualized by TEM at ×80,000. The photos show the response of the bacteria to the following treatments: **a** Drug-free and light-free (control). **b** AgNPs alone at 1/16 of its MIC. **c** Blue light exposure at 460 nm and 250 mW for 1 h. **d** Azithromycin alone at 0.25 μg/mL. **e** Triple combination of AgNPs, blue light and the azithromycin. Signs of membrane damage and cell lysis were more pronounced in cells treated with a combination of three agents compared to cells treated with each agent alone. *Small arrows* indicate the location of the AgNPs and the sites of the damage

[33], all isolates were found to be resistant to amoxicillin, azithromycin, clarithromycin, and linezolid, while they were susceptible to vancomycin (Table 2). With few exceptions, MRSA isolates are resistant to all beta-lactam antibiotics and commonly resistant to macrolides, with very rare resistance to glycopeptides antibiotics [33, 34]. Emergence of linezolid-resistance was previously reported in 0.05 % of *S. aureus* infections [35]. Antibiotics that are known to be ineffective against MRSA were used in this study to assess the possibility of enhancement of their antimicrobial activity by AgNPs and the blue light. This approach would be useful in "recycling" of these antibiotics that became useless against infections caused by MRSA to face the fast-growing drug-resistance with the slow development of new antimicrobial agents, and to preserve last resort antibiotics such as vancomycin.

Blue light has attracted increasing attention because of its intrinsic antimicrobial effect which does not involve the use of exogenous photosensitizers as in the photodynamic therapy (PDT), and the less damaging to mammalian cells than ultraviolet irradiation [13]. The biomedical applications of blue light at specific wavelengths and intensities against different pathogens have been reported earlier [36]. At 470 nm blue light was found to be efficient against MRSA strains associated with hospital-acquired and community-onset infections [37].

Double combinations of the AgNPs, at 1/2–1/128 of its MIC, with blue light were tested against selected MRSA isolates. The bactericidal activity of both agents was significantly enhanced ($p < 0.001$) when bacteria were treated with AgNPs with concurrent exposure to blue light for 1 h, compared to each of them alone (Fig. 1a–e). The combined therapy killed all bacteria after 8 h in all tested combinations while each of the silver compound and the blue light was less efficient in killing the organisms during the tested time. The mechanism of the antimicrobial effect of either AgNPs or blue light is still not fully understood. Several hypotheses have been suggested to explain such mechanisms. For example, it has been reported that AgNPs can damage bacterial cell membranes leading to structural changes, which render bacteria more permeable [38, 39]. AgNPs have unique optical, electrical, and thermal properties with high surface area to volume ratio resulting in the optimal possible interaction with bacterial surfaces leading to a higher antimicrobial activity [40]. The formation of free radicals by the silver nanoparticles is probably another mechanism that can lead to cell death [41, 42]. It has also been proposed that cationic silver is released from the nanoparticles when they are dissolved in water or when they penetrate into the cells [5]. Silver ions bind to the cellular membranes, proteins, and nucleic acids, causing structural changes and deformations of the bacterial cell [5]. They also deactivate many vital enzymes by interaction with thiol groups [31] and are involved in the generation of reactive oxygen species [32].

For blue light, the commonly accepted hypothesis is the production of highly cytotoxic reactive oxygen species (ROS) in a similar manner to PDT [43].

We have previously reported a similar synergistic interaction for a combination of AgNPs and blue light when both agents were tested against clinical isolates of *Pseudomonas aeruginosa* [44]. A possible mechanism of the observed synergy could be the transduction of the captured blue-light energy by blue light sensory proteins to the AgNPs resulting in the thermal destruction of the bacterial cells [45, 46].

Double combination of the AgNPs with five conventional antibiotics against the ten MRSA clinical isolates was investigated using checkerboard assay. Synergistic interactions were observed when the AgNPs were used with amoxicillin, azithromycin, clarithromycin or linezolid in 30–40 % of the combinations (Fig. 2). Other combinational activities were indifferent with no observed antagonistic interaction. Combination of the AgNPs with vancomycin, on the other hand, was indifferent against all isolates. Synergistic interactions between AgNPs and conventional antibiotics against different pathogens were previously reported. Ruden et al. [47] found synergistic interaction when AgNPs were combined with polymyxin B against gram-negative bacteria. Combination of AgNPs with ampicillin, chloramphenicol, and kanamycin against gram-positive and -negative pathogenic bacteria was also found to be synergistic [48]. Similarly, Smekalova et al. [49] observed synergistic effect when AgNPs were combined with penicillin G, gentamycin, and colistin against MDR bacteria.

Reversion of MRSA resistance to ineffective antibiotics by combination with AgNPs could be a novel strategy to combat infections caused by MDR pathogens. Biocompatible gold nanoparticles-amoxicillin complex was found to overcome the resistance of MRSA to the antibiotic [50]. The synergistic response of combination of AgNPs and ineffective antibiotics is probably due to an increase of the concentration of antibiotics at the site of bacterium–antibiotic interaction, and to facilitate binding of antibiotics to bacteria [51].

AgNPs combined with amoxicillin, azithromycin, clarithromycin or linezolid were tested against selected MRSA isolates with concurrent exposure to blue light for 1 h. The isolates were selected based on synergistic response, where they were most affected by the previous double combinations in the checkerboard assay. The antimicrobial activity of the three agents was significantly ($p > 0.001$) enhanced in the triple combinations compared to single- and double treatments with one or two of them. The bactericidal activity was more pronounced when azithromycin or clarithromycin was included in the triple therapy (Figs. 3, 4). The antimicrobial efficiency was also enhanced when linezolid (Fig. 5) or amoxicillin (data not shown) was included but with the same bactericidal effect in double and triple combinations.

The synergy observed in triple therapy might be explained by the combined mechanism of action of each agent alone, and the enhanced outcomes in their double combinations.

TEM images of isolate N8 that has been exposed to triple therapy (AgNPs, blue light and azithromycin) support the aforementioned suggestion that bacterial cell damage by the triple combination was more pronounced compared to the cells that were treated with each agent alone (Fig. 6a–e).

Conclusions

This study suggests a new strategy to combat serious infections caused by MDR bacteria. The triple combination of AgNPs, blue light, and antibiotics is a promising therapy for infections caused by MRSA. The triple therapy may include antibiotics, which are proven to be ineffective against MRSA. This approach would be useful to face the fast-growing drug-resistance with the slow development of new antimicrobial agents, and to preserve last resort antibiotics such as vancomycin. The study can be taken further by exploring the application of the triple therapy in patients infected with MRSA and other MDR bacteria, taking into consideration the best conditions for optimizing their synergistic effects and decreasing the harmful side effect.

Abbreviations

AgNPs: silver nano particles; AMX: amoxicillin; AZM: azithromycin; CFU/mL: colony forming units per milliliter; CLR: clarithromycin; CLSI: Clinical Laboratory Standard Institute; EUCAST: European Committee on Antimicrobial Susceptibility Testing; FIC: Fraction Inhibitory Index; LNZ: linezolid; MBC: minimum bactericidal concentration; MDR: multi-drug resistant; MHB: Mueller Hinton Broth; MIC: minimum inhibitory concentration; MLST: multiple locus sequence typing; MRSA: methicillin-resistant *Staphylococcus aureus*; mg/L: milligram per liter; mW: milliwatt; OXA: oxacillin; PDT: photodynamic therapy; PVP: polyvinylpyrrolidone; ROS: reactive oxygen species; TEM: transmission electron microscope; VAN: vancomycin.

Authors' contributions

FA performed the experimental work; TE prepared the nanomaterials, KA analyzed the results, guided FA for the experimental work and revised the final manuscript, ME designed the experiments, guided FA for the experimental work, generating the first draft, and finalized the manuscript. All authors read and approved the final manuscript.

Author details
[1] Department of Microbiology, Immunology, and Biotechnology, German University in Cairo, GUC, New Cairo City, Cairo, Egypt. [2] National Institute for Laser Enhanced Sciences, Cairo University, Cairo, Egypt.

Competing interests
The authors declare that they have no competing interests.

The authors declare that they did not have any funding source or grant to support their research work.

The authors declare that the research work has been approved by their university ethics committees, although it doesn't involve human subject or samples.

References

1. Chambers HF, DeLeo FR. Waves of resistance: *Staphylococcus aureus* in the antibiotic era. Nat Rev Microbiol. 2009;7(9):629–41.
2. Franklin DL. Antimicrobial resistance: the example of *Staphylococcus aureus*. J Clin Invest. 2003;111(9):1265–73.
3. Enright MC, Robinson DA, Randle G, Feil EJ, Grundmann H, Spratt BG. The evolutionary history of methicillin-resistant *Staphylococcus aureus* (MRSA). Proc Natl Acad Sci USA. 2002;99(11):7687–92.
4. Lara HH, Garza-Treviño EN, Ixtepan-Turrent L, Singh DK. Silver nanoparticles are broad-spectrum bactericidal and virucidal compounds. J Nanobiotechnology. 2011;9:30.
5. Franci G, Falanga A, Galdiero S, Palomba L, Rai M, Morelli G, Galdiero M. Silver nanoparticles as potential antibacterial agents. Molecules. 2015;20:8856–74.
6. Nowack B, Krug H, Height M. 120 years of nanosilver history: 609 implications for policy makers. Environ Sci Technol. 2011;45(4):1177–83.
7. Bogumiła R, Andrea H, Andreas L, Kenneth AD, Iseult L. Mechanisms of silver nanoparticle release, transformation and toxicity: a critical review of current knowledge and recommendations for future studies and applications. Materials. 2013;6:2295–350.
8. Ansari M, Khan H, Khan A, Malik A, Sultan A, Shahid M, et al. Evaluation of antibacterial activity of silver nanoparticles against MSSA and MRSA on isolates from skin infections. Biol Med. 2011;3(2):141–6.
9. Paredes D, Ortiz C, Torres R. Synthesis, characterization, and evaluation of antibacterial effect of Ag nanoparticles against *Escherichia coli* O157:H7 and methicillin-resistant *Staphylococcus aureus* (MRSA). Int J Nanomedicine. 2014;9:1717–29.
10. Abdel Rahim KA, Mohamed AM. Bactericidal and antibiotic synergistic effect of nanosilver against methicillin-resistant *Staphylococcus aureus*. Jundishapur J Microbiol. 2015;8(11):e25867.
11. Vrcek IV, Zuntar I, Petlevski R, Pavicic I, Dutour SM, Culin M, et al. Comparison of in vitro toxicity of silver ions and silver nanoparticles on human hepatoma cells. Environ Toxicol. 2016;31(6):679–92.
12. D'Britto V, Kapse H, Babrekar H, Pabhune AA, Bhoraskar SV, Premnath V, et al. Silver nanoparticle studded porous polyethylene scaffolds: bacteria struggle to grow on them while mammalian cells thrive. Nanoscale. 2011;3(7):2957–63.
13. Tianhong D, Asheesh G, Clinton KM, Mark SV, George PT, Michael RH. Blue light for infectious diseases: *Propionibacterium acnes, Helicobacter pylori*, and beyond. Drug Resist Updat. 2012;15(4):223–36.
14. Maclean M, McKenzie K, Anderson JG, Gettinby G, MacGregor SJ. 405 nm light technology for the inactivation of pathogens and its potential role for environmental disinfection and infection control. J Hosp Infect. 2014;88(1):1–11.
15. Enwemeka CS, Williams D, Enwemeka SK, Hollosi S, Yens D. Blue 470-nm light kills methicillin-resistant *Staphylococcus aureus* (MRSA) in vitro. Photomed Laser Surg. 2009;27(2):221–6.
16. Halstead FD, Thwaite JE, Burt R, Laws TR, Raguse M, Moeller R, et al. Antibacterial activity of blue light against nosocomial wound pathogens growing planktonically and as mature biofilms. Appl Environ Microbiol. 2016;82(13):4006–40016.
17. Jonas D, Grundmann H, Hartung D, Daschner FD, Towner KJ. Evaluation of the *mecA femB* duplex polymerase chain reaction for detection of methicillin resistant *Staphylococcus aureus*. Eur J Clin Microbiol Infect Dis. 1999;18(9):643–7.
18. Kapoor S. Preparation, characterization, and surface modification of silver particles. Langmuir. 1998;14(5):1021–5.
19. Clinical and Laboratory Standards Institute (CLSI): methods for dilution antimicrobial susceptibility tests for bacteria that grow aerobically—approved standards-seventh edition, in CLSI document M7-A7 2002, vol. 26 No. 2, Pennsylvania. p. 16–18.
20. Winston DJ, Ho WG, Bruckner DA, Champlin RE. Beta-lactam antibiotic therapy in febrile granulocytopenic patients. A randomized trial comparing cefoperazone plus piperacillin, ceftazidime plus piperacillin, and imipenem alone. Ann Intern Med. 1991;115(11):849–59.
21. Dykstra MJ, Reuss E. Biological electron microscopy theory, techniques and troubleshooting. 2nd ed. Berlin: Springer; 2003.
22. Gould SW, Cuschieri P, Rollason J, Hilton AC, Easmon S, Fielder MD. The need for continued monitoring of antibiotic resistance patterns in clinical isolates of *Staphylococcus aureus* from London and Malta. Ann Clin Microbiol Antimicrob. 2010;9:20.
23. Filice GA, Nyman JA, Lexau C, Lees CH, Bockstedt LA, Como-Sabetti K, et al. Excess costs and utilization associated with methicillin resistance for patients with *Staphylococcus aureus* infection. Infect Control Hosp Epidemiol. 2010;31(4):365–73.
24. Mauldin PD, Salgado CD, Hansen IS, Durup DT, Bosso JA. Attributable hospital cost and length of stay associated with healthcare-associated infections caused by antibiotic-resistant gram-negative bacteria. Antimicrob Agents Chemother. 2010;54(1):109–15.
25. Choi O, Hu Z. Size dependent and reactive oxygen species related nanosilver toxicity to nitrifying bacteria. Environ Sci Technol. 2008;42:4583–8.
26. von Eiff C, Heilmann C, Herrmann M, Peters G. Basic aspects of the pathogenesis of staphylococcal polymer associated infections. Infection. 1999;27(Suppl 1):S7–10.
27. Lowy FD. *Staphylococcus aureus infections*. N Engl J Med. 1998;339:520–32.
28. Khardori N, Yassien M, Wilson K. Tolerance of *Staphylococcus epidermidis* grown from indwelling vascular catheters to antimicrobial agents. J Ind Microbiol. 1995;15:148–51.
29. Costerton JW. Introduction to biofilm. Int J Antimicrob Agents. 1999;11:217–21.
30. Costerton JW, Stewart PS, Greenberg EP. Bacterial biofilms: a common cause of persistent infections. Science. 1999;284(5418):1318–22.
31. Gross M, Cramton SE, Götz F, Peschel A. Key role of teichoic acid net charge in *Staphylococcus aureus* colonization of artificial surfaces. Infect Immun. 2001;69:3423–6.
32. Donlan RM, Costerton JW. Biofilms: survival mechanisms of clinically relevant microorganisms. Clin Microbiol Rev. 2002;15:167–93.
33. The European Committee on Antimicrobial Susceptibility Testing (EUCAST): breakpoint tables for interpretation of MICs and zone diameters. Version 5.0. 2015. http://www.eucast.org. Accessed 3 Nov 2015
34. Gorwitz RJ, Jernigan DB, Powers JH, Jernigan JA. Participants in the CDC convened experts meeting on management of MRSA in the community. strategies for clinical management of MRSA in the community: summary of an experts' meeting convened by the centers for disease control and prevention. 2006.
35. Gu B, Kelesidis T, Tsiodras S, Hindler J, Humphries RM. The emerging problem of linezolid-resistant *Staphylococcus*. J Antimicrob Chemother. 2013;68(1):4–11.
36. Guffey JS, Wilborn J. Effects of combined 405-nm and 880-nm light on *Staphylococcus aureus* and *Pseudomonas aeruginosa* in vitro. Photomed Laser Surg. 2006;24(6):680–3.
37. Enwemeka CS, Williams D, Enwemeka SK, Hollosi S, Yens D. Blue 470-nm light kills methicillin-resistant *Staphylococcus aureus* (MRSA) *in vitro*. Photomed Laser Surg. 2008;27(2):221–6.
38. Lazar V. Quorum sensing in biofilms—how to destroy the bacterial citadels or their cohesion power? Anaerobe. 2011;17:280–5.
39. Periasamy S, Joo HS, Duong AC, Bach TH, Tan VY, Chatterjee SS, et al. How *Staphylococcus aureus* biofilms develop their characteristic structure. Proc Natl Acad Sci USA. 2012;109:1281–6.
40. Morones JR, Elechiguerra JL, Camacho A, Ramirez JT. The bactericidal effect of silver nanoparticles. Nanotechnology. 2005;16:2346.
41. Danilcauk M, Lund A, Saldo J, Yamada H, Michalik J. Conduction electron spin resonance of small silver particles. Spectrochim Acta Part A Mol Biomol Spectrosc. 2006;63:189–91.

42. Kim JS, Kuk E, Yu K, Kim JH, Park SJ, Lee HJ, et al. Antimicrobial effects of silver nanoparticles. Nanomedicine. 2007;3:95–101.
43. Maclean M, Macgregor SJ, Anderson JG, Woolsey GA. The role of oxygen in the visible-light inactivation of *Staphylococcus aureus*. J Photochem Photobiol B. 2008;92(3):180–4.
44. Nour ES, El-Tayeb TA, Abou-Aisha K, El-Azizi M. In vitro and in vivo antimicrobial activity of combined therapy of silver nanoparticles and visible blue light against *Pseudomonas aeruginosa*. Int J Nanomedicine. 2016;11:1749–58.
45. Wu L, McGrane RS, Beattie GA. Light regulation of swarming motility in *Pseudomonas syringae* integrates signaling pathways mediated by a bacteriophytochrome and a LOV protein. MBio. 2013;4(3):e00334.
46. Barkovits K, Schubert B, Heine S, Scheer M, Frankenberg-Dinkel N. Function of the bacteriophytochrome *BphP* in the *RpoS/Las* quorum sensing network of *Pseudomonas aeruginosa*. Microbiology. 2011;157(Pt 6):1651–64.
47. Ruden S, Hilpert K, Berditsch M, Wadhwani P, Ulrich AS. Synergistic interaction between silver nanoparticles and membrane-permeabilizing antimicrobial peptides. Antimicrob Agents Chemother. 2009;53(8):3538–40.
48. Hwang IS, Hwang JH, Choi H, Kim KJ, Lee DG. Synergistic effects between silver nanoparticles and antibiotics and the mechanisms involved. J Med Microbiol. 2012;61:1719–26.
49. Smekalova M, Aragon V, Panacek A, Prucek R, Zboril R, Kvitek L. Enhanced antibacterial effect of antibiotics in combination with silver nanoparticles against animal pathogens. Vet J. 2015;209:174–9.
50. Kalita S, Kandimalla R, Sharma KK, Kataki AC, Deka M, Kotoky J. Amoxicillin functionalized gold nanoparticles reverts MRSA resistance. Mater Sci Eng C Mater Biol Appl. 2016;61:720–7.
51. Allahverdiyev AM, Kon KV, Abamor ES, Bagirova M, Rafailovich M. Coping with antibiotic resistance: combining nanoparticles with antibiotics and other antimicrobial agents. Expert Rev Anti Infect Ther. 2011;9(11):1035–52.

15

Higher atypical enteropathogenic *Escherichia coli* (a-EPEC) bacterial loads in children with diarrhea are associated with PCR detection of the EHEC factor for adherence 1/lymphocyte inhibitory factor A (*efa1/lifa*) gene

Robert Slinger[2*], Kimberley Lau[1], Michael Slinger[2], Ioana Moldovan[2] and Francis Chan[2]

Abstract

Background: Typical enteropathogenic *Escherichia coli* (t-EPEC) are known to cause diarrhea in children but it is uncertain whether atypical EPEC (a-EPEC) do, since a-EPEC lack the bundle-forming pilus (*bfp*) gene that encodes a key adherence factor in t-EPEC. In culture-based studies of a-EPEC, the presence of another adherence factor, called EHEC factor for adherence/lymphocyte activation inhibitor (*efa1/lifA*), was strongly associated with diarrhea. Since a-EPEC culture is not feasible in clinical laboratories, we designed an *efa1/lifA* quantitative PCR assay and examined whether the presence of *efa1/lifA* was associated with higher a-EPEC bacterial loads in pediatric diarrheal stool samples.

Methods: Fecal samples from children with diarrhea were tested by qPCR for EPEC (presence of *eae* gene) and for shiga toxin genes to exclude enterohemorrhagic *E. coli,* which also contain the *eae* gene. EPEC containing samples were then tested for the bundle-forming pilus gene found in t-EPEC and *efa1/lifA*. The *eae* gene quantity in *efa1/lifA*-positive and negative samples was compared.

Results: Thirty-nine of 320 (12%) fecal samples tested positive for EPEC and 38/39 (97%) contained a-EPEC. The *efa1/lifA* gene was detected in 16/38 (42%) a-EPEC samples. The median *eae* concentration for *efa1/lifA* positive samples was significantly higher than for *efa1/lifA* negative samples (median 16,745 vs. 1183 copies/μL, respectively, $p = 0.006$).

Conclusions: Atypical enteropathogenic *E. coli*-positive diarrheal stool samples containing the *efa1/lifA* gene had significantly higher bacterial loads than samples lacking this gene. This supports the idea that *efa1/lifA* contributes to diarrheal pathogenesis and suggests that, in EPEC-positive samples, *efa/lifA* may be a useful additional molecular biomarker.

Keywords: Enteropathogenic *Escherichia coli*, Diarrhea, Real-time PCR, Gastroenteritis

*Correspondence: slinger@cheo.on.ca
[2] Department of Laboratory Medicine and Pathology, Children's Hospital of Eastern Ontario, University of Ottawa, 401 Smyth Rd, Ottawa, ON K1H 8L1, Canada
Full list of author information is available at the end of the article

Background

Enteropathogenic *Escherichia coli* (EPEC) is not detected with the standard stool culture methods used in clinical laboratories for bacterial pathogens, so its relative importance as a cause of diarrhea in children has been uncertain in the past [1]. With the recent increased use of molecular detection methods, however, EPEC has been found to be the most frequently detected bacterium in patients with diarrhea in developed countries [2, 3].

However, not all EPEC strains have the same ability to cause diarrhea. All EPEC and enterohemorrhagic *E. coli* (EHEC) contain the chromosomal *E. coli* attaching and effacing (*eae*) gene that encodes an outer membrane protein called intimin. Intimin mediates attachment to epithelial cells and leads to the attaching and effacing phenotype. EPEC can be differentiated from EHEC by the absence of the shiga toxin (*stx*) genes that are found in EHEC. EPEC is further classified into typical and atypical strains based on the presence or absence of the *E. coli* adherence factor containing the bundle-forming pilus (*bfp*) gene. EPEC containing the *bfp* gene are classified as typical EPEC (t-EPEC) [1]. Strains lacking *bfp* are classified as atypical EPEC (a-EPEC).

Typical enteropathogenic *E. coli* is accepted as a diarrhea pathogen, but the pathogenicity of a-EPEC is controversial. Some studies have shown an association with a-EPEC and diarrhea while others have not. In addition, a-EPEC can be found in asymptomatic children [4–6]. Diarrhea was seen in volunteers who ingested a-EPEC but to a lesser degree than in those who ingested t-EPEC [7, 8]. This controversy surrounding a-EPEC virulence has led to a search for additional gene markers in a-EPEC that might indicate pathogenicity. The *efa1/lifA* gene appears to be the leading virulence candidate. *Efa1/lifA* encodes for a large 385 kDa adhesion protein, called the EHEC factor for adherence (*Efa1*) since it was first described in an EHEC 0157:H7 strain [9]. *Efa1* was found to be identical to the lymphocyte inhibitory factor A protein (*lifA*) gene that lymphostatin, which inhibits lymphocyte proliferation and lymphokine production. The designation *efa1/lifA* was therefore given to the gene.

In study of 182 possible virulence markers in a-EPEC cultured strains from Norwegian children, the *efa1/lifA* gene had the strongest statistical association with diarrhea [9]. *Efa1/lifA* was present in 30% of a-EPEC strains from children with diarrhea and no strains from children without diarrhea ($p = 0.0008$). In a later study from Japan, *efa1/lifA* was detected in 33% of a-EPEC strains in individuals with diarrhea and 13% of those in a healthy control group [10]. This difference was statistically significant ($p < 0.05$), and *efa1/lifA* was the only gene examined which was significantly associated with diarrhea.

These studies demonstrating the importance of *efa1/lifA* were performed using stool cultures for EPEC, but this is a labor-intensive process that is not feasible in clinical microbiology laboratories, since it requires isolating multiple *E. coli* colonies in each specimen and then testing these individually for the genes of interest. We therefore developed a direct fecal *efa1/lifA* real-time quantitative PCR (qPCR) method to determine what proportion of fecal specimens containing a-EPEC also contained *efa1/lifA*. We then examined whether a-EPEC bacterial loads were higher in children when *efa1/lifA*-containing a-EPEC was present. Our hypothesis was that since the quantity of EPEC in fecal samples as measured by qPCR is associated with disease severity, infection with *efa1/lifA*-containing strains of a-EPEC might lead to higher bacterial loads [11].

Of note, work to clarify the pathogenicity of a-EPEC has become more crucial in recent years since EPEC are now detected by a commercially available molecular diarrheal panel, the Biofire FilmArray gastrointestinal panel (Biomerieux, Durham, NC) [2, 3]. This panel detects the *eae* gene, but not *bfp* or *efa1/lifA*. Since a-EPEC is much more likely than t-EPEC to be present in developed countries, clinicians seeing children with diarrhea whose samples test positive for EPEC will face uncertainty as to whether the organism detected is the cause of the illness. Additional molecular biomarkers that are associated with a-EPEC pathogenicity rather than the presence of the *eae* gene alone may therefore be useful.

Methods

Study site and ethics approval

This was a prospective observational study performed in the months June–Aug 2010–2013 at the Children's Hospital of Eastern Ontario, Ottawa, ON Canada, a 165 bed tertiary care hospital serving a catchment area of 1.5 million. It was decided to collect samples in the summer months since a seasonal predominance increasing in these months has been described for both EPEC and EHEC [1, 5].

Ethics approval was obtained for the study from the hospital Research Ethics Board (CHEOREB # 12/194X). Residual aliquots of fecal samples submitted for bacterial stool culture from patients with diarrhea that would otherwise have been discarded were tested by PCR for the target bacterial genes described below. All samples submitted to the laboratory for bacterial stool culture over the study period were included in the study.

The results of bacterial stool culture were recorded. Fecal samples were saved at −80 °C until nucleic acid extraction was performed. All patients were ≤18 years of age. According to the ethics approval received, in order to ensure patient anonymity, we did not record patient age or gender.

Outcome measures

Our main outcome measure was the difference, if any, in a-EPEC bacterial load in *efa1/lifA* positive vs. negative samples. The secondary outcome measures were the prevalence of a-EPEC and t-EPEC in fecal samples; the prevalence of *efa1/lifA* in samples in which a-EPEC was detected; and a comparison of EPEC prevalence to the prevalence of bacterial pathogens detected by culture.

Laboratory methods

Culture methods

Fecal samples were collected in Cary-Blair enteric transport medium. Samples were inoculated onto Blood agar plate, MacConkey agar plate, Hektoen enteric agar plate, Sorbitol MacConkey agar plate, *Campylobacter* agar plate and Selenite broth. The *Campylobacter* plate was placed in a microaerophilic environment at 42 °C. Other media were incubated in ambient air at 35 °C. After overnight incubation, the selenite broth was subcultured onto a Hektoen plate. Plates were examined for *Salmonella* species (spp.), *Shigella* spp., *Campylobacter* spp., *Yersinia enterocolitica, E. coli* 0157:H7, *Aeromonas* spp. *Plesiomonas shigelloides* and *Vibrio* spp. Possible pathogens were identified using standard laboratory methods [12].

PCR methods

DNA was extracted from fecal specimens using automated device (iPrep, Life Technologies, Carlsbad, CA). Extracted DNA was then treated to remove fecal PCR inhibitors using a commercial method (Zymo-Spin™ IV-μHRC Spin Filter Zymo Research, Irvine, CA).

Primer and 5′ exonuclease probe sequences for the study assays (*eae, stx*1, *stx*2, *bfp* and *efa1/lifA)* are shown in Table 1. The *efa1/lifA* assay was designed for this study while other assays had been previously published. *Efa1/lifA* assay design was performed using a commercial qPCR program (Allele ID, Premier Biosoft, Palo Alto CA). The limit of detection of the assay was measured by duplicate testing of 10-fold serial dilutions of a synthetic oligonucleotide target sequence (Ultramer, IDT, Coralville, IA).

Probe and primer specificity were checked using Basic Local Alignment Search Tool (BLAST) sequence searches and by testing the assay against the following bacterial organisms: *Streptococcus pneumoniae* American type culture collection (ATCC) 49,619, *Streptococcus salivarius* ATCC 13,419 *Escherichia coli* ATCC 25,922, *Haemophilus influenzae* ATCC 49,766, *H. influenzae* ATCC 49,247, *H. parainfluenzae* ATCC 7901, *Klebsiella pneumoniae* ATCC 700,603, *Moraxella catarrhalis* ATCC 25,238, *Staphylococcus aureus* ATCC 29,247, *Neisseria gonorrhoeae* ATCC 49,226, *N. lactamica* ATCC 23,970, *Pseudomonas aeruginosa* ATCC 27,853, *Enterococcus faecalis* ATCC 29,212, *S. dysgalactiae* subsp. *equisimilis, S. agalactiae* (Group B Streptococcus), *S. intermedius, S. constellatus,* and *S. anginosus.*

QPCR was performed on all samples for the *eae* gene and for the *stx*-1 and *stx*-2 genes to exclude EHEC [12, 14, 15]. *Eae*-positive; *stx*-negative samples were then tested for the *bfp* gene to differentiate t-EPEC and a-EPEC and for the *efa1/lifA* gene. Probes were of the 5-prime exonuclease type and were labelled with fluorescein amidite. Four probes were obtained from IDT (Coralville, IA) and contained an internal quencher as well as a 3-prime end quencher. One probe contained a minor groove binder and no internal quencher and was obtained from Life Technologies (Carlsbad, CA).

PCR assays were prepared in 20 μL volumes in 96-well qPCR plate. Positive and negative controls (no template) were performed with each qPCR plate run. QPCR plates were covered with MicroAmp® Optical Adhesive Film (Life Technologies Carlsbad, CA) to prevent cross-contamination. QPCR was performed with a 96 well fast cycling block on a ViiA7 thermocyler (Life Technologies) using 40 cycles of 2-temperature thermocyling (95 °C × 3 s and 60 °C × 30 s). QPCR was considered positive for the *eae, stx*1, *stx*2, and *efa1/lifA* genes if the cycle threshold value was ≤35 cycles and for the *bfp* gene if the cycle threshold value was ≤30 cycles. Specimens

Table 1 Gene targets PCR primer and probe sequences

Target gene/symbol	Forward primer	Reverse primer	Probe	Reference
Intimin (*eae*)	cattgatcaggatttttctggtgata	ctcatgcggaaatagccgtta	atagtctcgccagtattcgccaccaatacc	[11]
Shiga toxin 1(*stx*1)	gtggcattaatactgaattgtcatca	gcgtaatcccacggactcttc	tctgccggacacatag (MGB)	[12][a]
Shiga toxin 2 (*stx*2)	gggcagttattttgctgtgga	tgttgccgtattaacgaaccc	ctatcaggcgcgttttgaccatcttcg	[13]
Bundle-forming pilus (*bfp*)	gcatcattccgttgttgg	ggaccatgtattatcaaaaacctg	ccgccttctgacaagctgtgttgg	[14]
EHEC factor for adherence 1/lymphocyte inhibitory factor A (*efa1/lifA*)	tcacaccagaattattacgtcacaca	atggtagtcaggtatacatccgtatttc	accggcacaatactccagactccagaaga	This study

MGB minor groove binder

[a] Modified from published

were classified as containing EPEC if they were *eae*- positive and *stx*-negative, and then as t-EPEC (*bfp*-positive) or a-EPEC (*bfp*-negative). A-EPEC samples were further classified as being *efa1/lifA*-positive or negative.

Results

The limit of detection for the *efa1/lifA* assay was approximately 6 copies/PCR reaction. In comparison, the detection limit for the *eae* assay was one log higher at 60 copies/reaction. There was no cross-reactivity observed for the *efa1/lifA* assay with the non-*E. coli* bacterial species tested.

Three-hundred twenty fecal diarrheal samples were tested. The PCR and culture results are shown in Table 2. Thirty-nine of 320 (12%) fecal samples tested were found to have the EPEC marker profile (*eae*-positive, *stx*-negative). Of these EPEC samples, 38/39 (97%) were a-EPEC (*bfp*-negative), with only one t-EPEC (*bfp*-positive).

The *efa1/lifA* gene was detected in 16/38 (42%) a-EPEC samples. The median *eae* concentration in these samples was 16,745 copies/μL (range 26–3152,879 copies/μL). For the 22 *efa1/lifA*-negative a-EPEC samples, the median *eae* concentration was 1183 copies/μL (range 9–338,770 copies/μL). The difference in median copies/μL between the two groups was statistically significant ($p = 0.006$, Wilcoxon two-sample test two-sided).

Bacterial cultures were positive in 27/320 samples (8.4%), with 28 organisms detected in total. Other bacterial pathogens were detected in 4/38 (10%) a-EPEC-positive samples. The most common single bacterial type identified by culture was *Salmonella* spp., found in 13/320 (4%) samples. Only 1 EHEC (an *E. coli* O157:H7) was detected by culture, while one or both *stx* genes were detected by qPCR in five samples, including the one culture-positive sample.

Discussion

Our findings show that EPEC genes were present with relatively high frequency in fecal samples submitted for bacterial culture from children with diarrhea in Ontario, Canada. EPEC genes were detected in more samples than the most prevalent pathogen detected by stool culture, *Salmonella* spp. (12 vs. 4%, respectively). This relatively high rate of detection of EPEC in developed country settings when molecular testing is used has also been reported by others. For example, in a study of daycare attendees in the Netherlands using a qPCR method, EPEC was detected in 19.9% of stool samples [6]. Investigators using the Biofire Film Array GI panel (biomerieux) reported detecting eae in 15% of diarrheal samples in a European multicenter study and 29.49% of samples in a US study [2, 3]. The proportions of t-EPEC and a-EPEC were not stated in either study (the *bfp* gene is not included in the Biofire panel), but most are likely to have been a-EPEC, given the low prevalence of t-EPEC in developed countries [1].

However, as discussed previously, it remains uncertain whether a-EPEC caused the diarrhea seen in these patients. Other pathogens may have been present in our patients that were not detected by bacterial stool cultures performed. It is also possible that a-EPEC may be able to grow better in the diarrheic environment created by other organisms, but is not contributing to disease.

Volunteer studies have been performed to examine a-EPEC pathogenicity but the results of these studies

Table 2 PCR and culture results from diarrheal fecal samples

PCR	No. detected (%) n = 320
Eae positive	44 (14)
EPEC: *eae* positive/*stx*1 and *stx*2 negative	39 (12)
Atypical EPEC: *eae* positive/stx1 and *stx*2 negative/*bfp* negative	38 (12)
Typical EPEC: *eae* positive/*stx*1 and *stx*2 negative/*bfp* positive	1 (0.3)
EHEC: *eae* positive/*stx*1 or *stx*2 positive	5 (1.5)
eae positive/*stx* negative/*efa1/lifA* positive/*bfp* negative	16 (5)
eae positive/*stx* negative/*efa1/lifA* negative/*bfp* negative	22 (7)
Culture	
Salmonella spp.	13 (4)
Campylobacter spp.	5 (1.5)
Shigella spp.	3 (0.9)
Plesiomonas shigelloides	3 (0.9)
Yersinia enterocolitica	2 (0.6)
E. coli 0157:H7	1 (0.3)
Aeromonas spp.	1 (0.3)

Eae, E. coli attaching and effacing gene; *EPEC*, enteropathogenic *E. coli*; *stx*1, shigatoxin 1 gene; *stx*2, shigatoxin 2 gene; *bfp*, bundle-forming pilus gene; *EHEC*, enterohemorrhagic *E. coli*; *efa1/lifA*, EHEC factor for adherence 1/lymphocyte inhibitory factor A gene

were not conclusive. For example, diarrhea occurred in 9/10 volunteers who ingested a t-EPEC strain, but in 6/11 who ingested an a-EPEC strain [7]. In a second study, 11/13 adults developed diarrhea with t-EPEC ingestion, as compared to 5/30 who ingested *bfp*-negative mutant strains. Thus, strains lacking *bfp* show reduced virulence in adults [8]. However, interpreting these studies in the pediatric setting is difficult since these adult volunteers may have been exposed to EPEC strains earlier in life and developed some degree of immunity prior to the challenge study.

More recently, a strong statistical association between the presence of *efa1/lifA*-positive a-EPEC and the presence of diarrhea was noted in two studies, suggesting *efa1/lifA*-positive strains may be true diarrhea pathogens [9, 10]. Some research has been done that provides a biological basis for the contribution of *efa1/lifA* to a-EPEC pathogenicity. *Efa1/lifA* is known to be an adherence factor and, in a study by Badea, an *efa1/lifA* mutant EPEC was found to be significantly less adherent to epithelial cells than the parent *efa1/lifA*-positive strain. Additionally, human and rabbit hosts infected with an attaching and effacing (A/E) pathogens were found to produce antibodies to efa1 protein, and anti-efa1 antibodies reduced the adherence of *efa*-positive EPEC to epithelial cells [16]. These findings suggest that the *efa1/lifA* gene, in concert with the *eae* gene, may play a role in adherence of a-EPEC infections that could then lead to diarrhea.

We also observed that samples with *efa1/lifA* contained higher loads of a-EPEC (as measured by *eae* gene quantitation) than *efa1/lifA*-negative samples. Higher bacterial loads have been associated with occurrence of diarrhea in patients with a-EPEC, so our finding of this association between bacterial load and the presence of *efa1/lifA* suggests strains with *efa1/lifA* may be more pathogenic.

The source of a-EPEC detected in the gastrointestinal tract of children in our center is unknown. Interestingly, we detected over five times more samples with EPEC markers than EHEC markers (27 vs. 5), suggesting that children are exposed to a-EPEC than EHEC much more frequently in our region. A recent study reported that a-EPEC strains that have been associated with diarrhea were found frequently in chicken and chicken products, so it is possible that these foods may be one source of exposure [17].

There are several limitations to this pilot study that should be mentioned. First, samples from children without diarrhea were not tested, so the prevalence of a-EPEC or *efa1/lifA* in asymptomatic children in our region is unknown. As well, we studied samples collected over summer months, rather than year-round, so it is possible that the frequency of EPEC detection may have been different with sampling over the entire year. Our study also assumes that the genes detected by PCR belong to the same stool bacterium, rather than different bacterial strains. For example, stool samples positive for *eae* and *efa1/lifA* were assumed to contain an EPEC strain that possesses both genes. Another limitation is that PCR cannot differentiate live from dead bacteria. Thus, the detection EPEC genes could be due to dead bacteria that may have been ingested but perhaps killed during cooking. However, since methods to readily detect EPEC in culture in clinical laboratories are not available, molecular methods like PCR will likely be used as the method of choice for EPEC detection in clinical specimens, despite this drawback. Finally, we did not test fecal samples for viral or parasitic pathogens or for *Clostridium difficile.* Some children with EPEC detected may have had one of these micro-organisms in their fecal samples, which could suggest that EPEC may not have been the cause of the diarrhea in these cases. In future work, we plan to perform testing for these additional organisms as well as EPEC.

Our objective in the study was to assess whether *efa1/lifA* could be directly detected by qPCR in stool samples, and whether *efa1/lifA* status was related to bacterial load. We now hope to be able to perform a qPCR-based case–control study for a-EPEC and *efa1/lifA* that will deal with the limitations noted above.

Conclusion

Given our findings and previous reports regarding the significance of *efa1/lifA*, continued research into the role this gene plays in a-EPEC infection is needed. New volunteer studies comparing diarrheal symptoms in those ingesting *efa1/lifA*-positive and *efa1/lifA*-negative a-EPEC would be helpful. As noted, we hope to perform a case–control study in which *eae* and *efa1/lifA* will be examined and quantified by direct fecal qPCR in children with diarrhea and healthy controls.

As pointed out in a recent review, there are many other unanswered questions regarding EPEC [18], including the pathogenicity of a-EPEC and the optimum antibiotic treatment, if any, for patients with diarrhea in whom EPEC is detected. Historically, t-EPEC diarrhea in infants has been treated with a variety of oral antibiotics, such as gentamicin and colistin, with reported success [19] but randomized controlled trials of antibiotic treatment have not been performed. For a-EPEC, no information is available regarding antibiotic treatment. Given the ongoing shift in clinical microbiology laboratories from culture methods that do not detect EPEC to molecular detection panels that do, there is a pressing need to address these questions to help guide patient care.

Abbreviations

EPEC: enteropathogenic *Escherichia coli*; t-EPEC: typical EPEC; a-EPEC: atypical EPEC; EHEC: enterohemorrhagic *E. coli*; *eae*: *E. coli* attaching and effacing; *stx*: shigatoxin; *bfp*: bundle-forming pilus; *efa1/lifA*: EHEC factor for adherence/lymphocyte inhibitory factor A; qPCR: real-time quantitative PCR; species: spp..

Authors' contributions

RS drafted the primary manuscript. NB performed statistical analyses. IM, FC, and RS contributed to study design. KL, MS, and IM participated in the performance of the laboratory testing and data analysis. All authors contributed to the preparation and revision of the manuscript. All authors read and approved the final manuscript.

Author details

[1] McMaster University, Hamilton, ON, Canada. [2] Department of Laboratory Medicine and Pathology, Children's Hospital of Eastern Ontario, University of Ottawa, 401 Smyth Rd, Ottawa, ON K1H 8L1, Canada.

Acknowledgements

None.

Competing interests

The authors declare that they have no competing interests.

Funding

University of Ottawa Pathology and Laboratory Medicine Research Fund.

References

1. Ochoa TJ, Contreras CA. Enteropathogenic escherichia coli infection in children. Curr Opin Infect Dis. 2011;24:478–83.
2. Spina A, Kerr KG, Cormican M, Barbut F, Eigentler A, Zerva L, et al. Spectrum of enteropathogens detected by the FilmArray GI panel in a multicentre study of community-acquired gastroenteritis. Clin Microbiol Infect. 2015;21:719–28.
3. Buss SN, Leber A, Chapin K, Fey PD, Bankowski MJ, Jones MK, et al. Multicenter evaluation of the biofire FilmArray gastrointestinal panel for etiologic diagnosis of infectious gastroenteritis. J Clin Microbiol. 2015;53:915–25.
4. Olesen B, Neimann J, Böttiger B, Ethelberg S, Schiellerup P, Jensen C, et al. Etiology of diarrhea in young children in Denmark: a case–control study. J Clin Microbiol. 2005;43:3636–41.
5. Cohen MB, Nataro JP, Bernstein DI, Hawkins J, Roberts N, Staat MA. Prevalence of diarrheagenic Escherichia coli in acute childhood enteritis: a prospective controlled study. J Pediatr. 2005;146:54–61.
6. Enserink R, Scholts R, Bruijning-Verhagen P, Duizer E, Vennema H, de Boer R, et al. High detection rates of enteropathogens in asymptomatic children attending day care. PLoS ONE. 2014;9:e89496.
7. Levine MM, Nataro JP, Karch H, Baldini MM, Kaper JB, Black RE, et al. The diarrheal response of humans to some classic serotypes of enteropathogenic *Escherichia coli* is dependent on a plasmid encoding an enteroadhesiveness factor. J Infect Dis. 1985;152:550–9.
8. Bieber D, Ramer SW, Wu CY, Murray WJ, Tobe T, Fernandez R, et al. Type IV pili, transient bacterial aggregates, and virulence of enteropathogenic *Escherichia coli*. Science. 1998;280:2114–8.
9. Afset JE, Bruant G, Brousseau R, Harel J, Anderssen E, Bevanger L, et al. Identification of virulence genes linked with diarrhea due to atypical enteropathogenic *Escherichia coli* by DNA microarray analysis and PCR. J Clin Microbiol. 2006;44:3703–11.
10. Narimatsu H, Ogata K, Makino Y, Ito K. Distribution of non-locus of enterocyte effacement pathogenic island-related genes in *Escherichia coli* carrying *eae* from patients with diarrhea and healthy individuals in Japan. J Clin Microbiol. 2010;48:4107–14.
11. Barletta F, Ochoa TJ, Mercado E, Ruiz J, Ecker L, Lopez G, et al. Quantitative real-time polymerase chain reaction for enteropathogenic *Escherichia coli*: a tool for investigation of asymptomatic versus symptomatic infections. Clin Infect Dis. 2011;53:1223–9.
12. Garcia L, editor. Clinical Microbiology Procedures Handbook. 3rd ed. Washington: American Society for Microbiology; 2010.
13. Jenkins C, Lawson AJ, Cheasty T, Willshaw GA. Assessment of a real-time PCR or the detection and characterization of verocytotoxigenic *Escherichia coli*. J Med Microbiol. 2012;61:1082–5.
14. Jinneman KC, Yoshitomi KJ, Weagant SD. Multiplex real-time PCR method to identify Shiga toxin genes *stx*1 and *stx*2 and *Escherichia coli* O157:H7/H- serotype. Appl Environ Microbiol. 2003;69:6327–33.
15. Sharma VK, Dean-Nystrom EA, Casey TA. Semi-automated fluorogenic PCR assays (TaqMan) for rapid detection of *Escherichia coli* O157:H7 and other shiga toxigenic E. coli. Mol Cell Probes. 1999;13:291–302.
16. Badea L, Doughty S, Nicholls L, Sloan J, Robins-Browne RM, Hartland EL. Contribution of *efa1/lifA* to the adherence of enteropathogenic *Escherichia coli* to epithelial cells. Microb Pathog. 2003;34:205–15.
17. Alonso MZ, Sanz ME, Irino K, Krüger A, Lucchesi PMA, Padola NL. Isolation of atypical enteropathogenic *Escherichia coli* from chicken and chicken-derived products. Brit Poultry Sci. 2016;57:161–4.
18. Donnenberg MS, Finlay BB. Combating enteropathogenic *Escherichia coli* (EPEC) infections: the way forward. Trends Microbiol. 2013;21:317–9.
19. South MA. Enteropathogenic *Escherichia coli* disease: new developments and perspectives. J Pediatr. 1971;79:1–11.

16

Smear positive pulmonary tuberculosis and associated factors among homeless individuals in Dessie and Debre Birhan towns, Northeast Ethiopia

Tsedale Semunigus[1], Belay Tessema[2], Setegn Eshetie[2*] and Feleke Moges[2]

Abstract

Background: Tuberculosis (TB) remains one of the globe's deadliest communicable diseases. The homeless individuals are at high risk to acquire TB and multi-drug resistant TB (MDR-TB), because of their poor living conditions and risky behaviors. Tuberculosis and MDR-TB in the homeless individuals can pose a risk to entire communities. However, the magnitude of the problem is not known in Ethiopia. Therefore, the aim of this study was to determine the prevalence and associated factors of smear positive pulmonary TB (PTB) and MDR-TB among homeless individuals in Dessie and Debre Birhan towns, Northeast Ethiopia.

Methods: A community based cross-sectional study design was conducted from September 2014 to June 2015. Using an active screening with cough of ≥2 weeks, 351 TB suspects homeless individuals were participated in this study. Data were collected by using pre-tested and structured questionnaire. Spot-morning-spot sputum sample was collected and examined for acid-fast bacilli (AFB) using fluorescence microscopy by Auramine O staining technique. All AFB positive sputum was further analyzed by GeneXpert for detection of *Mycobacterium tuberculosis* complex and rifampicin resistant gene. Univariate and multivariate logistic regressions were applied to identify factors associated with smear positive PTB and P value <0.05 was considered as statistically significant.

Results: The prevalence of smear positive PTB was 2.6 % (95 % CI 1.3–5) among TB suspect homeless individuals. Extrapolation of this study finding implies that there were 505 smear positive PTB per 100,000 homeless individuals. All smear positive PTB sputum specimens were further analyzed by GeneXpert assay, the assay confirmed that all were positive for MTBC but none were resistant to RIF or MDR. Smoking cigarette regularly for greater than 5 years (AOR 10.1, 95 % CI 1.1, 97.7), body mass index lower than 18.5 (AOR 6.9, 95 % CI 1.12, 41.1) and HIV infection (AOR 6.8, 95 % CI 1.1, 40.1) were significantly associated with smear positive PTB.

Conclusion: The prevalence of smear positive PTB among TB suspect homeless individuals was 2.6 %. Among smear positive PTB, prevalence of HIV co-infection was very high 5 (55.5 %). Smoking cigarette regularly for greater than 5 years, BMI lower than 18.5 and HIV infection were factors associated with smear positive PTB. Special emphasis is needed for homeless individuals to exert intensive effort to identify undetected TB cases to limit the circulation of the disease into the community.

Keywords: Homeless individuals, Tuberculosis, Associated factors, Northeast Ethiopia

*Correspondence: wolet03.2004@gmail.com
[2] School of Biomedical and Laboratory Sciences, Department of Medical Microbiology, University of Gondar, P.O. Box: 196, Gonder, Ethiopia
Full list of author information is available at the end of the article

Background

Tuberculosis (TB) is an airborne chronic infectious disease mainly caused by *Mycobacterium tuberculosis* (MTB). The tubercle bacilli are obligate aerobes; grow most successfully in areas of the body with lots of blood and oxygen and commonest point of entry into the body is via the lungs, pulmonary TB (PTB), but may also affect any organ or tissue outside of the lungs, extra pulmonary TB (EPTB) [1]. Tuberculosis is mostly transmitted by inhalation of infected droplet nuclei, which are discharged in the air when a person with untreated PTB coughs, sneezes, spits and sings [2]. Globally PTB accounts for 85 % of all TB cases; among them smear positive PTB comprises 75–80 %. Smear positive PTB is the most infectious and most likely transmit from human to human and the infection prevention and control programs are air borne precautions. Therefore, the identification of TB suspects (cough for 2 weeks and more duration) and screening them by examination of sputum allows discovering those who are transmitting the disease and to start early treatment [3].

Poverty, malnutrition, over-crowded or unsanitary living conditions, low socioeconomic status, drug abuse, cigarette smoking, alcoholism, close contact with active TB cases, human immunodeficiency virus/acquired immune deficiency syndrome (HIV/AIDS) and increasing numbers of homeless people are the greatest risk factors for the acquisition of active TB [1]. Homelessness is a global problem; an estimated one hundred million to one billion people are homeless worldwide [4]. Homelessness is becoming a common feature of cities and fast growing towns of the poor countries in Africa, mainly due to a very high increasing rate of rural–urban migration and poverty [5]. Similarly, homeless people are also increasingly encountered in different area of Ethiopian cities [6]. Because of poor living conditions and as they indulge in risky behaviors, homeless people are exposed to many communicable diseases [7]. The death rate among this group of people is about 4 times higher than the general population [8]. Homeless people are included in the high-risk classification for developing TB disease by Centers for Disease Control and prevention (CDC) as they suffer disproportionately from a variety of health problems and emergency shelters remain volatile TB transmission sites [9].

In addition, being homelessness are creating favorable conditions for the development and transmission of MDR-TB because these groups are hard-to-reach groups, poor diagnostic and treatment services, more likely to incomplete and inadequate TB treatment and poor management of the disease including infection control [10, 11]. Many homeless TB patients often could not regard their health as a high priority and may prioritize substance needs such as food, shelter and providing for any addiction [12]. Globally, PTB in homeless individuals is especially problematic because it may be highly contagious and can present as advanced disease with poor outcomes, including mortality [13].

Generally 72 % of domestic TB outbreaks investigated by CDC in the year 2002–2010 involved homelessness in developed countries [14]. Therefore, appropriate health interventions should be done for homeless individuals to reduce the adverse outcomes of these communicable diseases [15]. Currently, Ethiopia is working towards interrupting transmission of TB, and preventing the emergence and spread of MDR-TB in the general population. In spite of these efforts, the problem remained a continuous challenge in the country [16]. Although, homelessness is one of the greatest risk factors for the acquisition of TB, and homelessness is a problem in Ethiopian cities, tuberculosis prevalence and associated factors among homeless individuals in Ethiopia has not been well reported. Therefore the aim of this study was to determine smear positive pulmonary tuberculosis and associated factors among homeless individuals in Dessie and Debre Birhan towns, Northeast Ethiopia.

Methods

Study area, study design and study participants

A community based cross-sectional study was conducted in Dessie and Debre Birhan towns from September 2014 to June 2015. Homeless individuals, who were aged ≥15 years, and had cough of 2 weeks and more duration were included in the study, whereas those who were unable to produce sputum were excluded from the study.

Variables

Dependent variable

Smear positive PTB and MDR-TB.

Independent variable

Socio demographic factors: age, sex, marital status, religion, educational status. Behavioral factors: smoking, duration of smoking, alcohol drinking, duration of alcohol drinking, khat chewing, duration of khat chewing, drug using, duration of drug usage. Environmental factors: duration of being homeless, number of homeless individuals slept/live together in one restricted place, close contact with known TB patients, close contact with chronically cougher patients. Morbidity history and status: current TB suggestive symptoms, past TB history, past TB treatment starting, completion of TB treatment, body mass index (BMI), HIV infection.

Sample size determination and sampling technique

A total of 351 individuals were enrolled in the study using active screening strategies to identify PTB suspects. Approximately 1780 homeless individuals were screened during the study period for symptoms suggestive of TB, such as cough of 2 weeks or more duration according to the National TB manual [17]. Out of the total screened, 351/1780 (19.7 %) homeless individuals were having cough of $\geq$2 weeks duration, were included into the study.

Questionnaire

A structured and pre-tested questionnaire was completed by 4 trained data collectors (2 laboratory technologists and 2 nurses) by face-to-face interview. The questionnaire had four parts; socio demographic characteristics, behavioral characteristics, environmental factors and morbidity history and status of the study participants. A questionnaire was first developed in English and then translated into Amharic language for appropriateness and clarity so; the participants were interviewed with their mother languages and finally retranslated to English by another language expert to check its consistency.

Sputum sample collection and florescence microscopy examination

About 3–10 ml of spot- morning-spot sputum samples were collected using coded and new, translucent, screw-capped specimen collection containers by laboratory technologist from the study participants. The sputum samples were placed in cold boxes immediately upon receipt and delivered to Dessie and Debre Birhan referral hospitals laboratory on the day of collection. Sputum-smear microscopy was performed using Primo Star iLED, light emitting diode (LED)—florescence microscopy (FM) by using Auramine O staining procedure as follows; a smear was prepared and dried, then heat-fixed. Stained the smear with filtered 0.1 % Auramine O solution and kept the staining reagent for 20 min and washed well. Decolorized with 0.5 % acid-alcohol and kept for 3 min and gently rinsed with water. Counterstained with 0.5 % potassium permanganate solution for 1 min, then gently rinsed with water and drained. Finally, the back of the slide cleaned, air-dried and the stained slides were observed under 20×, 40× magnifications of FM for AFB. The AFB was appeared bright yellow against dark background materials [18].

GeneXpert examination

All AFB positive sputum samples were subjected to GeneXpert MTB/RIF system (Cepheid, USA) in Dessie and Debre Birhan referral hospitals laboratory. The system is a fully automated nested real-time polymerase chain reaction (PCR), which simultaneously detects *M. tuberculosis* complex (MTBC) and mutations in the ribonucleic acid polymerase Beta subunit gene (rpoB), which are responsible for the resistance to rifampin (RIF) [19–21].

Rapid HIV test

To determine the HIV status of the study participants, pre-test counseling was provided by trained nurses. Then whole blood was collected by finger stick. The presence of HIV-1 and HIV-2 antibodies was determined by using rapid test kits, HIV (1 + 2) antibody Colloidal Gold (KHB, Shanghai Kehua Bio-engineering Co Ltd, China) as a screening test, followed by HIV 1/2 STAT-PAK® (Chembio Diagnostics, USA), when the KHB result was reactive. Where the result of STAT-PAK® was discordant with KHB, a third test, Unigold™ HIV (Trinity Biotech, Ireland), was also used as a tiebreaker to determine the test result following the manufacturers' instruction. After testing, post test counseling was provided for all participants.

Nutritional assessment

The participants' body weight and height were measured by digital scale to the nearest 0.1 kg and 0.1 cm respectively. Body mass index is defined as the weight in kilogram by the individual divided by the square of the height in meter. It is used to determine the nutritional status of study participants into malnutrition (BMI = less than 18.5 kg/m^2), normal (BMI = 18.5–24.9 kg/m^2) and overweight (BMI = 25.0–29.9 kg/m^2) as recommended by CDC [22].

Quality assurance

A pre-test was done in Kombolcha town in 20 (5 %) homeless individuals who were similar with study participants prior to the data collection to check the clarity and consistency of the questionnaires and acceptability of laboratory procedure. Necessary correction was taken before the actual data collected. The data collectors, who can speak the local language (Amharic), were trained for 1 day on data collection procedures for this study to attain standardization and maximize interview reliability. The purpose of the study was informed to study participants for the quality of the data. In addition the study participants were instructed on how to produce an appropriate sputum specimen. Instruments and reagents were checked for reliability and reproducibility of the test before any test started. All new lots of reagents were tested with known positive and negative control. All positive microscopy slides and 10 % percent of negative slides were double checked by second experienced laboratory technologists for confirmation. The data collections, application of standard laboratory test procedures and test result were checked by senior laboratory technologist and principal investigator. Filled questionnaire and laboratory test result were collected after checking consistency and completeness. The overall data collection process was supervised by the principal investigator.

Data processing and analysis

Following the data collection, data were checked, coded and entered using EPI-INFO version 3.5 and exported to SPSS version 20 for analysis. Both descriptive and analytical statistical procedures were utilized. Descriptive statistics like percentage, mean and standard deviation were used for presentation of data and prevalence of smear positive PTB and MDR-TB. All variables of the study were initially tested for association with smear positive PTB by using binary logistic regression model. Those variables which have a p-value less than 0.2 by univariate analysis were put in the multivariable analysis model to control the possible effect of confounders. Finally the variable which has independent association with smear positive PTB was identified on the basis of odd ratio (OR) with 95 % confidence interval (CI) and P value less than 0.05. The variable was entered into multivariate model using the forward stepwise (likelihood ratio) regression method. Model fitness was checked using Hosmer and Lemeshow goodness of a fit test (0.70).

Results

Socio-demographic characteristics of the study participants

A total of 351 individuals were enrolled, who had cough of 2 weeks or more duration. Out of the total study participants, 190 were from Dessie town that constituted 54.1 % of the total participants and 161 were from Debre Birhan town that comprised 45.9 % of the 351 participants. Majority of study participants were males, 324 (92.7 %), and 333 (95.9 %) were between 15 and 44 years of old. The mean age of the participants were 26.7 (SD ±7.96) years. About 163 (46.4 %) of the study participants were illiterate and most of the participants 308 (87.7 %) were single and 301 (85.7 %) of the participants followed Orthodox Christians religion (Table 1).

Table 1 Socio-demographic characteristics of homeless individuals with smear positive PTB prevalence, Dessie and Debre Birhan towns, Northeast Ethiopia, September 2014 to June 2015 (N = 351)

Variables	Smear positive PTB		Total N (%)
	Negative n (%)	Positive n (%)	
Age			
15–24	158 (46.2)	3 (33.3)	161 (45.9)
25–34	138 (40.3)	4 (44.4)	142 (40.5)
35–44	28 (8.2)	2 (22.3)	30 (8.5)
45–60	18 (5.3)	0 (0)	18 (5.1)
Sex			
Male	316 (92.4)	8 (88.9)	324 (92.3)
Female	26 (7.6)	1 (11.1)	27 (7.7)
Marital status			
Single	300 (87.7)	8 (88.9)	308 (87.8)
Married	11 (3.2)	1 (11.1)	12 (3.4)
Divorced	17 (4.9)	0 (0)	17 (4.8)
Widowed	14 (4.1)	0 (0)	14 (4.0)
Educational status			
Illiterate	158 (46.2)	5 (55.6)	163 (46.4)
Primary school	176 (51.5)	4 (44.4)	180 (51.3)
Secondary school	8 (2.3)	0 (0)	8 (2.3)
Religion			
Orthodox	293 (85.7)	8 (88.9)	301 (85.8)
Muslim	47 (13.7)	1 (11.1)	48 (13.7)
Protestant	2 (0.6)	0 (0)	2 (0.5)

Prevalence of smear positive PTB and MDR-TB in homeless individuals

Out of the total study participants, smear positive PTB was detected in 9 of the participants (8 males and 1 female) by LED-FM. All smear positive PTB sputum specimens were further analyzed by GeneXpert assay, the assay confirmed that all were positive for MTBC but none were resistant to RIF or MDR. Therefore, the prevalence of smear positive PTB was 2.6 % (95 % CI 1.3, 5 %) among the study participants. The point prevalence of smear positive PTB was extrapolated to be 505/100,000 homeless individuals. All smear positive PTB cases were found in the age group (17–44 years) of the participants. Eight (88.9 %) smear positive PTB cases were found in the study participants who smoke cigarettes, drink alcohol and chew khat (flowering plant and leaves are chewed, contains cathinone, an amphetamine-like stimulant, which is said to cause excitement) during the study periods. Five (55.5 %) smear positive PTB cases were found in the study participants who were malnourished during the study periods. In addition, among the total smear positive PTB participants, 5 (55.5 %) were co-infected with HIV infection.

Behavioral characteristics of the study participants

Out of the total study participants 169 (48.1 %) had smoking cigarette during the study periods, of these, 67 (39.6 %) regularly used cigarette for greater than 5 years. The mean smoking periods of the participants was 64.7 (SD ±43.6) months. Besides, 263 (74.9 %) participants had experience with drinking alcohol, from these individuals, 164 (62.4 %) were regular alcohol drinkers for greater than 5 years. The mean alcohol drinking periods of the participants was 81.9 (SD ±56.9) months. More than half of the respondents, 195 (55.6 %) were also khat chewers, during the study periods. The mean khat chewing periods of the participants was 64.1 (SD ±46.2) months. About 10 (2.8 %) of the participants were using drugs during the study periods (Fig. 1).

Living conditions of the homeless study participants

The participants mean duration of being homelessness was 65.9 (SD ±49.16) months and about 148 (42.2 %) of the participants were homelessness for greater than 5 years. The average number of homeless individuals slept/live together in one restricted homeless shelter were 5 (SD ±2.99) and almost half 163 (46.4 %) of the participants were sleeping/living together in one restricted homeless shelter by being more than 5 persons. Among the study participants 17 (4.8 %) and 114 (32.5 %) had close contact with known TB patients and chronically cougher patients respectively (Table 2).

Morbidity history and status of the study participants

Out of the total study participants 10 (2.8 %) participants had a past history of TB disease, all of these were diagnosed during being homelessness and all were starting anti-TB treatment but more than half of them 6 (60 %) were defaulted anti-TB treatment. Out of the total study participants 25 (7.1 %) participants were malnourished, BMI less than 18.5. Out of the total study participants 22 (6.3 %) participants were HIV infected (Table 3).

Factors associated with smear positive tuberculosis in homeless individuals

In multivariable logistic regression, smoking cigarette regularly for greater than 5 years, BMI less than 18.5 and HIV infection were statistically significant association with

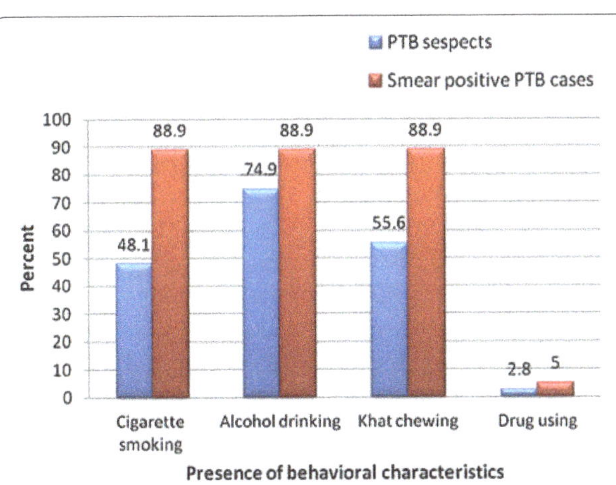

Fig. 1 Behavioral characteristics of homeless individuals, Dessie and Debre Birhan towns, Northeast Ethiopia, September 2014 to June 2015 (N = 351)

Table 2 Environmental factors of homeless individuals with smear positive PTB prevalence, Dessie and Debre Birhan towns, Northeast Ethiopia, September 2014 to June 2015 (N = 351)

Variables	Smear positive PTB		Total N (%)
	Negative n (%)	Positive n (%)	
Duration of being homelessness			
>5 years	141 (41.2)	7 (77.8)	148 (42.2)
≤5 years	201 (58.8)	2 (22.2)	203 (57.8)
Average number of homeless			
>5 persons	157 (45.9)	6 (66.7)	163 (46.4)
≤5 persons	185 (54.1)	3 (33.3)	188 (53.6)
Close contact with known TB patients			
Yes	15 (4.4)	2 (22.2)	17 (4.8)
No	327 (95.6)	7 (77.8)	334 (95.2)
Close contact with chronically cougher			
Yes	108 (31.6)	6 (66.7)	114 (32.5)
No	234 (68.4)	3 (33.3)	237 (67.5)

Table 3 Morbidity history and status of homeless individuals with smear positive PTB prevalence, Dessie and Debre Birhan towns, Northeast Ethiopia, September 2014 to June 2015 (N = 351)

Variables	Smear positive PTB		Total N (%)
	Negative n (%)	Positive n (%)	
Past history of PTB			
Yes	9 (2.6)	1 (11.1)	10 (2.8)
No	333 (97.4)	9 (88.9)	341 (97.2)
Past anti-TB treatment			
Defaulted	5 (55.6)	1 (100)	6 (60)
Completed	4 (44.4)	0 (0)	4 (40)
BMI (kg/m^2)			
<18.5	20 (5.8)	5 (55.6)	25 (7.1)
≥18.5	322 (94.2)	4 (44.4)	326 (92.9)
HIV antibody test			
Reactive	17 (5)	5 (55.6)	22 (6.3)
Non-reactive	325 (95)	4 (44.4)	329 (93.7)

smear positive PTB. Participants who smoke cigarette regularly for greater than 5 years were 10.1 times more likely to have smear positive PTB than those who smoke cigarette regularly for less than 5 years. The study also showed that statistically significant association between smear positive PTB and BMI. Participants who had BMI less than 18.5 were 6.9 times more likely to have smear positive PTB as compared to those who had BMI greater than 18.5. Furthermore, HIV infected homeless individuals were 6.8 times more likely to have smear positive PTB than those HIV uninfected homeless individuals (Table 4).

Table 4 Factors associated with smear positive pulmonary tuberculosis in homeless individuals Dessie and Debre Birhan towns, Northeast Ethiopia, September 2014 to June 2015 (N = 351)

Variables	Smear positive PTB		Crude odds ratio (95 % CI)	Adjusted odds ratio (95 % CI)	P value
	Negative	Positive			
Smoking					
>5 years	60	7	11.8 (1.4–98.1)	10.1 (1.1–97.7)	0.046
≤5 years	101	1	1	1	
BMI (kg/m^2)					
<18.5	20	5	20.1 (5.0–80.8)	6.9 (1.2–41.1)	0.033
≥18.5	322	4	1	1	
HIV status					
Positive	17	5	23.9 (5.9–97.1)	6.8 (1.1–40.1)	0.036
Negative	325	4	1	1	

Discussion

This study showed that the prevalence of smear positive PTB among TB suspect homeless individuals was 2.6 %. This finding is in line with studies conducted in USA (3.28 %) [23], Japan (1.5 %) [24] and Rome (3.86 %) [25]. This is also supported by systematic review and meta-analysis of prevalence of active TB among homeless individuals, estimated to be 0.2–7.7 % [8]. In this study all TB cases are found in young and productive age group (17–44 years) of the participants. This finding is consistent with reports from similar socio-economical settings, highest among young adults, which lead to grave socio-economic consequences in a country [26]. This high TB burden may also attribute to an aggressive transmission of TB in the homeless individuals and to the surrounding community.

Moreover, TB prevalence in this study is to some extent higher than studies conducted among homeless individuals in Marseilles (1 %) [27] and Iran (1.2 %) [15], the lower prevalence of TB in those countries could be due to high socio-economic status and low overall TB prevalence in the countries. In addition, relatively lower prevalence of TB in Iran might be due to lower prevalence of HIV infection (3.4 %) [15]. However, TB prevalence in this study is lower than studies conducted among homeless individuals in USA (6.1 %) [28], Seoul, South Korea (24.86 %) [13], North-eastern Poland (4.13 %) [29] and Colombia (7.9 %) [30], the difference might be due to difference in study design and setting, sample size and laboratory diagnosis method used. Particularly a study in USA, the analysis covered a wide geographic area with large sample size and the cases were either smear positive PTB or culture confirmed other form of TB [28]. On the other hand, in South Korea the prevalence of active TB was not based on sputum smear AFB but, it is based on chest radiography [13] this could be over sensitive and not specific enough as FM thus, might be increase the prevalence of TB than this study. In North-eastern Poland, the participants were first screened by chest radiography, then molecular testing and culture were performed [29], the use of an advanced diagnostic technique might be not underestimated the actual prevalence. In Colombia all reported cases were culture positive for MTB [30], could be revealed all types of TB in addition to smear positive PTB.

Several studies indicated that higher prevalence of TB in homeless individuals than the general population [24, 31, 32]. For example, in USA compared to the general population, homeless individuals had an approximately tenfold increase in TB prevalence [33]. Extrapolation of this study finding also indicated that about 4.67 times higher burdens of smear positive PTB in homeless individuals than the general population (108/100,000) in Ethiopia [34]. This study point prevalence of smear positive PTB is comparable to a study conducted in Greater London (780/100,000) [32]. Furthermore, despite the overall decline in TB incidence in the general population, 28 outbreaks of TB occurred in Illinois among homeless individuals, indicating that ongoing transmission of TB to the homeless individuals and the entire community [35]. This disproportionate burden of TB in homeless individuals might be due to that these groups are the most neglected and live in under-privileged social conditions such as poverty, malnutrition and overcrowd unhygienic environment with relatively limited access to health care [10].

In this study RIF resistant or MDR-TB was not found. However, studies conducted in USA (2.7 %) [28], USA (1.1 %) [33], Busan Medical Center, Korea (11.5 %) [10] and London (6.5 %) [32] MDR–TB was found among homeless individuals. Absence of MDR-TB in this study might be due to the small number of smear positive PTB cases enrolled in the study. However well known risk factors for the development of MDR-TB, previous anti-TB treatment defaulter rate is high (60 %) in this study.

In this study, participants who smoke cigarette regularly for greater than 5 years were 10.1 times more likely to have smear positive PTB than those who smoke cigarette regularly for less than 5 years. Even though there were no other studies considered the duration of smoking in homeless individuals, the role of smoking in the development of active TB is well established [36] either through increased susceptibility to new infection with MTB or increase the risk of developing active TB [37]. Thus, increasing duration of smoking might be increase the development of TB disease. Smoking cigarette by itself has also reported as a risk factor for acquisition of active TB in Rome [25] and Montreal, Canada [38] but in this study it was not significantly associated. However, in this study about 88.9 % smear positive PTB cases were found among cigarette smokers.

In addition, this study showed that participants who had BMI less than 18.5 were 6.94 times more likely to have smear positive PTB as compared to those who had BMI greater than 18.5. This finding also supported by studies conducted in Seoul, South Korea [13] and Rome [25]. In fact, malnutrition is adversely affecting the immune status of individuals; it makes individuals more susceptible to TB infection and progression of active TB disease [39]. Moreover, in this study, HIV infected homeless individuals were 6.75 times more likely to have smear positive PTB than those HIV uninfected homeless individuals. This is in line with studies conducted in USA [23, 28] and Montreal, Canada [38]. It has well known that HIV infection often leads to a greater rate of TB either through reactivation or increased susceptibility to new infection with MTB thus, the main driving factor which aggravates TB. The lifetime risk of HIV infected individuals to develop TB is 20-37 times higher than HIV uninfected individuals [17]. In addition, in this study HIV infection was found in 22 (6.3 %) of the study participants. This high HIV burden might be due to risky behaviors of homeless individuals to acquire the disease. In this study TB–HIV co-infection were also considerably high (55.56 %).

In contrast to studies conducted in USA [28], Rome [25] and Montreal, Canada [38], in this study alcohol drinking was not significantly associated with smear positive PTB. The reason might be more or less homeless individuals in this study, exhibit similar alcohol drinking characteristics (about three quarters of the participants were drunk alcohol during the study periods), this might reduce the individual variation and make it difficult to see its effect on outcomes of smear positive PTB. However, about 88.9 % smear positive PTB cases were found among alcohol drinker study participants. In addition, in contrast to a study conducted in Seoul, South Korea [13], in this study past history of TB disease is not significantly associated with smear positive PTB. The reason might be participants who had a past history of TB disease were small in number in this study, might be not enough to show the effect of past history of TB on smear positive PTB.

Limitation of study

Smear negative PTB didn't look for, as well as extra pulmonary TB. Probably the 2 weeks cough can be misdetermined by persons living on streets with limited date and time remembrance and others.

Conclusion

The prevalence of smear positive PTB among TB suspect homeless individuals was high. Extrapolation of this study finding also indicates that the point prevalence of smear positive PTB in homeless individuals was 4.67 times higher than the general population in Ethiopia. It indicates that there is high transmission of TB in the homeless individuals and also become a risk to the entire community. Although MDR-TB was not found, well known risk factors for MDR-TB, previous anti-TB treatment defaulter rate is higher in the study participants. Smoking cigarette regularly for greater than 5 years, malnutrition and HIV infection were significantly associated factors with smear positive PTB among homeless individuals. Special emphasis is needed for homeless individuals to exert intensive effort to identify undetected TB cases to limit circulation of the disease into the community. Developing and implementing specific TB prevention and control strategies with integrated risk reduction approach is needed for homeless individuals.

Abbreviations

AFB: acid fast bacilli; BMI: body mass index; CDC: Center for Disease Control and prevention; FM: fluorescence microscopy; HIV: human immunodeficiency virus; INH: isoniazid; MDR-TB: multidrug resistant tuberculosis; MTB: *M. tuberculosis*; PCR: polymerase chain reaction; PTB: pulmonary tuberculosis; RIF: rifampicin; TB: tuberculosis.

Authors' contributions

TS conception of research idea, study design, data collection, analysis and interpretation. BT, SE, and FM supervision, data collection, analysis, interpretation and the drafting of manuscript. All authors read and approved the final manuscript.

Author details

[1] Amhara Regional Health Bureau, North Shewa Zonal Health Bureau, Debre Birhan, Ethiopia. [2] School of Biomedical and Laboratory Sciences, Department of Medical Microbiology, University of Gondar, P.O. Box: 196, Gonder, Ethiopia.

Acknowledgements

We would like to thank study participants and University of Gondar, Dessie and Debre Birhan hospitals for allowing us to use the laboratory facilities.

Competing interests

The authors declare that they have no competing interests.

Consent for publication

Not applicable.

Funding

Partial funding of the research was obtained from Amhara health regional bureau.

References

1. Bhowmik D, Chandira R, Jayakar B, Kumar K. Recent trends of drug used treatment of tuberculosis. J Chem Pharm Res. 2009;1(1):113–33.
2. Abebe DS, Bjune G, Ameni G, Biffa D, Abebe F. Prevalence of pulmonary tuberculosis and associated risk factors in Eastern Ethiopian prisons. Int J Tuberc Lung Dis. 2011;15(5):668–73.
3. Federal Ministry of Health Ethiopia. Tuberculosis, leprosy and TB/HIV prevention and control programme manual. 4th ed. Addis Ababa: Ministry of Health; 2008.
4. Fekadu A, Hanlon C, Gebre-Eyesus E, Agedew M, Solomon H, Teferra S, et al. Burden of mental disorders and unmet needs among street homeless people in Addis Ababa, Ethiopia. BMC Med. 2014;12(1):138.
5. Dube-D K. The status, challenges, and expectations of homeless people in Ethiopia: a case study of Bahir Dar. Eur Acad Res. 2014;2(2):3027–44.
6. Ali M. Status of homeless population in urban Ethiopia: a case study of Amhara region. Int J Manag Soc Sci Res Rev. 2014;3(1):61–8.
7. Badiaga S, Raoult D, Brouqui P. Preventing and controlling emerging and reemerging transmissible diseases in the homeless. Emerg Infect Dis. 2008;14(9):1353–9.
8. Beijer U, Wolf A, Fazel S. Prevalence of tuberculosis, hepatitis C virus, and HIV in homeless people: a systematic review and meta-analysis. Lancet Infect Dis. 2012;12(11):859–70.
9. Chintan B, Bhatt M. Tuberculosis prevention and control guidelines for homeless service agencies in Miami Dade County, Florida. Florida Health Department: Florida; 2013.
10. Heo D-J, Min HG, Lee HH. The clinical characteristics and predictors of treatment success of pulmonary tuberculosis in homeless persons at a public hospital in Busan. Korean J Fam Med. 2012;33(6):372–80.
11. Tankimovich M. Barriers to and interventions for improved tuberculosis detection and treatment among homeless and immigrant populations: a literature review. J Community Health Nurs. 2013;30(2):83–95.
12. Khan K, Rea E, McDermaid C, Stuart R, Chambers C, Wang J, et al. Active tuberculosis among homeless persons, Toronto, Ontario, Canada, 1998–2007. Emerg Infect Dis. 2011;17(3):357–65.
13. Lee C-H, Jeong YJ, Heo EY, Park JS, Lee JS, Lee BJ, et al. Active pulmonary tuberculosis and latent tuberculosis infection among homeless people in Seoul, South Korea: a cross-sectional study. BMC Public Health. 2013;13(1):1–6.
14. Center for Disease Control and prevention. Management of TB in the homeless: CDC's experience with outbreaks. National Center for HIV/AIDS, Viral Hepatitis, STD, and TB Prevention Division of TB Elimination; 2013.
15. Bagheri AF, Gouya MM, Saifi M, Rohani M, Tabarsi P, Sedaghat A, et al. Vulnerability of homeless people in Tehran, Iran, to HIV, tuberculosis and viral hepatitis. PLOS ONE. 2014;9(6):1–7.
16. Seyoum B, Demissie M, Worku A, Bekele S, Aseffa A. Prevalence and drug resistance patterns of *Mycobacterium tuberculosis* among new smear positive pulmonary tuberculosis patients in Eastern Ethiopia. Tuberc Res Treat. 2014;2014:1–7.
17. Federal Democratic Repuplic of Ethiopia Ministry of Health. Guidelines for clinical and programmatic management of TB, leprosy and TB/HIV in Ethiopia. 5th ed. Addis Abeba: Ministry of Health; 2012.
18. Foundation for Inovative New Diagnostics. Training Manual for Floresence-Based AFB microscopy. Geneva: Foundation for Inovative New Diagnostics; 2008.
19. World Health Organisation. Xpert MTB/RIF implementation manual. Geneva: World Health Organization; 2014. WHO/HTM/TB/2014.1.
20. Federal Democratic Republic of Ethiopia Ministry of Health/Ethiopian Public Heath Institute. Implementation guideline for GeneXpert MTB/RIF Assay in Ethiopia. Addis Ababa: Ethiopian Public Health Institute; 2014.
21. Kalokhe AS, Shafiq M, Lee JC, Ray SM, Wang YF, Metchock B, et al. Multidrug-resistant tuberculosis drug susceptibility and molecular diagnostic testing: a review of the literature. Am J Med Sci. 2013;345(2):143–8.
22. Department of Health and Human Services. Body mass index: considerations for practitioners. USA: Center for Disease Control and Prevention; 2011. https://www.cdc.gov/obesity/downloads/BMIforPactitioners.pdf.
23. Notaro SJ, Khan M, Kim C, Nasaruddin M, Desai K. Analysis of the health status of the homeless clients utilizing a free clinic. J Community Health. 2013;38(1):172–7.
24. Tabuchi T, Takatorige T, Hirayama Y, Nakata N, Harihara S, Shimouchi A, et al. Tuberculosis infection among homeless persons and caregivers in a high-tuberculosis-prevalence area in Japan: a cross-sectional study. BMC Infect Dis. 2011;11(22):1–8.
25. Laurenti P, Bruno S, Quaranta G, La Torre G, Cairo AG, Nardella P, et al. Tuberculosis in sheltered homeless population of rome: an integrated model of recruitment for risk management. Sci World J. 2012;2012:1–7.
26. World Health Organization. Global tuberculosis report 2012. Geneva: World Health Organization; 2012. WHO/HTM/TB/2012.6.
27. Badiaga S, Richet H, Azas P, Zandotti C, Rey F, Charrel R, et al. Contribution of a shelter-based survey for screening respiratory diseases in the homeless. Eur J Public Health. 2009;19(2):157–60.
28. Haddad MB, Wilson TW, Ijaz K, Marks SM, Moore M. Tuberculosis and homelessness in the United States, 1994–2003. JAMA. 2005;293(22):2762–6.
29. Romaszko J, Buciński A, Kuchta R, Bednarski K, Zakrzewska M. The incidence of pulmonary tuberculosis among the homeless in North-eastern Poland. Cent Eur J Med. 2013;8(2):283–5.
30. Herna´ndez Sarmiento JM, Correa N, Franco JG, Alvarez M, et al. Tuberculosis among homeless population from Medellín, Colombia: associated mental disorders and socio-demographic characteristics. J Immigr Minor Health. 2013;15(4):693–9.
31. Wrezel O. Respiratory infections in the homeless. UWO Med J. 2009;78(2):61–5.
32. Story A, Murad S, Roberts W, Verheyen M, Hayward AC. Tuberculosis in London: the importance of homelessness, problem drug use and prison. Thorax. 2007;62(8):667–71.
33. Bamrah S, Yelk Woodruff R, Powell K, Ghosh S, Kammerer J, Haddad M. Tuberculosis among the homeless, United States, 1994–2010. Int J Tuberc Lung Dis. 2013;17(11):1414–9.
34. Kebede A, Alebachew Z, Tsegaye F, Lemma E, Abebe A, Agonafir M, et al. The first population-based national tuberculosis prevalence survey in Ethiopia, 2010–2011. Int J Tuberc Lung Dis. 2014;18(6):635–9.
35. Centers for Disease Control and prevention. Tuberculosis outbreak associated with a homeless shelter-Kane County, Illinois, 2007–2011. MMWR Morb Mortal Wkly Rep. 2012;61(11):186–9.
36. Davies PD, Yew WW, Ganguly D, Davidow AL, Reichman LB, Dheda K, et al. Smoking and tuberculosis: the epidemiological association and immunopathogenesis. Trans R Soc Trop Med Hyg. 2006;100(4):291–8.
37. Hassmiller KM. The association between smoking and tuberculosis. Salud Publica Mex. 2006;48(1):201–16.
38. de Bibiana JT, Rossi C, Rivest P, Zwerling A, Thibert L, McIntosh F, et al. Tuberculosis and homelessness in Montreal: a retrospective cohort study. BMC Public Health. 2011;119(833):1–10.
39. Kim HJ, Lee CH, Shin S, Lee JH, Kim YW, Chung HS, et al. The impact of nutritional deficit on mortality of in-patients with pulmonary tuberculosis. Int J Tuberc Lung Dis. 2010;14(1):79–85.

17

Antibiotic consumption in laboratory confirmed vs. non-confirmed bloodstream infections among very low birth weight neonates in Poland

A. Różańska[1*], J. Wójkowska-Mach[1], P. Adamski[2], M. Borszewska-Kornacka[3], E. Gulczyńska[4], M. Nowiczewski[4], E. Helwich[5], A. Kordek[6], D. Pawlik[7] and M. Bulanda[1]

Abstract

Background: Newborns are a population in which antibiotic consumption is extremely high. Targeted antibiotic therapy should help to reduce antibiotics consumption. The aim of this study was an assessment of antibiotic usage in bloodstream infections treatment in the Polish Neonatology Surveillance Network (PNSN) and determining the possibility of applying this kind of data in infection control, especially for the evaluation of standard methods of microbiological diagnostics.

Methods: Data were collected between 01.01.2009 and 31.12.2013 in five teaching NICUs from the PNSN. The duration of treatment in days (DOT) and the defined daily doses (DDD) were used for the assessment of antibiotics consumption.

Results: The median DOT for a single case of BSI amounted to 8.0 days; whereas the median consumption expressed in DDD was 0.130. In the case of laboratory confirmed BSI, median DOT was 8 days, and consumption—0.120 DDD. Median length of therapy was shorter for unconfirmed cases: 7 days, while the consumption of antibiotics was higher—0.140 DDD ($p < 0.0001$). High consumption of glycopeptides expressed in DOTs was observed in studied population, taking into account etiology of infection.

Conclusions: Even application of classical methods of microbiological diagnostics significantly reduces the consumption of antibiotics expressed by DDD. However, the high consumption of glycopeptides indicates the necessity of applying rapid diagnostic assays. Nevertheless, the assessment of antibiotic consumption in neonatal units represents a methodological challenge and requires the use of different measurement tools.

Keywords: Antimicrobial consumption, Infection surveillance, Bloodstream infections, Neonatal infections

Background

Infection control in neonatal intensive care units (NICUs) should have high priority, because its incidence is among the highest in different patient populations. Bloodstream infections (BSI) are the most common clinical form of infections in NICUs. The incidence of early-onset BSI (diagnosed <3 days after delivery) is 7% in Poland [1] and in Norway [2], 6% in the USA [3] and 2.4% in Israel [4].

In contrast, risk of late-onset BSI reaches 14.9/1000 patient days (pds) worldwide [5]; in the German NeoK-ISS: 8.3/1000 pds [6] and in Poland—6.7/1000 pds [7]. However, in the USA (for infants born at 28 weeks gestation or earlier)—36% [8], while in Israel, 39% [9].

Numerous studies show that newborns are a population in which antibiotic usage is extremely high [10, 11]. Those studies were performed mainly in West European

*Correspondence: rozanska@ifb.pl
[1] Chair of Microbiology, Jagiellonian University Medical College, 18 Czysta Street, 31-121 Krakow, Poland
Full list of author information is available at the end of the article

countries and in the United States, but there are no such reports from Poland or Central Europe.

Assessment of antibiotic usage in neonatal intensive care units encounters significant difficulties connected with the lack of standardized methods for this specific patient population. Defined daily dose (DDD), an international standard measure used for drug consumption assessment, is a technical unit of measurement which reflects the average maintenance dose per day for a drug used for its main indication in adults [12]. For this reason, this parameter has certain limitations for the analysis in the child population. However, defined daily dose was used in some studies, especially for comparative purposes in homogenous patient population [13]. Other parameters used for antibiotic usage assessment are as follows: LOT—the number of days during which at least one dose of any antibiotic was received, DOT—the aggregate sum of LOT or PDD—prescribed daily dose or proportion of patients with antibiotic treatment in a specific period [14–16].

Antibiotics consumption assessment can have numerous implications. In the area of infection control it can serve as a relatively simple indicator for assessing the effectiveness of methods of microbiological diagnostics. Microbiological diagnostics of blood stream infections in hospital practice still remains a challenge.

The aims of this study were:

- an assessment of antibiotic usage in bloodstream infection (BSI) treatment, taking into account etiology, in the Polish Neonatal Surveillance Network wards using two kinds of parameters, that is DDD and DOT,
- determining the possibility of applying this kind of data in infection control, especially for the evaluation of standard methods of microbiological diagnostics.

Methods

Data were collected prospectively between 01.01.2009 and 31.12.2013 in five teaching neonatal intensive care units (NICU) that took part in the Polish Neonatology Surveillance Network (PNSN). The PNSN is a prospective national surveillance system for the most relevant infections in the group of very low birth weight (birth weight <1500 g, VLBW) infants in Poland. The PNSN recorded severe infections, including BSI, observed during hospitalization: from admission to discharge, transfer or death. Participation in PNSN was voluntary and confidential for wards. Detailed description of data collection system, study wards, epidemiology of early- and late-onset BSI and its microbiology have been already published elsewhere [1, 7]. The study was approved by the Bioethics Committee of Jagiellonian University Medical College—no. KBET/221/B/2011. All data entered into the electronic database and analyzed retrospectively during the preparation of this article were previously de-identified. BSI (both: early- and late-onset) were defined according to Gastmeier et al. [17] with modifications. BSI was detected when at least two of the following signs were observed:

Temperature >38 or <36.5 °C or temperature instability, tachycardia or bradycardia, apnea, prolonged capillary refill, metabolic acidosis, hyperglycemia, the other sign of bloodstream infections, such as: lethargy; and one of the following criteria: C-reactive protein (CRP) >2.0 mg/dL, immature/total neutrophil ratio (I/T ratio) >0.2, leukocytes <5000/μL, platelets <10,000/μL.

Early-onset BSI was defined as septicemia diagnosed <3 days after delivery.

Laboratory confirmed BSI (LC-BSI) were those cases in which positive results of the microbiological testing were obtained, that means etiological factor was isolated. All blood specimens of at least 1 mL (taken prior to implementing antibiotic treatment) were injected into an aerobic blood culture bottle. Isolates were identified by the automated identification system (VITEK 2, bioMérieux, Poland). In the studied wards, molecular methods for identification of etiological factors were not used. BSI cases in which samples for microbiological testing were not collected or etiological factor was not isolated were classified as not confirmed ones.

Antibiotic usage for BSI treatment (until cure) was assessed for 767 cases. The analysis of antibiotic use included only the cases in which treatment was successful—13 records concerning infants who had died within 7 days of starting the therapy were excluded from the study (all of them were laboratory confirmed).

Two kinds of indicators were used for the description of antibiotic usage:

1. DOT, expressed in days—the aggregate (for every separate type of antibiotics) sum of number of days during which at least one dose of any antibiotic was received, and
2. DDD, expressed in grams—the defined daily dose, according to the ATC/DDD system of the World Health Organization (Anatomical Therapeutic Chemical, group "J01") [12].

Both measures were taken into account in reference to one case of infection. Data on the medicine type, dose, and the length of therapy were derived from individual records in the chart of each individual patient.

Antibiotic consumption were calculated for all antimicrobials used in therapy, and for the following classes: beta-lactams (ampicillin, cloxacillin, piperacillin, cefotaxime, ceftriaxone, ceftazidime, meropenem, imipenem), aminoglycosides (amikacin, netilmicin, gentamicin), glycopeptides (vancomycin), antimycotics (fluconazole, amphotericin B) and others (ciprofloxacin, clindamycin, erythromycin, clarithromycin, sulfamethoxazole with trimethoprim). Etiological factors were assigned to the following groups: Gram-negative (*Enterobacteriaceae* and other rods), Gram-positive (staphylococci, streptococci), candida. While conducting treatment with the application of drugs from several groups, used in parallel or consecutively, all of them were included into analysis. When, during treatment, positive microbiological cultures were obtained from different samples, or samples taken at different times (within 5 days), growth of microorganisms belonging to various groups (e.g. *Escherichia coli* and *Candida albicans*) was defined as cases of changing etiology (group "changing").

Due to DDD and DOT distribution significantly different from the normality, the statistical analysis based on the Kruskal–Wallis test. If the significance had been obtained, analysis was suplemented by the post hoc Steel–Dwass test, with critical value $p = 0.05$. All analysis were provided with SAS JMP package.

Results

In the study period, records of 2003 VLBW newborns and 780 BSI cases (regardless of the date of recognition of first BSI symptoms) were filled with all data.

Laboratory confirmed BSI (LC-BSI) constituted 84.9% (662) of all recognized cases of BSI.

In the analyzed population of VLBW neonates with BSI, in whom the etiological agent was isolated, combination therapy was used in 67% of cases, while in the group without microbiological confirmation, in 74% of cases.

The total duration of antibiotic therapy for 767 cases of BSI, which are incorporated into the present analysis, amounted to 14,056 DOTs or 381.6 DDDs. The median length of antibiotic therapy for a single case of BSI, regardless of microbiological confirmation or its lack, amounted to 8.0 days; whereas the median consumption expressed in DDD was 0.130. In the case of LC-BSI, median DOT was also 8.0 days, and consumption—0.120 DDD. Median length of therapy was shorter for unconfirmed cases: 7.0 days, while the consumption of antibiotics was higher—0.140 DDD ($p < 0.0001$) (Table 1).

Antibiotic consumption expressed by the DDD index was higher in the case of BSI caused by Gram-positive cocci than Gram-negative bacilli (0.140 vs. 0.136 DDD, Table 2), and the differences concerned 2× higher consumption of aminoglycosides (0.109 vs. 0.056 DDD, Table 2; $p = 0.0092$, Table 3).

Highest DOT values for beta-lactams concerned fungal infections and for the "changing" group, similarly to the consumption of antibiotics expressed by DDD.

Median length of therapy for BSI infections caused by Gram-positive cocci was longer than the ones caused by Gram-negative bacilli (9.0 vs. 7.5 DOT, Table 2), and the differences were mainly associated with the employment of glycopeptides (8.0 vs. 10.0 DOT, Table 2, $p = 0.0004$, Table 3).

Detailed data on antibiotic consumption expressed by DDD and DOT (values of medians per one infection case), taking into account groups of antibiotics, are presented in Table 2.

The results of statistical analysis regarding the consumption of the individual groups of antibiotics depending on the etiology of infection are shown in Table 3.

Depending on the applied indicator assessing the consumption of antibiotics in the treatment of BSI: DOT or DDD, the percentage share for individual groups of antibiotics varied.

Table 1 Values (median) of DOT and DDD in bloodstream infections treatment in microbiologically confirmed (LC) vs. unconfirmed cases (Not-LC)

Antimicrobial group	DOT (days)		p value	DDD		p value
	Microbiologically confirmed N = 649	Microbiologically unconfirmed N = 118		Microbiologically confirmed N = 649	Microbiologically unconfirmed N = 118	
	Median (IQR)	Median (IQR)		Median (IQR)	Median (IQR)	
Aminoglycosides	7.0 (5.0; 9.3)	7.0 (6.0;7.0)	0.5265	0.101 (0.050; 0.171)	0.095 (0.045; 0.179)	<0.0001
Antimycotic	12.5 (9.0;16.0)	10.0 (7.8;14.3)		0.210 (0.132; 0.040)	0.198 (0.073; 0.463)	
Beta-lactams	8.0 (5.0;11.0)	7.0 (6.8;8.8)		0.254 (0.136; 0.438)	0.300 (0.210; 0.420)	
Glycopeptides	10.0 (8.0;11.0)	9.0 (7.0;11.0)		0.120 (0.080; 0.168)	0.120 (0.083; 0.146)	
Other	9.0 (6.0;14.8)	8.0 (5.0;15.5)		0.210 (0.105; 0.530)	0.098 (0.060; 0.410)	
Total	8.0 (5.0; 16.0)	7.0 (5.0; 15.5)		0.120 (0.050; 0.530)	0.143 (0.045; 0.463)	

DOT days of therapy (per one infection case), *DDD* defined daily dose (per one infection case), *IQR* interquartile range, *N* number of BSI cases

Table 2 Values (median) of DOT and DDD in bloodstream infections treatment according to etiological factors

Etiology	DOT (days) Median (IQR)	DDD Median (IQR)
Gram+ N = 452		
Aminoglycosides	7.0 (5.0; 9.0)	0.109 (0.560; 0.180)
Antimycotics	12.0 (9.3; 16.0)	0.195 (0.131; 0.341)
Beta-lactams	7.0 (5.0; 10.0)	0.252 (0.180; 0.420)
Glycopeptides	10.0 (8.0; 11.0)	0.128 (0.088; 0.168)
Other	9.0 (5.0; 15.0)	0.211 (0.096; 0.452)
Total	9.0 (5.0; 15.0)	0.140 (0.056; 0.453)
Gram− N = 103		
Aminoglycosides	6.0 (4.3; 8.0)	0.056 (0.036; 0.137)
Antimycotics	12.0 (8.2; 17.0)	0.228 (0.131; 0.360)
Beta-lactams	8.0 (4.0; 11.0)	0.244 (0.096; 0.448)
Glycopeptides	8.0 (4.0; 9.0)	0.098 (0.039; 0.149)
Other	8.5 (5.3; 10.8)	0.229 (0.099; 0.608)
Total	7.5 (4.0; 17.0)	0.136 (0.036; 0.447)
Changing N = 76		
Aminoglycosides	7.0 (5.0; 10.0)	0.105 (0.061; 0.180)
Antimycotics	12.0 (10.0; 16.0)	0.250 (0.158; 0.735)
Beta-lactams	7.0 (6.5; 11.0)	0.281 (0.169; 0.495)
Glycopeptides	10.0 (7.0; 11.0)	0.085 (0.056; 0.167)
Other	9.0 (6.0; 14.5)	0.187 (0.120; 2.580)
Total	9.0 (5.0; 16.0)	0.149 (0.056; 2.580)
Candida N = 18		
Aminoglycosides	8.5 (4.8; 12.8)	0.140 (0.070; 0.210)
Antimycotics	10.5 (9.0; 15.8)	0.225 (0.092; 0.353)
Beta-lactams	12.0 (9.0; 19.5)	450 (192.9; 2175)
Glycopeptides	10.0 (7.3; 10.8)	0.087 (0.063; 0.161)
Other	13.5 (10.0; 17.0)	3.276 (0.153; 6.400)
Total	10.0 (4.8; 19.5)	0.164 (0.063; 6.400)

Changing—when, during treatment, positive microbiological cultures were obtained from different samples, or samples taken at different times (within 5 days), growth of microorganisms belonging to various groups (e.g. *Escherichia coli* and *Candida albicans*) was defined as cases of changing etiology (group "changing")

DOT days of therapy (per one case), *DDD* defined daily dose (per one case), *IQR* interquartile range, *N* number of cases

In treatment of BSI as a whole, according to the DOT index, glycopeptides were used the longest: 42.1%, and, after taking into account the etiology of infection, it was the predominant group also in infections caused by Gram-positive cocci: 51%, in the event of changes in the etiological agent: 40.6%. In treatment of microbiologically unconfirmed BSI, glycopeptides were used in 33.8% DOT (Fig. 1).

The largest share in total consumption of antibiotics in all analyzed cases of BSI expressed by DDD was represented by beta-lactams: 32.6%, especially with microbiologically unconfirmed BSI: 53.2% (Fig. 2).

In the event when antibiotic consumption was evaluated by DDD, antifungal medication constituted almost one-fourth of the applied drugs, and when the unit of measurement was DOT—13.3% (Figs. 1, 2).

Discussion

BSI represent a critical complication associated with hospitalization of very low birth weight (VLBW) infants, contributing to longer stay, and different long-term adverse outcomes. This phenomenon is well-understood and described [3, 7, 18–21], contrary to the subject under discussion, in which, unfortunately, data concerning antibiotic consumption are sparse and incomplete.

The proportion of microbiologically confirmed cases of BSI observed in the present study indicates similarity, but not identicalness, with other national programs. In the analysis of differences, attention should be paid to the applied definition of infections and different significance of microbiological findings for various types of surveillance. In American NHSN, in which to confirm LC-BSI, it was necessary to obtain at least 2 identical blood cultures, clinical sepsis was observed in 6.7–12.7% of infections [22], i.e. twice less frequently than in this study—significantly less restrictive in evaluating microbiological results. It unfortunately, indicates too rare application of the capabilities of contemporary microbiology in everyday clinical practice of the studied NICUs. This is confirmed by the results of a Cypriot study, in which LC-BSI constituted 96% of all BSIs [23]. Another matter is the debated problem of legitimacy of repeated blood drawing for cultures from VLBW newborns. Currently, it is more and more frequently assumed that, in this patient population, it is more justifiable to draw a single full-volume sample than to take two or more—even in the event of a result revealing typical skin contaminants, i.e. coagulase-negative staphylococci [24]. This is confirmed by the definitions adopted in the Netherlands [25], in NICHD Vermont Oxford Network [3] and the ones employed in the German national program called Neo-KISS [17].

The obtained data show that the use of diagnostics, even based on the standard, basic level, meaning culture, is a proceeding effectively affecting the consumption of antibiotics, and therefore, the costs of therapy, i.e. they reduce the consumption of antibiotics expressed by DDD.

The indicator most commonly used to assess the consumption of drugs, including antibiotics, is defined daily dose. This recognized international standard applicable in measuring the consumption of antibiotics is based on the average dose for the treatment of adults. For this reason, it is an indicator which, in relation to children, should be used with caution and one should take into account its limitations [26, 27].

Table 3 Statistical significance of antibiotic consumption expressed in DOT and DDD in bloodstream infections treatment according to etiological factor

	Candida	Gram–	Gram+	Changing
DOT aminoglycosides (H = 6.5939, df = 4; p = 0. 590)				
Not LC	0.7346	0.4524	0.9929	0.2733
Candida	na	0.6917	0.9235	0.9962
Gram–		na	0.4358	0.2780
Gram+			na	0.8323
Total DDD aminoglycosides (H = 31.7944, df = 4; p < 0.0137)				
Not LC	0.7980	0.3370	0.5284	0.9576
Candida	na	0.3438	0.9582	0.9757
Gram–		na	0.0092	0.3480
Gram+			na	1.0000
DOT antifungals (H = 2.5563, df = 4; p = 0.6346)				
Not LC	0.9978	0.9978	0.8403	0.7241
Candida	na	0.9995	0.9155	0.8539
Gram–		na	0.9885	0.8474
Gram+			na	0.9753
Total DDD antifungals (H = 16.5505, df = 4; p = 0.4042)				
Not LC	0.1485	0.7166	0.9926	0.7086
Candida	na	0.3429	0.4524	0.9454
Gram–		na	0.2909	0.9236
Gram+			na	0.1509
DOT beta-lactams (H = 15.0687, df = 4; p = 0.0046)				
Not LC	0.0286	0.8176	0.7340	0.0039
Candida	na	0.2451	0.1935	0.3721
Gram–		na	0.9978	0.2494
Gram+			na	0.1390
Total DDD beta-lactams (H = 11.2708, df = 4; p = 0.1930)				
Not LC	0.6238	0.3438	0.2861	0.3044
Candida	na	0.9999	0.9852	1.0000
Gram–		na	0.6380	1.0000
Gram+			na	0.7880
DOT glycopeptides (H = 19.0396, df = 4; p = 0.0008)				
Not LC	0.9986	0.0481	0.4925	0.9997
Candida	na	0.4196	0.9989	0.9992
Gram–		na	0.0004	0.1049
Gram+			na	0.6125
Total DDD glycopeptides (H = 0.4767, df = 4; p = 0.0010)				
Not LC	0.8227	0.5865	0.4612	0.5951
Candida	na	1.0000	0.4731	0.9998
Gram–		na	0.0498	0.9802
Gram+			na	0.0157
DOT other (H = 2.2959, df = 4; p = 0.6815)				
Not LC	0.6828	0.9978	0.9220	0.9922
Candida	na	0.7617	0.8871	0.9772
Gram–		na	0.9735	0.9984
Gram+			na	0.9999
Total DDD other (H = 3.8955, df = 4; p = 0.3787)				
Not LC	0.9707	0.9538	0.8169	0.9981
Candida	na	0.9986	0.4667	0.5815
Gram–		na	0.8990	0.9884
Gram+			na	0.9910

p values for each pair of etiological factor groups are given in the table cells

Changing—when, during treatment, positive microbiological cultures were obtained from different samples, or samples taken at different times (within 5 days), growth of microorganisms belonging to various groups (e.g. *Escherichia coli* and *Candida albicans*) was defined as cases of changing etiology (group "changing")

DOT days of therapy, *DDD* defined daily dose, *IQR* interquartile range, *na* not applicable, *Not LC* not laboratory confirmed

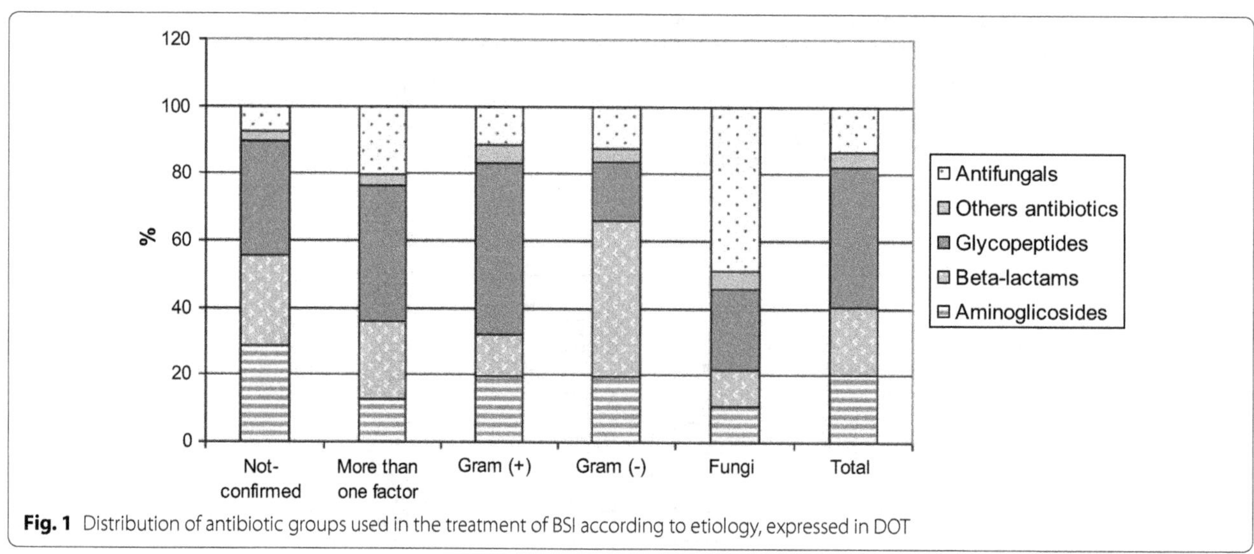

Fig. 1 Distribution of antibiotic groups used in the treatment of BSI according to etiology, expressed in DOT

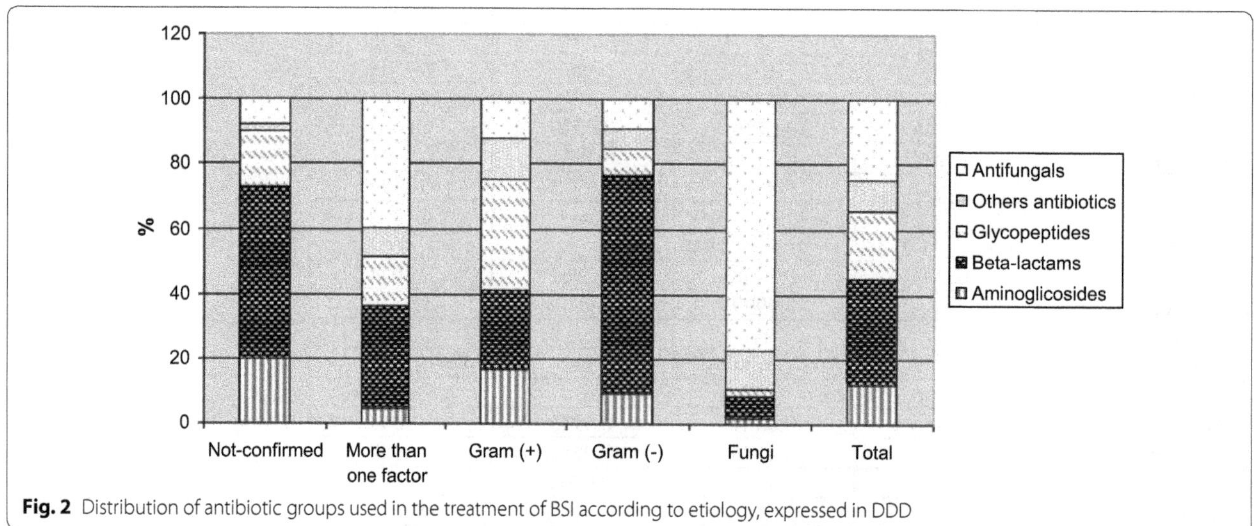

Fig. 2 Distribution of antibiotic groups used in the treatment of BSI according to etiology, expressed in DDD

Howether, both measures: DDD and the length of therapy were used by different authors with the application of various denominators—the number of admissions, number of person days or with respect to the treatment of a single patient [13, 15].

To evaluate the consumption of antibiotics in pediatric wards, particularly neonatal units, Gerber et al. employed DOT [15]. Depending on the type of neonatal unit, they found the length of treatment to be in the range from 5.7 in medical NICUs to 34.3 DOT in surgical NICUs. Median DOT in this study was about forty percent higher than in the medical NICUs in the study by Gerber; however, due to distinct populations and different degrees of detail, it is difficult to explicitly compare these values. Studies concerning antibiotic consumption in the neonatal population are not numerous, but what is more important: the published papers present a differentiated approach to the subject and are carried out with the use of diverse methodology and for various needs [5, 11, 13, 26, 28].

However, the main objective of this study was the analysis of the evaluation of antibiotic consumption in the treatment of one form of infection in a narrow and specific patient population, giving special consideration to the possibility of its use in the evaluation of the effectiveness and accuracy of microbiological diagnostics as an element of surveillance of infections in NICU.

And so, in NICUs covered by the study, significantly lower consumption of antibiotics expressed by DDD was observed in the case of LC-BSI treatment, compared to those in which the etiological agent was not isolated. On this basis, it can be concluded that the microbiological diagnosis of BSI in newborns treated in NICU was conducted properly and the results of microbiological tests were used in targeted therapy, what made it possible to obtain a reduction in the consumption of antimicrobial drugs and, consequently, the cost of treatment. In Polish NICUs, costs of medication account for nearly one-fifth of the total cost of treatment, the amount of which is inversely proportional to a child's birth weight and directly proportional to the length of hospitalization [20].

A different situation was observed in the population of the PNSN neonates, who developed necrotising enterocolitis, wherein the length of therapy and consumption rates were not affected by the isolation of the potential etiological agent [29]. But with NEC, difficulties present themselves as regards obtaining material for microbiological examination, which would enable the isolation of the etiological agent. The quoted results concerning antibiotic consumption in NEC cases and the ones demonstrated in the present study regarding BSI illustrate the possibilities of how analyses in this respect could be utilized in infection control and, in particular, in evaluation of adequacy and effectiveness of microbiological diagnostics.

On the other hand, no significant differences in DOT values in cases of LC-BSI and microbiologically unconfirmed BSI were observed. This is contradictory to the current approach to modern antimicrobial stewardship: in newborn population, with suspected BSI, it is recommended to terminate antibiotic treatment after 48 h since the identification of symptoms, if the infection was not confirmed microbiologically. Even traditional diagnostics based on the culture method ensures obtaining a positive result (information on microbial etiology of infection) within 48 h [30, 31].

For antimicrobial stewardship to efficiently and effectively influence the reduction of antibiotic consumption, but not to decrease patient safety, in neonatal units, a principle of daily detailed review of the situation of neonates treated with antibiotics should be introduced, so as to minimize the intake of antibiotics in children, whose blood cultures and other clinical specimens tested negative and symptoms of infection are no longer observed or infectious origin of the disease was excluded. The lack of significant differences in DOT values of laboratory confirmed vs. not-confirmed BSI cases would point to the fact that these recommendations are not applied in the PNSN wards.

It should also be noted that rapid diagnostic molecular methods (which enable rapid assessment of the need to implement or discontinue therapy with vancomycin) could be implemented to decrease glycopeptides consumption, because glycopeptides are not easy to use in neonates [32, 33]. For it has been observed that the use of glycopeptides in the case of BSI caused by *Enterobacteriaceae* was lower by only approx. 20% in comparison with BSI caused by Gram-positive cocci. Generally, in our study, in treatment of BSI as a whole glycopeptides were used the longest. Similar situation was reported in study of Sameer et al. [34].

As for aminoglycosides, only the use of the DDD indicator permitted the demonstration of their significantly increased consumption in BSI caused by Gram-positive cocci (109 DDD), in comparison with BSI that were caused by Gram-negative bacilli (56.1 DDD).

Also noteworthy is the fact that there is a large share of antifungal drugs in the treatment of the analyzed cases of BSI, 25% of the entire consumption expressed by DDD (13.3% DOT), with simultaneous, lower than anticipated, participation of yeast-like fungi isolated in microbiological testing [35, 36]. This coincides with the trends observed in other studies. According to Fridkin, the application of fluconazole in infection prophylaxis contributed to this fact, which is also confirmed by other authors [6]. Thus, the high level of antimycotic medication consumption in PNSN wards fulfilled the task of reducing the incidence of fungal infections.

Antibiotic consumption assessment using at least two different measures, as presented in our study, can be a useful tool in antibiotic stewardship [27]. In presenting case, the results of the analysis indicate the need of implementing more sensitive and faster methods of microbiological diagnostics (PCR and/or MALDI-TOF) as a first step of reducing antibiotics consumption due to faster identification of etiological factor of infection. PCR increases the sensitivity of diagnostics test and shortens the time of identification of microorganisms without culture. MALDI-TOF improves the specificity and shortens the time of identification after receiving microorganism grow in culture method [37, 38]. These diagnostics techniques are still very rarely used in Polish hospital. They are considered as expensive procedures by hospitals' management, because complex cost-effectiveness analysis in the field of infection control, taking into account at least the cost of prolonged hospital stay, are not performed. In the study patient population occurrence of BSI significantly increases length of stay in NICU, by approximately 20 days [21].

Conclusions

Analysis of antibiotic consumption is an essential component of infection control, especially for NICU patients—for effective planning and reliable evaluation of interrelationships between individual elements of control programs.

Application of classical methods of microbiological diagnostics based on blood cultures significantly reduces the consumption of antibiotics expressed by DDD.

High consumption of glycopeptides marked by DOT indicates the necessity of applying rapid diagnostic assays.

Nevertheless, the assessment of antibiotic consumption in neonatal units represents a methodological challenge and requires the use of different measurement tools.

Abbreviations

BSI: bloodstream infection; DOT: days of therapy; DDD: defined daily dose; LC-BSI: laboratory confirmed bloodstream infection; LOT: length of therapy; NICU: neonatal intensive care unit; PDD: prescribed daily dose; PNSN: Polish Neonatal Surveillance Network; VLBW: very low birth weight; PCR: polymerase chain reaction; MALDI-TOF: matrix assisted laser desorption ionisation, MALDI; time of flight, TOF.

Authors' contributions

AR designed the study and was a major contributor in writing the manuscript; JWM drafted the first version of this manuscript; PA performed statistical analysis; MBK, EG, MN, AK, DP collected the data on the wards; MB have given final approval of the version to be published. All authors read and approved the final manuscript.

Author details

[1] Chair of Microbiology, Jagiellonian University Medical College, 18 Czysta Street, 31-121 Krakow, Poland. [2] Institute of Nature Conservation Polish Academy of Sciences, Krakow, Poland. [3] Clinic of Neonatology and Intensive Neonatal Care, Warsaw Medical University, Warsaw, Poland. [4] Clinic of Neonatology, Polish Mother's Memorial Hospital-Research Institute, Lodz, Poland. [5] Clinic of Neonatology and Intensive Neonatal Care, Institute of Mother and Child, Warsaw, Poland. [6] Department of Neonatal Diseases, Pomeranian Medical University, Szczecin, Poland. [7] Clinic of Neonatology, Jagiellonian University Medical College, Krakow, Poland.

Acknowledgements

Not applicable.

Competing interests

The authors declare that they have no competing interests.

Ethics approval

The study was approved by the Bioethics Committee of Jagiellonian University Medical College-No. KBET/221/B/2011.

Funding

The project of the Polish Neonatology Surveillance Network was funded by the Polish Ministry of Science and Higher Education (Decision No. 669/E-215-BSWN-0180/2008). The funder had no impact on the design of the study and collection, analysis and interpretation of data and writing the manuscript.

References

1. Wójkowska-Mach J, Borszewska-Kornacka M, Domańska J, Gadzinowski J, Gulczyńska E, Helwich E, et al. Early-onset Infections of very-low-birth-weight infants in Polish neonatal intensive care units. Pediatr Infect Dis J. 2012;31(7):691–5.
2. Ronnestad A, Abrahamsen TG, Medbo S, Reigstad H, Lossius K, Kaaresen PI, et al. Septicemia in the first week of life in a Norwegian National Cohort of extremely premature infants. Pediatrics. 2005;115:e262–8. doi:10.1542/peds.2004-1834.
3. Stoll BJ, Hansen NI, Bell EF, Shankaran S, Laptook AR, Walsh MC, et al. The Eunice Kennedy Shriver National Institute of Child Health and Human Development Neonatal Research Network: neonatal outcomes of extremely preterm infants from the NICHD Neonatal Research Network. Pediatrics. 2010;123(3):443–56. doi:10.1542/peds.2009-2959.
4. Klinger G, Levy I, Sirota L, Boyko V, Lerner-Geva L, Reichman B. Outcome of early-onset sepsis in a national cohort of very low birth weight infants. Pediatrics. 2010;125(4):e736–40. doi:10.1542/peds.2009-2017.
5. Versporten A, Sharland M, Bielicki J, Drapier N, Vankerckoven V, Goossens H. The antibiotic resistance and prescribing in European children project. A neonatal and pediatric antimicrobial web-based point prevalence survey in 73 hospitals worldwide. Pediatr Infect Dis J. 2013;32(6):242–53.
6. Fridkin SK, Kaufman D, Edwards JR, Shetty S, Horan T. Changing incidence of Candida bloodstream infections among NICU patients in the United States: 199502994. Padiatrics. 2006;117(5):1680–7.
7. Wojkowska-Mach J, Borszewska-Kornacka M, Domanska J, Gadzinowski J, Gulczynska E, Nowiczewski M, et al. Late-onset bloodstream infections of very-low-birth-weight infant. Data from the Polish Neonatology Surveillance Network in 2009–2011. J BMC Infect Dis. 2014;14(1):339. doi:10.1186/1471-2334-14-339.
8. Schwab F, Geffers C, Barwolff S, Ruden H, Gastmeier P. Reducing neonatal nosocomial bloodstream infections through participation in a national surveillance system. J Hosp Infect. 2007;65:319–25.
9. Makhoul IR, Sujov P, Smolkin T, Lusky A, Reichman B. Pathogen-specific early mortality in very low birth weight infants with late-onset sepsis: a national survey. Clin Infect Dis. 2005;40:218–24.
10. Grohskopf LA, Huskins WC, Sinkowitz-Cochran RL, Levine GL, Goldmann DA, Jarvis WR. Use of antimicrobial agents in United States neonatal and pediatric intensive care patients. Pediatr Infect Dis J. 2005;24:766–73.
11. Liem Y, van den Hoogen A, Rademaker C, Egberts TC, Fleer F, Krediet TG. Antibiotic weight-watching: slimming down on antibiotic use in a NICU. Acta Peadiatr. 2010;99:1900–2.
12. WHO Collaborating Centre for Drug Statistics Methodology, Guidelines for ATC classification and DDD assignment 2010. Oslo, 2009. ISSN 1726-4898, ISBN 978-82-8082-369-4
13. Porta A, Hsia Y, Doerholt K, Menson E, Spyridis N, Bielicki J, et al. Comparing neonatal and paediatric antibiotic prescribing between hospitals: a new algorithm to help international benchmarking. J Antimicrob Chemother. 2012;67:1278–86.
14. Berrington A. Antimicrobial prescribing in hospitals: be careful what you measure. J Antimicrob Chemother. 2010;65:163–8.
15. Gerber JS, Kronman MP, Ross RK, Hersh AL, Newland JG, Metjian TA, et al. Identifying targets for antimicrobial stewardship in children's hospitals. Infect Control Hosp Epidemiol. 2013;34(12):1252–8.
16. Haug JB, Reikvam A. WHO defined daily doses versus hospital-adjusted defined daily doses: impact on results of antibiotic use surveillance. J Antimicrob Chemother. 2013;68:2940–7.
17. Gastmeier P, Geffers C, Schwab F, Fitzner J, Oblader M, Ruden H. Development of a surveillance system for nosocomial infections: the component for neonatal intensive care in Germany. J Hosp Infect. 2004;57:126–31.
18. Brodie SB, Sands KE, Gray JE, Parker RA, Goldmann DA, Davis RB, Richardson DK. Occurrence of nosocomial bloodstream infections in six neonatal intensive care units. Pediatr Infect Dis J. 2000;19:56–65.
19. Drews MB, Ludwig AC, Leititis JU, Daschner FD. Low birth weight and nosocomial infection of neonates in a neonatal intensive care unit. J Hosp Infect. 1995;30:65–72.
20. Krawczyk-Wyrwicka I, Piotrowski A, Rydlewska-Liszkowska I, Hanke W. Costs of intensive care of newborns born prematurely. Prz Epidemiol. 2006;60:155–62.
21. Różańska A, Wójkowska-Mach J, Adamski P, Borszewska-Kornacka M, Gulczyńska E, Nowiczewski M, et al. Infections and risk-adjusted length of stay and hospital mortality in Polish neonatology intensive care units. Int J Infect Dis. 2015;35:87–92.
22. Edwards JR, Peterson KD, Mu Y, Banwrjee S, Allen-Bridson K, Morrell G, et al. National healthcare safety network (nhsn) report: data summary for 2006 through 2008, issued december 2009. Am J Infect Control. 2009;37:783–805. doi:10.1016/j.ajic.2009.10.001.

23. Gikas A, Roumbelaki M, Bagatzouni-Pieridou D, Alexandrou M, Zinieri V, Dimitriadis I, et al. Device-associated infections in the intensive care units of Cyprus: results of the first national incidence study. Infection. 2010;38:165–71.
24. Huang YC, Wang YH, Chou YH, Lien RI. Significance of coagulase-negative staphylococci isolated from a single blood culture from neonates in intensive care. Ann Trop Paediatr. 2006;26(4):311–8.
25. Van der Zwet WC, Kaiser AM, van Elburg RM, Berkhof J, Fetter WP, Parlevliet GA, et al. Nosocomial infections in a Dutch neonatal intensive care unit: surveillance study with definitions for infection specifically adapted for neonates. J Hosp Infect. 2005;61:300–11.
26. Liem Y, Heerdink A, Egberts A, Rademaker CM. Quantifying antibiotic use in peadiatrics: a proposal for neonatal DDDs. Eur J Clin Microbiol Infect Dis. 2010;29:1301–3.
27. Barlam T, Cosgrove S, Abbo L, MacDougall C, Schuetz AN, Septimus EJ, et al. Implementing an antibiotic stewardship program: guidelines by the Infectious Diseases Society of America and the Society for Healthcare Epidemiology of America. Clin Infect Dis. 2016;62(10):e51–77.
28. Różańska A, Wójkowska-Mach J, Borszewska-Kornacka M, Ćmiel A, Gadzinowski J, Gulczyńska E, et al. Antibiotic consumption and its costs of purchase in Polish Neonatology Networks Units. Przegl Epidemiol. 2012;66:513–9.
29. Wójkowska-Mach J, Różańska A, Borszewska-Kornacka M, Domańska J, Gadzinowski J, Gulczyńska E, et al. Necrotizing enterocolitis in preterm infants: epidemiology and antibiotic consumption in the Polish Neonatology Network neonatal intensive care units in 2009. PLoS ONE. 2014;9(3):e92865. doi:10.1371/journal.pone.0092865.
30. Garcia-Prats JA, Cooper TR, Schneider VF, Stager CE, Hansen TN. Rapid detection of microorganisms in blood cultures of newborn infants utilizing an automated blood culture system. Pediatrics. 2000;105(3):523–7.
31. Kaiser JR, Cassat JE, Lewno MJ. Should antibiotics be discontinued at 48 hours for negative late-onset sepsis evaluations in the neonatal intensive care unit? J Perinatol. 2002;22(6):445–7.
32. Lim HS, Chong YP, Noh YH, Jung JA, Kim YS. Exploration of optimal dosing regimens of vancomycin in patients infected with methicillin-resistant *Staphylococcus aureus* by modeling and simulation. J Clin Pharm Ther. 2014;16.39(2):196–203.
33. Ampe E, Delaere B, Hecq JD, Tulkens PM, Glupczynski Y. Implementation of a protocol for administration of vancomycin by continuous infusion: pharmacokinetic, pharmacodynamic and toxicological aspects. Int J Antimicrob Agents. 2013;41(5):439–46.
34. Sameer J, Oshoudi A, Prasad P, Delamona P, Larson E, Zaoutis T, et al. Antibiotic use in neonatal intensive care units and adherence with Centers for Disease Control and Prevention 12 step campaign to prevent antimicrobial resistance. Pediatr Infect Dis J. 2009;28(12):1047–51.
35. Friedman S, Richardson SE, Jacobs SE, O'Brien K. Systemic Candida infection in extremely low birth weight infants: short term morbidity and long term neurodevelopmental outcome. Pediatr Infect Dis J. 2000;19:499–504.
36. Manzoni P, Stolfi I, Pugni L, Decembrio L, Magnani C, Vetrano G, et al. A multicenter, randomized trial of prophylactic fluconazole in preterm neonates. N Engl J Med. 2007;356:2483–95.
37. Nieman AE, Savelkoul PH, Beishuizen A, Henrich B, Lamik B, MacKenzie CR, et al. A prospective multicenter evaluation of direct molecular detection of blood stream infection from a clinical perspective. BMC Infect Dis. 2016;16:314. doi:10.1186/s12879-016-1646-4.
38. Chen Y, Porter V, Mubareka S, Kotowich L, Simor AE. Rapid identification of bacteria directly from positive blood cultures by use of a serum separator tube, smudge plate preparation, and matrix-assisted laser desorption ionization-time of flight mass spectrometry. J Clin Microbiol. 2015;53(10):3349–52. doi:10.1128/JCM.01493-15.

18

Molecular characterization of clinical IMP-producing *Klebsiella pneumoniae* isolates from a Chinese Tertiary Hospital

Kaisheng Lai†, Yanning Ma†, Ling Guo, Jingna An, Liyan Ye and Jiyong Yang*

Abstract

Background: IMP-producing *Klebsiella pneumoniae* (IMPKpn) exhibits sporadic prevalence in China. The mechanisms related to the spread of IMPKpn remain unclear.

Methods: Carbapenem non-susceptible *K. pneumoniae* isolates were collected from our hospital. The genetic relatedness, antimicrobial susceptibility, as well as sequence types (ST) were analyzed by pulsed-field gel electrophoresis (PFGE), VITEK 2 AST test Kit, and multilocus sequence typing (MLST), respectively. S1-PFGE, Southern blot analysis and multiple PCR amplification were used for plasmid profiling.

Results: Between October 2009 and June 2016, 25 non-repetitive IMPKpn isolates were identified. PFGE results showed that these isolates belonged to 20 genetically unrelated IMPKpn strains. Diverse STs were identified by MLST. Most strains carried $bla_{IMP\text{-}4}$, followed by $bla_{IMP\text{-}1}$. Four incompatibility types of bla_{IMP}-carrying plasmids were identified, which included A/C (n = 2), B/O (n = 2), L/M (n = 1) and N (n = 14), while type of other one plasmid failed to be determined.

Conclusions: The IMPKpn isolates exhibited sporadic prevalence in our hospital. IncN types of plasmids with various sizes have emerged as the main platform mediating the spread of the bla_{IMP} genes in our hospital.

Keywords: IMP, *Klebsiella pneumoniae*, Sequence type

Background

The spread of carbapenemase-producing *Enterobacteriaceae* has been a major challenge both for treatment of individual patients and for policies of infection control [1]. IMP-1 is the first identified metallo-β-lactamase conferring carbapenem resistance and was described in 1988 in a *Pseudomonas aeruginosa* strain in Japan [2]. IMP-type carbapenemases can hydrolyze almost all β-lactams. The popular IMP-type carbapenemases have been widespread in non-fermenting Gram-negative bacilli, including *Pseudomonas aeruginosa, Acinetobacter* spp., and members of the *Enterobacteriaceae* family [3]. The bla_{IMP} genes are usually located on large plasmids with different replicon types or incompatibility (Inc) types, such as IncA/C, L/M, N, and HI2, which have been commonly associated with the carriage and transmission of various bla_{IMP} genes [4–7].

Klebsiella pneumoniae is an important pathogen causing various infections. IMP-producing *K. pneumoniae* (IMPKpn) isolates have been identified worldwide and caused a few small-scale outbreaks [3, 5, 6, 8, 9]. Up to now, diverse sequence types (ST) of IMPKpn have been reported, including STs 15, 37, 107, 133, 252, 323, 340, 476, 478, 626, 686, 889, 903, 1114 and 1306 [5–11].

In China, IMP-producing *Enterobacteriaceae* isolates have been found across the country [3, 6, 7, 9–21]. Variants of bla_{IMP} have been identified in *K. pneumoniae, Escherichia coli* and *Enterobacter cloacae*. Among IMPKpn, IMP-4 is the most commonly encountered isoform in clinical isolates, followed by IMP-8, IMP-26 and IMP-38 [6, 9–18, 22]. Meanwhile, the IMPKpn isolates exhibit high diversity of sequence type (ST), and IMPKpn STs15,

*Correspondence: yangjy301@hotmail.com
†Kaisheng Lai and Yanning Ma contributed equally to this work
Department of Microbiology, Chinese PLA General Hospital, 301 Hospital, 28# Fuxing Road, Beijing 100853, China

37, 107, 133, 323, 476, 686, 889, 1114 and 1306 have been recovered [6, 7, 10, 11].

In the present study, a retrospective study of clinical carbapenem-non-susceptible *enterobacteriaceae* isolates from our hospital was performed. In total, 25 IMPKpn isolates were identified in this study. Phenotypic and genotypic characteristics of these isolates were further analyzed.

Methods

Bacterial isolates

All clinical *Enterobacteriaceae* isolates were collected from a 4000-bed tertiary-care hospital and were identified by VITEK® MS (bioMérieux SA, Marcy-l'Etoile, France). The isolates exhibiting resistance or intermediate to any one of ertapenem or imipenem or meropenem will be defined as carbapenem non-susceptibility strain, and will be screened for bla_{IMP} by PCR and subsequent amplicon sequencing using the primers IMP-1F: 5′-TGAGCAAGTTATCTGTATTC and IMP-1R: 5′-TTAGTTGCTTGGTTTTGATG [11]. *E. coli* ATCC 25922 was used as a quality control strain for antimicrobial susceptibility testing. The *Salmonella* ser. Braenderup strain H9812 was used as a reference standard for pulsed-field gel electrophoresis (PFGE). No ethical approval was obtained for using the clinical samples, because they were collected during routine bacteriologic analyses in public hospitals, and the data were anonymously analyzed.

Antimicrobial susceptibility testing

The MICs of clinical commonly used antimicrobial agents (listed in Fig. 1) were measured using VITEK 2 AST-GN09 and AST-GN13 test Kit (bioMérieux, Inc.) according to the manufacturer's instructions. All susceptibility results were interpreted according to the 2017 CLSI performance standards [23].

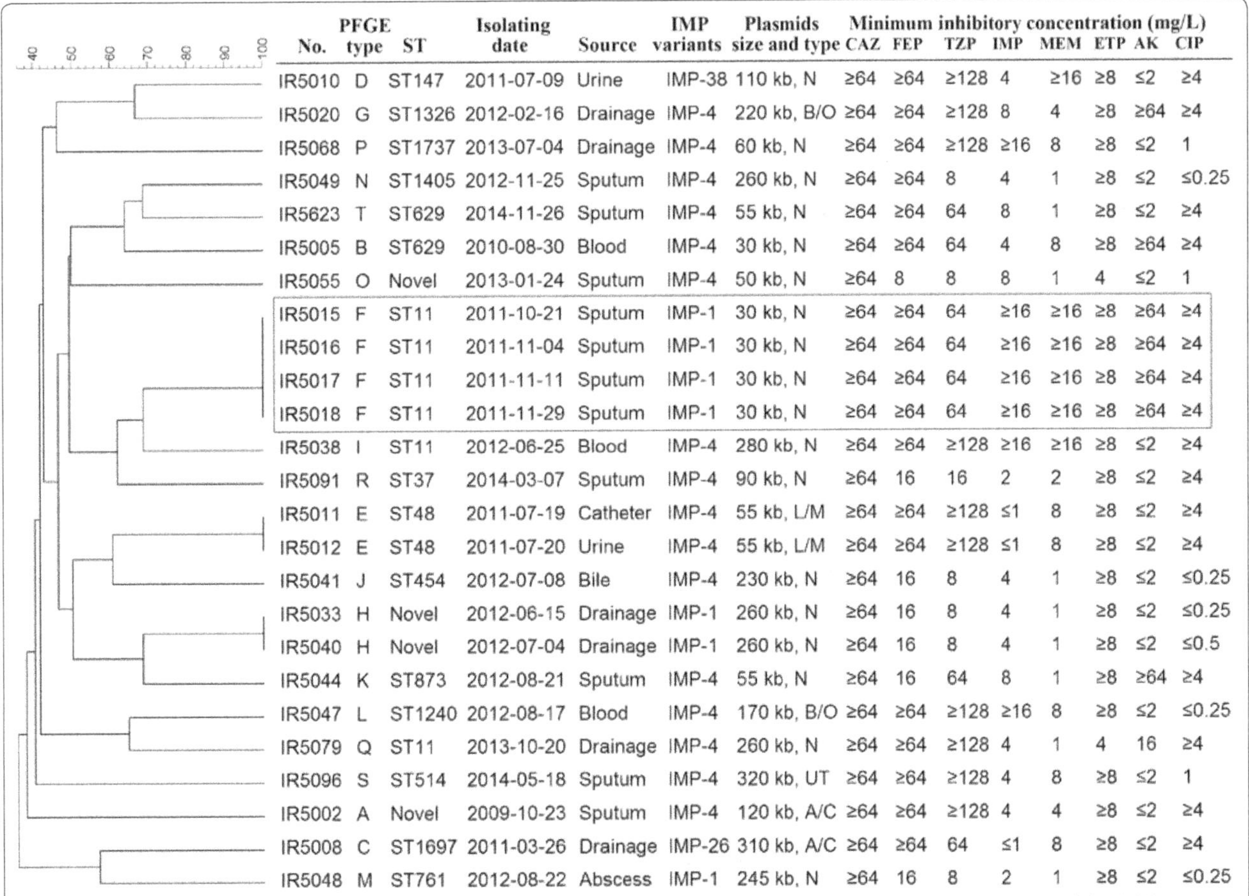

No.	PFGE type	ST	Isolating date	Source	IMP variants	Plasmids size and type	CAZ	FEP	TZP	IMP	MEM	ETP	AK	CIP
IR5010	D	ST147	2011-07-09	Urine	IMP-38	110 kb, N	≥64	≥64	≥128	4	≥16	≥8	≤2	≥4
IR5020	G	ST1326	2012-02-16	Drainage	IMP-4	220 kb, B/O	≥64	≥64	≥128	8	4	≥8	≥64	≥4
IR5068	P	ST1737	2013-07-04	Drainage	IMP-4	60 kb, N	≥64	≥64	≥128	≥16	8	≥8	≤2	1
IR5049	N	ST1405	2012-11-25	Sputum	IMP-4	260 kb, N	≥64	≥64	8	4	1	≥8	≤2	≤0.25
IR5623	T	ST629	2014-11-26	Sputum	IMP-4	55 kb, N	≥64	≥64	64	8	1	≥8	≤2	≥4
IR5005	B	ST629	2010-08-30	Blood	IMP-4	30 kb, N	≥64	≥64	64	4	8	≥8	≥64	≥4
IR5055	O	Novel	2013-01-24	Sputum	IMP-4	50 kb, N	≥64	8	8	8	1	4	≤2	1
IR5015	F	ST11	2011-10-21	Sputum	IMP-1	30 kb, N	≥64	≥64	64	≥16	≥16	≥8	≥64	≥4
IR5016	F	ST11	2011-11-04	Sputum	IMP-1	30 kb, N	≥64	≥64	64	≥16	≥16	≥8	≥64	≥4
IR5017	F	ST11	2011-11-11	Sputum	IMP-1	30 kb, N	≥64	≥64	64	≥16	≥16	≥8	≥64	≥4
IR5018	F	ST11	2011-11-29	Sputum	IMP-1	30 kb, N	≥64	≥64	64	≥16	≥16	≥8	≥64	≥4
IR5038	I	ST11	2012-06-25	Blood	IMP-4	280 kb, N	≥64	≥64	≥128	≥16	≥16	≥8	≤2	≥4
IR5091	R	ST37	2014-03-07	Sputum	IMP-4	90 kb, N	≥64	16	16	2	2	≥8	≤2	≥4
IR5011	E	ST48	2011-07-19	Catheter	IMP-4	55 kb, L/M	≥64	≥64	≥128	≤1	8	≥8	≤2	≥4
IR5012	E	ST48	2011-07-20	Urine	IMP-4	55 kb, L/M	≥64	≥64	≥128	≤1	8	≥8	≤2	≥4
IR5041	J	ST454	2012-07-08	Bile	IMP-4	230 kb, N	≥64	16	8	4	1	≥8	≤2	≤0.25
IR5033	H	Novel	2012-06-15	Drainage	IMP-1	260 kb, N	≥64	16	8	4	1	≥8	≤2	≤0.25
IR5040	H	Novel	2012-07-04	Drainage	IMP-1	260 kb, N	≥64	16	8	4	1	≥8	≤2	≤0.5
IR5044	K	ST873	2012-08-21	Sputum	IMP-4	55 kb, N	≥64	16	64	8	1	≥8	≥64	≥4
IR5047	L	ST1240	2012-08-17	Blood	IMP-4	170 kb, B/O	≥64	≥64	≥128	≥16	8	≥8	≤2	≤0.25
IR5079	Q	ST11	2013-10-20	Drainage	IMP-4	260 kb, N	≥64	≥64	≥128	4	1	4	16	≥4
IR5096	S	ST514	2014-05-18	Sputum	IMP-4	320 kb, UT	≥64	≥64	≥128	4	8	≥8	≤2	1
IR5002	A	Novel	2009-10-23	Sputum	IMP-4	120 kb, A/C	≥64	≥64	≥128	4	4	≥8	≤2	≥4
IR5008	C	ST1697	2011-03-26	Drainage	IMP-26	310 kb, A/C	≥64	≥64	64	≤1	8	≥8	≤2	≥4
IR5048	M	ST761	2012-08-22	Abscess	IMP-1	245 kb, N	≥64	16	8	2	1	≥8	≤2	≤0.25

(Columns CAZ–CIP: Minimum inhibitory concentration (mg/L))

Fig. 1 Dendrogram of patterns generated by PFGE of IMP-producing *K. pneumoniae* isolates. The PFGE types, ST, isolating date of the IMPKpn isolates, IMP variants, the size and type of bla_{IMP}-carrying plasmids and the MICs of common-used antimicrobial agents were list in this figure. The frame indicated the characterization of IMP-producing *K. pneumoniae* isolates causing an outbreak. *ST* sequence type, *CAZ* ceftazidime, *FEP* cefepime, *TZP* piperacillin–tazobactam, *IMP* imipenem, *MEM* meropenem, *ETP* ertapenem, *AK* amikacin, *CIP* ciprofloxacin, *UT* unable type

PFGE and MLST analyses

PFGE with *Xba*I was performed for IMPKpn isolates as previously described [24]. MLST was carried out for IMPKpn according to protocols provided on their MLST websites (http://www.pasteur.fr/recherche/genopole/PF8/mlst/Kpneumoniae).

Plasmid and southern blot analyses

A bla_{NDM} probe was generated by labeling the PCR product using the PCR DIG Probe Synthesis Kit (Roche Applied Sciences, Mannheim, Germany). The size and incompatibility types of bla_{IMP}-carrying plasmids were analyzed by the S1-PFGE, Southern blot and multiple PCR as previously described [24, 25]. The whole genomic DNA including the plasmid of the isolates was digested with 20 U of S1 nuclease at 37 °C for 20 min, and separated by PFGE. Then, the DNA fragments were transferred to positively charged nylon membranes (Roche Applied Science). Hybridization was carried out with the DIG Easy Hyb Granules (Roche Applied Sciences), and the detection was performed using the DIG Nucleic Acid Detection Kit (Roche Applied Sciences).

Results

Prevalence and genetic relatedness of IMPKpn

The first IMPKpn isolate in our hospital was identified in October 2009. Since then until June 2016, 25 non-repetitive IMPKpn isolates have been recovered. The source of the IMPKpn isolates included 11 sputum, 6 drainges, 3 bloods, 2 urines, 1 catheter, 1 bile and 1 abscess. The 25 IMPKpn isolates were categorized into 20 PFGE types (type A to T). Type F contained 4 isolates, and types E and H contained 2 isolates, other 16 types contained only 1 isolate (Fig. 1). Isolates with same PFGE type were considered as the same strain. Therefore, a total of 20 IMPKpn strains with no genetic relationship were further analyzed.

Antimicrobial susceptibility

The antimicrobial susceptibility patterns of the isolates were listed in Fig. 1. All isolates presented resistance to ceftazidime, cefepime and piperacillin–tazobactam, and exhibited heterogeneous resistance patterns to carbapenem, amikacin and ciprofloxacin (Fig. 1).

bla_{IMP} variants

PCR and subsequent amplicon sequence alignment revealed that most strains carried bla_{IMP-4}, and several bla_{IMP} gene sequences displayed 100% identity with the published sequence of the bla_{IMP-1} (for 3 strains), bla_{IMP-26} (for 1 strains) and bla_{IMP-38} (for 1 strains) genes, respectively (Fig. 1).

MLST

Among 20 IMPKpn strains, a diversity of STs was identified. Three strains were identified as ST11, two strains were defined as ST629, and 12 strains belonged to independent STs. Three novel STs were identified with the allelic profile 18-71-26-125-115-2-51 (type A strain), 42-22-25-96-115-20-49 (type H strain) and 71-1-1-83-16-121-5 (type O strain), respectively (Fig. 1).

Plasmid analysis

The bla_{IMP} genes were located on plasmids with sizes ranged from approximately 30 to 320 kb (Fig. 1). Four incompatibility types of bla_{IMP}-carrying plasmids including A/C, B/O, L/M and N were identified, whereas type of one plasmid was unable to be determined. In total, 14 IMPKpn strains carried the IncN plasmids with sizes ranging from 30 to 280 kb, while two A/C (120- and 310-kb), two IncB/O (170- and 220-kb) and one IncL/M (55 kb) plasmids were characterized.

Discussion

The worldwide spread of carbapenemase-producing *K. pneumoniae* has been a growing clinical problem and threat to public health [1]. In this study, 25 non-duplicated IMPKpn isolates were collected between October 2009 and June 2016. During this period, 8.5% (537 of 6310) of clinical *K. pneumoniae* isolates exhibited carbapenem-resistant phenotypes, and only 0.19% (25/537) of carbapenem-non-susceptible *K. pneumoniae* strains produced IMP. Further analysis showed that the majority of carbapenemase-producing *K. pneumoniae* was the KPC-2-producing *K. pneumoniae*, followed by OXA-48- and NDM-producing *K. pneumoniae* [24–26]. Therefore, IMPKpn exhibited sporadic prevalence in our hospital. In China, IMPKpn isolates have been identified across the country, and the main variants are IMP-4 and IMP-8 [3, 6, 7, 9–21], while IMP-26 and IMP-38 have also been identified [16, 18]. In this study, besides the scattered emergence of IMP-1, IMP-26 and IMP-38, we found that the majority of IMPKpn isolates produced IPM-4 (Fig. 1) which was different from the prevalence of IMP variants that were reported from other Asian regions, where IMP-1 accounted for the majority [3]. Taken together, the source, evolution and dissemination of IMPKpn may be different in different regions.

In this study, PFGE analysis revealed that the majority of IMPKpn isolates belonged to different types, while an outbreak at small scales (type F strain) that covered only four patients was observed (Fig. 1), suggesting that the majority of IMPKpn isolates analyzed in this study were genetically unrelated strains. Meanwhile, most strains exhibited high ST diversity. Only three and two clones of IMPKpn strains belonged to ST11 and ST629, respectively, while other STs were only identified in single strain. Three strains were identified as new clones with novel STs (Fig. 1). Other reports also showed that the STs of IMPKpn are highly dispersed [5–11], suggesting the clonal diversity of IMPKpn isolates. Thus, the IMPKpn exhibited a significant sporadic prevalence across the world. Under the same medical condition and selective pressure, the KPC-2-producing *K. pneumoniae* spread throughout our hospital [24]. However, the IMPKpn strains only exhibited low prevalence and small scale of outbreaks at the same time. A study revealed that some biological characteristics, such as cell motility, secretion, DNA repair and modification, may contribute to the rapid spread of KPC-producing *K. pneumoniae* ST258 and ST11 [27]. Recent genomic analysis of *K. pneumoniae* has established that the genomic background was closely related to the pathogenicity of *K. pneumoniae* [28]. Therefore, the virulence characteristics, rather than their drug-resistant phenotype, may be the major driving force responsible for the emergence and widely spread of antibiotic-resistant pathogens. The urgent efforts are needed to reveal the genetic background of these pathogens, as well as its relationship with their pathogenic and transmission abilities, which is the essential first step to design intervention strategies preventing their spread.

In this study, most of the clinical isolates exhibited low-level resistance or even sensitivity to imipenem and meropenem, but high-level resistance to ertapenem (Fig. 1). Similar results have also been reported in other studies from China [9, 13, 14, 16, 20]. These studies showed that the effects of IMP hydrolase on different carbapenems may be diverse, and therefore, the carbapenem-sensitive phenotype does not mean negative for carbapenemase. In most laboratories in China, the production of carbapenemases was not usually detected by modified Hodge test [23] in clinical IMPKpn isolates with carbapenem-sensitive phenotype. The weak hydrolytic ability of IMPs to carbapenems may lead to an underestimation of the prevalence of IMPKpn isolates. It was reported that some IMP variants (such IMP-26) exhibited increased carbapenem-hydrolyzing activity [29]. However, the IMP-26-producing IMPKpn were sensitive to imipenem in this study (Fig. 1). Another study also showed that the IMP-26-producing IMPKpn displayed only low-level resistance to imipenem [14]. Therefore, the production of IMPs was not the only factor responsible for high-level carbapenem resistance, other resistance mechanisms may also confer this process, which include hyperexpression of efflux systems, and loss of the outer membrane channel OprD that allows the entry of carbapenems into the cell [30]. For clinical IMPKpn isolates, it is less clear to what extent the different resistant mechanisms have impact on the carbapenem-resistant phenotype.

Plasmid analysis in this study showed that the majority (13 of 20) of bla_{IMP}-carrying plasmids belonged to IncN. Another study in China found the dissemination of IncN bla_{IMP}-coding plasmids among *K. pneumoniae* of different genotypes [7]. These results suggested that IncN plasmids have a unique advantage and fitness in the spread of bla_{IMP} genes. However, because most of the IncN plasmids had different sizes in this study (Fig. 1), it was possible that the dissemination of bla_{IMP} genes in our hospital may not mediated by transfer of plasmids but other mechanisms.

The present study has several limitations. First, because this study was retrospective analysis and only limited patient information was available, thus the study focused on the characterization of phenotype and genotype of clinical IMPKpn isolates. Second, the genetic environment of bla_{IMP} genes remained to be characterized in our future study. Another limitation of the study included the absence of analyzing other resistance-related determinants, the outer-membrane permeabilities, and efflux systems of IMPKpn isolates. Further studies are needed to address these limitations.

Authors' contributions

KL, YM, LG, JA and LY performed the phenotypic and genotypic analysis of clinical isolates. JY designed the study, performed data analysis and drafted the manuscript. All authors read and approved the final manuscript.

Acknowledgements

Not applicable.

Competing interests

The authors declare that they have no competing interests.

Consent for publication

We give our permission for the above material to appear in the print, online, and licensed versions of *Annals of Clinical Microbiology and Antimicrobials.*

Funding

This study was supported by the China Mega-Project on Infectious Disease Prevention (Grant No. 2017ZX10103002-002-002).

References

1. van Duin D. Doi Y. The global epidemiology of carbapenemase-producing Enterobacteriaceae. Virulence. 2016;11:1–10. doi:10.1080/21505594.2016.1222343.
2. Watanabe M, Iyobe S, Inoue M, Mitsuhashi S. Transferable imipenem resistance in *Pseudomonas aeruginosa*. Antimicrob Agents Chemother. 1991;35(1):147–51.

3. Zhao WH, Hu ZQ. IMP-type metallo-beta-lactamases in Gram-negative bacilli: distribution, phylogeny, and association with integrons. Crit Rev Microbiol. 2011;37(3):214–26.
4. Ho PL, Lo WU, Chan J, Cheung YY, Chow KH, Yam WC, Lin CH, Que TL. pIMP-PH114 carrying bla IMP-4 in a *Klebsiella pneumoniae* strain is closely related to other multidrug-resistant IncA/C2 plasmids. Curr Microbiol. 2014;68(2):227–32.
5. Peirano G, Lascols C, Hackel M, Hoban DJ, Pitout JD. Molecular epidemiology of Enterobacteriaceae that produce VIMs and IMPs from the SMART surveillance program. Diagn Microbiol Infect Dis. 2014;78(3):277–81.
6. Wang JT, Wu UI, Lauderdale TL, Chen MC, Li SY, Hsu LY, Chang SC. Carbapenem-nonsusceptible Enterobacteriaceae in Taiwan. PLoS ONE. 2015;10(3):e0121668.
7. Feng W, Zhou D, Wang Q, Luo W, Zhang D, Sun Q, Tong Y, Chen W, Sun F, Xia P. Dissemination of IMP-4-encoding pIMP-HZ1-related plasmids among *Klebsiella pneumoniae* and *Pseudomonas aeruginosa* in a Chinese teaching hospital. Sci Rep. 2016;6:33419.
8. Fukigai S, Alba J, Kimura S, Iida T, Nishikura N, Ishii Y, Yamaguchi K. Nosocomial outbreak of genetically related IMP-1 beta-lactamase-producing *Klebsiella pneumoniae* in a general hospital in Japan. Int J Antimicrob Agents. 2007;29(3):306–10.
9. Yu F, Ying Q, Chen C, Li T, Ding B, Liu Y, Lu Y, Qin Z, Parsons C, Salgado C, et al. Outbreak of pulmonary infection caused by *Klebsiella pneumoniae* isolates harbouring blaIMP-4 and blaDHA-1 in a neonatal intensive care unit in China. J Med Microbiol. 2012;61(Pt 7):984–9.
10. Wang Y, Cao W, Zhu X, Chen Z, Li L, Zhang B, Wang B, Tian L, Wang F, Liu C, et al. Characterization of a novel *Klebsiella pneumoniae* sequence type 476 carrying both bla KPC-2 and bla IMP-4. Eur J Clin Microbiol Infect Dis. 2012;31(8):1867–72.
11. Ho PL, Cheung YY, Wang Y, Lo WU, Lai EL, Chow KH, Cheng VC. Characterization of carbapenem-resistant *Escherichia coli* and *Klebsiella pneumoniae* from a healthcare region in Hong Kong. Eur J Clin Microbiol Infect Dis. 2016;35(3):379–85.
12. Yan JJ, Ko WC, Wu JJ. Identification of a plasmid encoding SHV-12, TEM-1, and a variant of IMP-2 metallo-beta-lactamase, IMP-8, from a clinical isolate of *Klebsiella pneumoniae*. Antimicrob Agents Chemother. 2001;45(8):2368–71.
13. Yang Q, Wang H, Sun H, Chen H, Xu Y, Chen M. Phenotypic and genotypic characterization of Enterobacteriaceae with decreased susceptibility to carbapenems: results from large hospital-based surveillance studies in China. Antimicrob Agents Chemother. 2010;54(1):573–7.
14. Xia Y, Liang Z, Su X, Xiong Y. Characterization of carbapenemase genes in Enterobacteriaceae species exhibiting decreased susceptibility to carbapenems in a university hospital in Chongqing, China. Ann Lab Med. 2012;32(4):270–5.
15. Chen S, Feng W, Chen J, Liao W, He N, Wang Q, Sun F, Xia P. Spread of carbapenemase-producing enterobacteria in a southwest hospital in China. Ann Clin Microbiol Antimicrob. 2014;13:42.
16. Jian Z, Li Y, Liu W, Li H, Zhang Y, Gu X, Peng W. Detection of the novel IMP-38 among carbapenemase-producing Enterobacteriaceae in a university hospital, China. J Infect Dev Ctries. 2014;8(8):1044–8.
17. Li H, Zhang J, Liu Y, Zheng R, Chen H, Wang X, Wang Z, Cao B, Wang H. Molecular characteristics of carbapenemase-producing Enterobacteriaceae in China from 2008 to 2011: predominance of KPC-2 enzyme. Diagn Microbiol Infect Dis. 2014;78(1):63–5.
18. Hu L, Zhong Q, Shang Y, Wang H, Ning C, Li Y, Hang Y, Xiong J, Wang X, Xu Y, et al. The prevalence of carbapenemase genes and plasmid-mediated quinolone resistance determinants in carbapenem-resistant Enterobacteriaceae from five teaching hospitals in central China. Epidemiol Infect. 2014;142(9):1972–7.
19. Wei Z, Yu T, Qi Y, Ji S, Shen P, Yu Y, Chen Y. Coexistence of plasmid-mediated KPC-2 and IMP-4 carbapenemases in isolates of *Klebsiella pneumoniae* from China. J Antimicrob Chemother. 2011;66(11):2670–1.
20. Li B, Xu XH, Zhao ZC, Wang MH, Cao YP. High prevalence of metallo-beta-lactamase among carbapenem-resistant *Klebsiella pneumoniae* in a teaching hospital in China. Can J Microbiol. 2014;60(10):691–5.
21. Lo WU, Cheung YY, Lai E, Lung D, Que TL, Ho PL. Complete sequence of an IncN plasmid, pIMP-HZ1, carrying blaIMP-4 in a *Klebsiella pneumoniae* strain associated with medical travel to China. Antimicrob Agents Chemother. 2013;57(3):1561–2.
22. Cao XL, Cheng L, Zhang ZF, Ning MZ, Zhou WQ, Zhang K, Shen H. Survey of clinical extended-spectrum beta-lactamase-producing enterobacter cloacae isolates in a Chinese Tertiary Hospital, 2012–2014. Microb Drug Resist. 2017;23(1):83–9.
23. CLSI. Performance standards for antimicrobial susceptibility testing. 27th ed. Wayne: Clinical and Laboratory Standards Institute, 950 West Valley Road, Suite 2500; 2017.
24. Yang J, Ye L, Guo L, Zhao Q, Chen R, Luo Y, Chen Y, Tian S, Zhao J, Shen D, et al. A nosocomial outbreak of KPC-2-producing *Klebsiella pneumoniae* in a Chinese hospital: dissemination of ST11 and emergence of ST37, ST392 and ST395. Clin Microbiol Infect. 2013;19(11):E509–15.
25. An J, Guo L, Zhou L, Ma Y, Luo Y, Tao C, Yang J. NDM-producing Enterobacteriaceae in a Chinese hospital, 2014–2015: identification of NDM-producing Citrobacter werkmanii and acquisition of blaNDM-1-carrying plasmid in vivo in a clinical *Escherichia coli* isolate. J Med Microbiol. 2016;65(11):1253–9.
26. Guo L, An J, Ma Y, Ye L, Luo Y, Tao C, Yang J. Nosocomial outbreak of OXA-48-producing *Klebsiella pneumoniae* in a Chinese hospital: clonal transmission of ST147 and ST383. PLoS ONE. 2016;11(8):e0160754.
27. Chmelnitsky I, Shklyar M, Hermesh O, Navon-Venezia S, Edgar R, Carmeli Y. Unique genes identified in the epidemic extremely drug-resistant KPC-producing *Klebsiella pneumoniae* sequence type 258. J Antimicrob Chemother. 2013;68(1):74–83.
28. Brisse S, Fevre C, Passet V, Issenhuth-Jeanjean S, Tournebize R, Diancourt L, Grimont P. Virulent clones of Klebsiella pneumoniae: identification and evolutionary scenario based on genomic and phenotypic characterization. PLoS ONE. 2009;4(3):e4982.
29. Tada T, Nhung PH, Miyoshi-Akiyama T, Shimada K, Tsuchiya M, Phuong DM, Anh NQ, Ohmagari N, Kirikae T. Multidrug-resistant sequence type 235 *Pseudomonas aeruginosa* clinical isolates producing IMP-26 with increased carbapenem-hydrolyzing activities in vietnam. Antimicrob Agents Chemother. 2016;60(11):6853–8.
30. Zavascki AP, Carvalhaes CG, Picao RC, Gales AC. Multidrug-resistant *Pseudomonas aeruginosa* and *Acinetobacter baumannii*: resistance mechanisms and implications for therapy. Expert Rev Anti Infect Ther. 2010;8(1):71–93.

19

The efficacy and safety of tigecycline for the treatment of bloodstream infections: a systematic review and meta-analysis

Jian Wang, Yaping Pan, Jilu Shen* and Yuanhong Xu

Abstract

Patients with bloodstream infections (BSI) are associated with high mortality rates. Due to tigecycline has shown excellent in vitro activity against most pathogens, tigecycline is selected as one of the candidate drugs for the treatment of multidrug-resistant organisms infections. The purpose of this study was to evaluate the effectiveness and safety of the use of tigecycline for the treatment of patients with BSI. The PubMed and Embase databases were systematically searched, to identify published studies, and we searched clinical trial registries to identify completed unpublished studies, the results of which were obtained through the manufacturer. The primary outcome was mortality, and the secondary outcomes were the rate of clinical cure and microbiological success. 24 controlled studies were included in this systematic review. All-cause mortality was lower with tigecycline than with control antibiotic agents, but the difference was not significant (OR 0.85, [95% confidence interval (CI) 0.31–2.33; $P = 0.745$]). Clinical cure was significantly higher with tigecycline groups (OR 1.76, [95% CI 1.26–2.45; $P = 0.001$]). Eradication efficiency did not differ between tigecycline and control regimens, but the sample size for these comparisons was small. Subgroup analyses showed good clinical cure result in bacteremia patients with CAP. Tigecycline monotherapy was associated with a OR of 2.73 (95% CI 1.53–4.87) for mortality compared with tigecycline combination therapy (6 studies; 250 patients), without heterogeneity. Five studies reporting on 398 patients with *Klebsiella pneumoniae* carbapenemase-producing *K. pneumoniae* BSI showed significantly lower mortality in the tigecycline arm than in the control arm. The combined treatment with tigecycline may be considered the optimal option for severely ill patients with BSI.

Background

Bloodstream infections (BSI) are potentially life-threatening diseases. BSI was defined as at least 1 positive blood culture for a recognized pathogen and clinical symptoms consistent with bacteraemia. They can cause serious secondary infections, such as infective endocarditis and osteomyelitis, and may result in severe sepsis. Meanwhile, BSI due to multidrug-resistant (MDR) organisms has been associated with multiple poor outcomes, including increased length of hospital stay, health care costs and a high rate of morbidity and mortality.

Tigecycline is a glycylcycline with a broad spectrum of antibacterial activity. The emergence of MDR strains infections has been extensively observed worldwide and has become a priority issue over past decade. Tigecycline is a useful alternative to face the challenges of many MDR organisms. Tigecycline has a large volume of distribution of 7–10 l/kg [1], penetrating well into different tissues, it has been approved for the treatment of complicated skin and soft-structure infections (cSSSI), complicated intra-abdominal infections (cIAI), and community-acquired bacterial pneumonia (CAP). Tigecycline is not indicated for treatment of diabetic foot infection or for hospital-acquired or ventilator-associated pneumonia [2]. The use of tigecycline in bacteremia is controversial because of its low serum levels with standard dosing [3].

Attention should be paid by clinicians, because tigecycline was associated with higher mortality than comparator antibiotics [4–6]. However, a recent meta-analysis showed that the drug was not associated with

*Correspondence: shenjilu@126.com
Department of Clinical Laboratory, The First Affiliated Hospital of Anhui Medical University, Anhui Medical University, Hefei 230022, Anhui, China

significantly higher mortality than comparator antibiotics and was as effective as comparators when the analysis was restricted to patients who received tigecycline for approved indications [7]. A prospective study demonstrates that tigecycline plus prolonged infusion standard-dose imipenem/cilastatin, showed good clinical efficacy on VAP patients with XDR-Ab VAP bacteremia [8]. The increased mortality associated with tigecycline is not yet well understood in the treatment of BSI. Therefore, we systemically searched and analysed the current available evidence to assess clinical effectiveness of tigecycline for the treatment of BSI.

Methods

Literature search

Relevant studies were identified through PubMed, Embase and hand-searched from inception until October 2016.The search terms were:"(tigecycline OR TGC OR tygacil) and (bacteraemia OR bacteremia OR bloodstream infection OR sepsis OR septicaemia)". No language restrictions were applied.

Study selection

Any article providing the clinical outcomes of patients treated for bloodstream infections caused by any etiological agent was considered eligible for inclusion in the review. Prospective and retrospective observational cohort studies examining the association between tigecycline use (on hospital admission or previous users) and the outcomes of bacteremic patients were included. The outcome of interest was overall hospital mortality at the longest follow-up at each single study. Case reports and case series including fewer than 10 infected patients treated with tigecycline were excluded from the review.

Data extraction

The extracted data consisted of the main characteristics of a study (first-author name, year of publication, country, study period, and design), main characteristics and underlying diseases of the study population, number of patients with infections BSI, the causative pathogen(s), sites of infections, and antibiotic treatment (combination therapy or monotherapy). Clinical outcomes (mortality, treatment failure) of patients in each treatment group were recorded as well.

Statistical analysis

We chose mortality as the primary outcome, because of the high mortality rates among patients with BSI, while the secondary outcomes were: clinical response, microbiological response, adverse effects, and emergence of resistance. Microbiological response was defined as successful when eradication or sterile culture results were obtained during or after the antibiotic therapy. Because there are no standard criteria to assess clinical response and adverse events, we accepted the criteria as reported in each study.

All statistical analyses were performed using the comprehensive meta-analysis V2.2 (BioStat, Englewood, NJ). Among the controlled studies, the between-study heterogeneity was assessed using the I^2 test, whereby I^2 values >50% were defined as indicating heterogeneity. Either fixed-effects (Mantel–Haenszel method) or random-effects (DerSimonian and Laird method) models were used, depending on the heterogeneity result. If no heterogeneity was found, meta-analysis was done using the Mantel–Haenszel fixed-effects model. Binary outcomes from controlled studies were expressed as odds ratios (OR) with their 95% confidence intervals (CI), and continuous outcomes were expressed as the mean difference between 2 groups. Egger regression, as well as the Begg methods, was used to evaluate publication bias. All P values were two-tailed, and a P value of ≤ 0.05 was considered statistically significant. Some statistical analysis was performed by using the SPSS statistical software (version 19; SPSS Inc., Chicago, IL). Categorical variables were evaluated by using the χ^2 test or 2-tailed Fisher's exact test, as appropriate. Subgroup analyses for mortality and clinical cure were planned for bacteraemic patients. Comparisons were subcategorized by the type of infection. A funnel plot was used to assess small-study effects.

Results

Literature search results

1540 potential articles were identified; 56 case reports and clinical series including less than 10 infected patients were excluded; 41 duplicates and 18 single-arm studies were excluded; 22 studies were ruled out because they did not present clear treatment regimens or detailed clinical outcomes; 24 articles were excluded due to few patients in each group. Ultimately 24 studies met the inclusion criteria, 24 controlled studies (1961 patients) included in this systematic review.

Study characteristics

The features of the 24 trials are described in Table 1. Five of them were prospective cohort studies, 7 were retrospective studies. All of the included controlled studies had an NOS score >3. Most patients in the included studies were critically ill, with most of them in ICU.

Mortality

As shown in Fig. 1, no significant difference was noted when tigecycline was compared with control groups in terms of all-cause mortality (14 studies; 1502 patients) [OR 0.841, 95% confidence interval (CI) 0.517–1.367;

Table 1 Characteristics of included studies

Reference	Study years	Location	Type of study	Type of infection	Causative pathogen(s)	Mortality assessed	Sample size(no.of tigecycline/control patients)	Concomitant antibiotics administeredin tigecycline group	Compatator	Tigecycline dose	Control regimen dose
Oliva et al. [22]	Na	Multicenter	Prospective, double-blind phase 3	cIAI with bacteremia	Mix	Undetermined	14/27	None	Imipenem cilastatin	Initial dose of 100 mg, followed by 50 mg every 12 h	500 mg followed by 500 mg per 6 h combined imipenem and cilastatin
McGovern et al. [11]	2001–08	USA	Comparative studies, phase 3 and 4	Bacteremia	Mix	Overall	162/163	Na	Na	Na	Na
Daikos et al. [23]	2009–10	Greece	Retrospective	BSI	CP-Kp	At 28 days	94/81	Colistin aminoglycoside carbapenem	Colistin aminoglycoside carbapenem	For tigecycline the total daily dose was 100–200 mg administered in two divided dosages	1 g imipenem and meropenem every 8 h, 5 mg/kg gentamicin and amikacin once daily
Jean et al. [8]	2013	Taiwan	Prospective	VAP with bacteremia	XDR-Ab	At 14 days	28/56	Ipipenem/cilasta	Sulbactam + imipenem/cilastatin	Na	Na
Florescu et al. [24]	2003–05	Multicenter	Double-blind, phase 3	Bacteremia	MRSA VRE	At 12–37 days after the last dose	14/20	None	Vancomycin or linezolid	Initial dose of 100 mg, followed by 50 mg every 12 h	1 g per 12 h followed by 600 mg per 12 h vancomycin plus linezolid
Sacchidanand et al. [25]	Na	Multicenter	Randomized, double-blind, phase 3	cSSSI with bacteremia	XDR-Ab	Overall	8/22	None	Vancomycin plus aztreonam	Initial dose of 100 mg, followed by 50 mg every 12 h	1 g per 12 h followed by 2 g per 12 h vancomycin plus aztreonam
Liou et al. [26]	2007–13	Taiwan	Retrospective	Secondary bacteremia	Acinetobacter	At 14 days	17/65	Ampicillin-sulbactam sulbactam levofloxacin ceftazidime	Na	Standard dose of tigecycline	Na
Cheng et al. [27]	2010–13	Taiwan	Prospective	Bacteremia	XDR-Ab	At discharge	29/55	Colistin	Colistin carbapenem	Initial dose of 100 mg, followed by 50 mg every 12 h	2.5–5 mg/kg/d of colistin base divided over 8 or 12 h

Table 1 continued

Reference	Study years	Location	Type of study	Type of infection	Causative pathogen(s)	Mortality assessed	Sample size(no.of tigecycline/control patients)	Concomitant antibiotics administeredin tigecycline group	Compatator	Tigecycline dose	Control regimen dose
Tanaseanu et al. [28]	2003–05	Multicenter	Randomized, double-blind, phase 3	CAP with bacteremia	*Streptococcus pneumoniae*	At 7–23 days after the last dose	22/40	None	Levofloxacin	Initial dose of 100 mg, followed by 50 mg every 12 h	500 mg every 24 h levofloxacin
Tumbarello et al. [29]	2010–11	Italy	Retrospective	BSI	KPC-Kp	At 30 days	70/48	Colistin gentamicin meropenem	Colistin gentamicin meropenem	Every 12 h (100–200 mg/day)	Every 8–12 h for a total daily dose of 6,000,000–9,000,000 IU colistin; 4–5 mg/kg every 24 h gentamicin; 2 g every 8 h meropenem
Zarkotou et al. [30]	2008–10	Greece	Observational	BSI	KPC-Kp	Overall	22/13	Colistin gentamicin carbapenem amikacin	Colistin gentamicin carbapenem	Na	Na
Bucaneve et al. [31]	2008–10	Multicenter	Prospective, open-label	Bacteremia	Mix	Overall	86/94	Piperacillin/tazobactam	Piperacillin/tazobactam	Initial dose of 100 mg, followed by 50 mg every 12 h	4.5 g piperacillin/tazobactam every 8 h
Papadimitriou-Olivgeris et al. [32]	Na	Greece	Single-centre observational study	BSI	KPC-Kp	At 30 days	27/9	Colistin gentamicin	Colistin gentamicin	Na	Na
Gardiner et al. [19]	Na	Multicenter	Retrospective, randomized, 7 double-blind and 1 open-label, phase 3	Bacteremia	Mix	Na	91/79	Na	Na	Na	Na
Breedt et al. [33]	2002–03	Multicenter	Randomized, double-blind, phase 3	cSSSI with bacteremia	Mix	Overall	15/10	None	Vancomycin-aztreonam	Initial dose of 100 mg, followed by 50 mg every 12 h	1 g vancomycin plus 2 g aztreonam per 12 h

Table 1 continued

Reference	Study years	Location	Type of study	Type of infection	Causative pathogen(s)	Mortality assessed	Sample size(no.of tigecycline/ control patients)	Concomitant antibiotics administeredin tigecycline group	Compatator	Tigecycline dose	Control regimen dose
Babinchak et al. [34]	2002–04	Multicenter	Randomized, double-blind, phase 3	cIAI with bacteremia	Mix	Overall	40/50	None	Imipenem-cilastatin	Initial dose of 100 mg, followed by 50 mg every 12 h	500 mg followed by 500 mg per 6 h combined imipenem and cilastatin
Ellis-Grosse et al. [35]	2001–04	Multicenter	Randomized, double-blind, phase 3	cSSSI with bacteremia	Mix	Overall	23/24	None	Vancomycin-aztreonam	Initial dose of 100 mg, followed by 50 mg every 12 h	1 g vancomycin plus 2 g aztreonam per 12 h
Fomin et al. [36]	Na	Multicenter	Double-blind, phase 3	cIAI with bacteremia	Mix	Na	26/23	None	Imipenem-cilastatin	Initial dose of 100 mg, followed by 50 mg every 12 h	500 mg followed by 500 mg per 6 h combined imipenem and cilastatin
Dartois et al. [37]	Na	Multicenter	Double-blind, phase 3	CAP with bacteremia	Mix	Overall	32/31	None	Levofloxacin	Initial dose of 100 mg, followed by 50 mg every 12 h	500 mg per 24 h or per 12 h levofloxacin
Qureshi et al. [38]	2005–09	USA	Retrospective	Bacteremia	KPC-Kp	At 28 days	11/23	Carbapenem aminoglycoside	Carbapenem gentamicin cefepime et al.	Na	Na
Lauf et al. [39]	2006–09	Multicenter	Randomized, double-blind, phase 3	Bacteremia	Mix	Na	7/14	None	Ertapenem ± vancomycin	150 mg once-daily tigecycline	1 g once-daily ertapenem ± vancomycin
Gomez-Simmonds et al. [40]	2006–13	USA	Retrospective	BSI	CR-Kp	At 30 days	26/42	Beta-lactam antibiotic	Polymyxin b aminoglycoside	Initial dose of 100 mg, followed by 50 mg every 12 h	Na
Maki et al. [41]	2007	USA	Prospective	Bacteremia	CVC-CoNS	Na	8/23	Na	Vancomycin	50 mg every 12 h	Na
Oliveira et al. [42]	2009–13	Brazil	Retrospective	Bacteremia	KPC-Enterobacteriaceae	At 30 days	15/62	Carbapenem polymyxin aminoglycoside	Carbapenem polymyxin aminoglycoside	Na	Na

BSI, bloodstream infection; cIAI, complicated intra-abdominal infections; cSSSI, complicated skin and skin-structure infections; CAP, community-acquired pneumonia; CR-Kp, carbapenem-resistant *K. pneumoniae*; CVC-CoNS, central venous catheter-related coagulase-negative staphylococcal; KPC-Kp, *Klebsiella pneumoniae* carbapenemase-producing *K. pneumoniae*; MRSA, methicillin-resistant *Staphylococcus aureus*; Na, not available; VAP, ventilator-associated pneumonia; VRE, vancomycin-resistant enterococci; XDR-Ab, extensively drug-resistant *Acinetobacter baumannii*

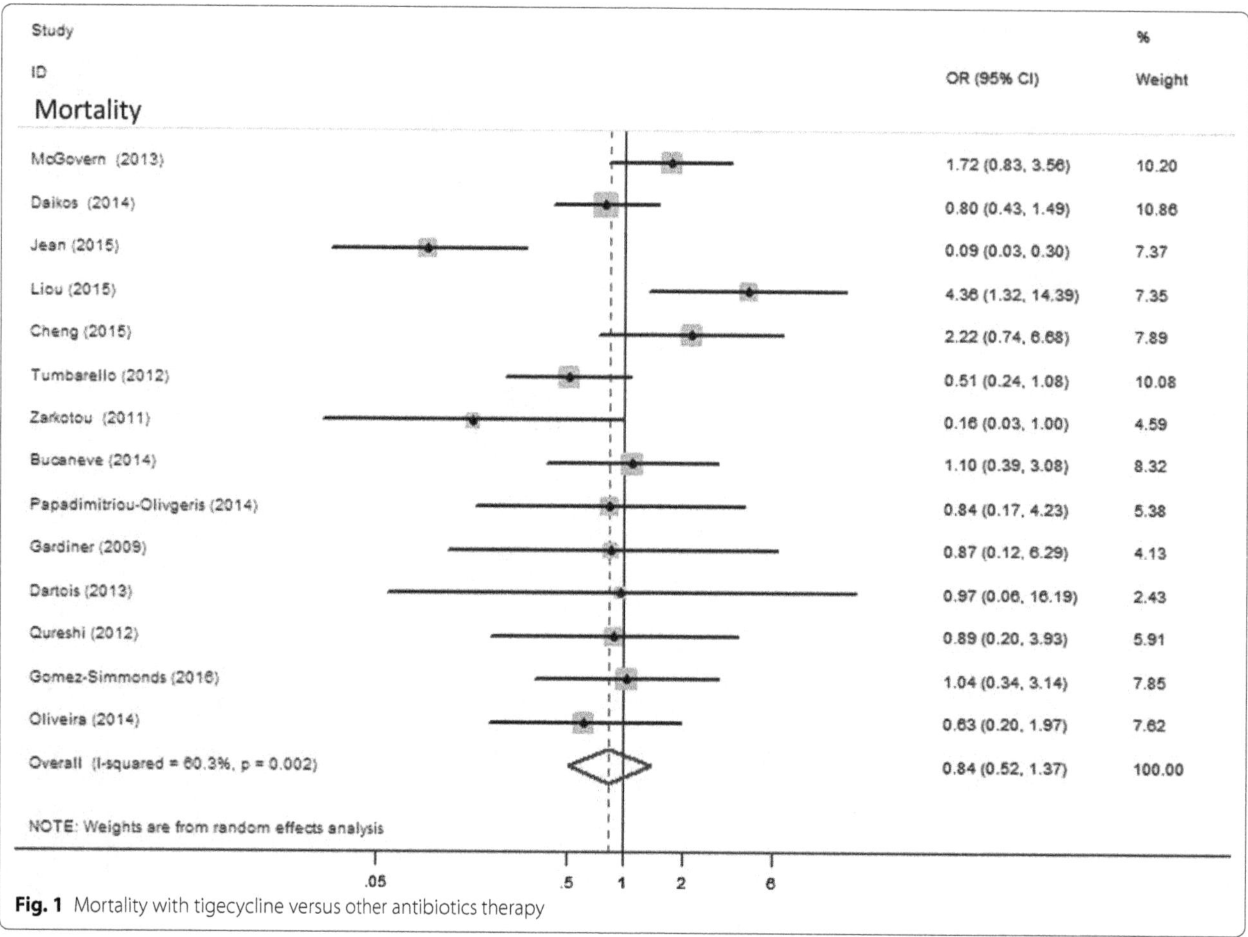

Fig. 1 Mortality with tigecycline versus other antibiotics therapy

P = 0.485]. Because statistical heterogeneity existed among studies (X^2 = 32.76, df = 13, (P = 0.002), I^2 = 60.3%), a random-effects model of analysis was used. No publication bias was detected by Egger regression (t = −0.39; df = 12.0; P = 0.701) or Begg (z = 0.55; df = 12.0; P = 0.584).

Table 2 shows the subgroup analysis of the controlled studies. A significant difference was observed between the tigecycline monotherapy therapy group and the tigecycline combination therapy group in terms of mortality (6 studies; 250 patients) (OR 2.733, [95% CI 1.533–4.873; P = 0.001]; I^2 = 8.7%). A significantly higher mortality was noted in the monotherapy group than in the combination therapy group in cases of blood stream infection. The mortality in the combination of tigecycline plus colistin based group was not significantly lower than that in the other antibiotics combination group (OR 0.68, [95% CI 0.407–1.135; P = 0.14]; I^2 = 0.0%).

Table 2 Subgroup analysis of overall mortality with tigecycline versus other antibiotics for treatment of bloodstram infections in controlled studies

Variables	Studies, no. (patients, no.)	Mortality of tigecycline compared with control OR (95% CI); P	Heterogeneity of studies
Monotherapy vs combination	6 (250)	2.733 (1.533–4.873); 0.001	X^2 = 5.47, df = 5, (P = 0.361), I^2 = 8.7%
Tigecycline plus polymyxins based vs other antibiotics combination	5 (289)	0.680 (0.407–1.135); 0.140	X^2 = 2.88, df = 4, (P = 0.578), I^2 = 0.0%
Kp BSI	6 (466)	0.678 (0.457–1.006); 0.054	X^2 = 3.95, df = 5, (P = 0.556), I^2 = 0.0%
KPC-Kp BSI	5 (398)	0.636 (0.417–0.971); 0.036	X^2 = 3.31, df = 4, (P = 0.507), I^2 = 0.0%
Acinetobacter BSI	3 (221)	0.967 (0.096–9.759); 0.978	X^2 = 23.76, df = 2, (P = 0.001), I^2 = 91.6%

CI, confidence interval; OR, odds ratio

In the patients infected with *Klebsiella pneumoniae* (Kp) BSI, tigecycline seemed to have a lower mortality than comparator drugs, but the difference was not significant (OR 0.678, [95% CI 0.457–1.006; P = 0.054]; I^2 = 0.0%; [P = 0.556]). Five studies (398 patients) reported data on carbapenemase-producing Kp BSI, and a significant difference with respect to overall mortality was observed between the tigecycline therapy group and the controls (OR 0.636, [95% CI 0.417–0.971; P = 0.036]; I^2 = 0.0%; [P = 0.507]). Three controlled studies (221 patients) reported Acinetobacter BSI, no difference was seen between patients who received tigecycline as therapy and others in mortality (OR 0.967, [95% CI 0.096–0.759; P = 0.978]; I^2 = 91.6%; [P = 0.001]).

Clinical cure

There was a significant differences were observed between the tigecycline and control groups in this regard (OR 1.76, [95% CI 1.26–2.45; P = 0.001]; I^2 = 29.2%; [P = 0.159]; Fig. 2). Clinical cure was significantly higher in the tigecycline population. In the subgroup analysis, for analysis by type of infection, without statistical significance was found in patients with cIAI (OR 0.97, [95% CI 0.52–1.80; P = 0.919]; I^2 = 0.0%; [P = 0.953]) and cSSSI (OR 0.71, [95% CI 0.26–1.90; P = 0.494]; I^2 = 0.0%; [P = 0.821]), but in trials assessing patients with CAP, for the rate of clinical cure, the efficacy of tigecycline was better than that of comparator regimens (OR 2.44, [95% CI 1.20–4.94; P = 0.013]; I^2 = 0.0%; [P = 0.821]). As shown in Fig. 2.

Microbiological response

As shown in Fig. 2, tigecycline group did not differ significantly compared with the comparators in the rate of microbiological success (OR 2.07, [95% CI 0.56–7.70; P = 0.279]; I^2 = 0.0%; [P = 0.854]) (Fig. 2).

Adverse effects

There were not sufficiently effective data to be recoded, so that the common adverse effects of tigecycline (nausea, vomiting, and diarrhea) could not be extracted in any of the studies.

Discussion

We conducted this systematic review and meta-analysis to investigate the effectiveness and safety of tigecycline for the treatment of BSI. Numerous studies have established bacteremia as a marker of severe infection and a

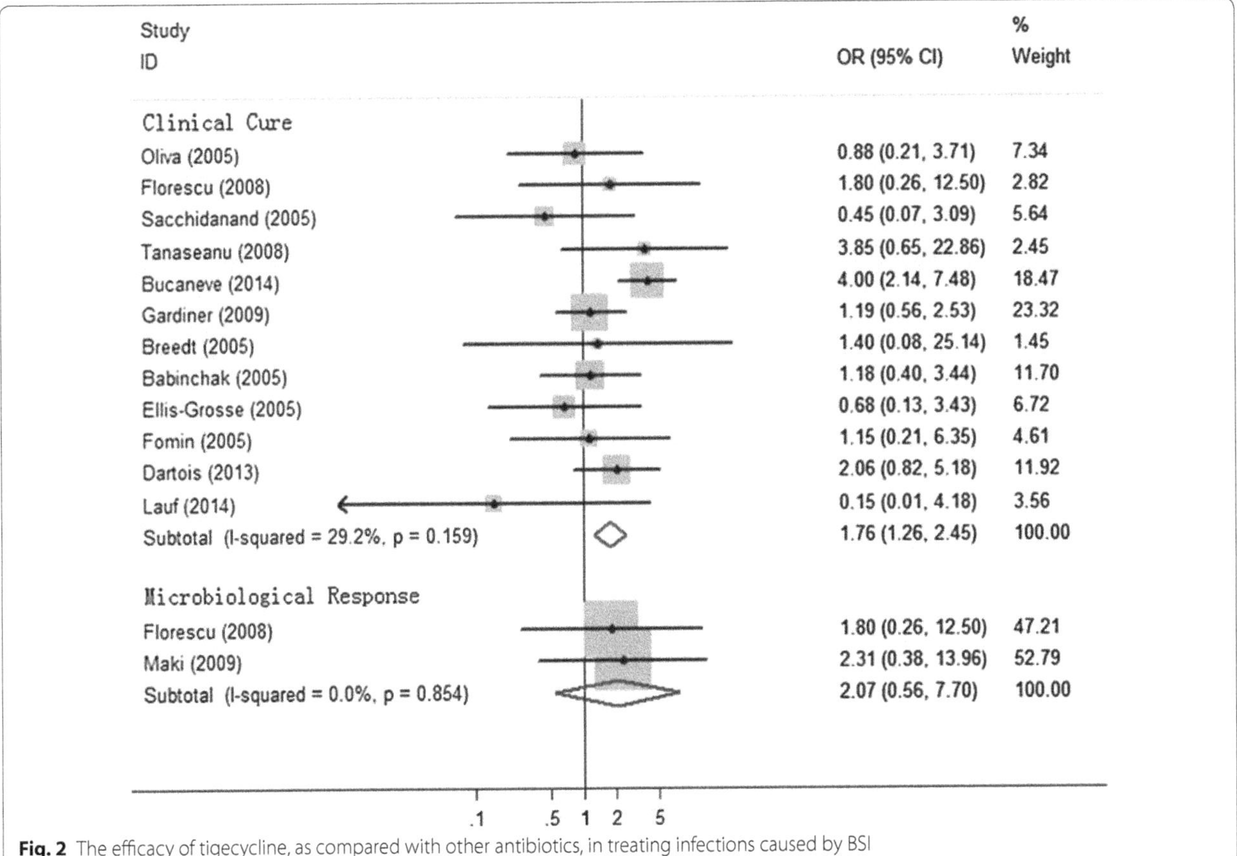

Fig. 2 The efficacy of tigecycline, as compared with other antibiotics, in treating infections caused by BSI

risk for adverse outcomes in multiple treatment settings [9, 10], but there were some positive elements about the treatment of BSI with tigecycline.

To our knowledge, this was the first systematic review to assess the efficacy of tigecycline in treating BSI. Although all-cause mortality was lower with tigecycline than with the control regimens, the difference was not significant. Tigecycline seemed to be better than levofloxacin for treatment of community-acquired pneumonia, and worse than control regimens for cIAI and cSSSI, but these differences were not significant. However, drug safety guidelines published by the FDA refer to an increased mortality risk associated with intravenous tigecycline compared with other drugs used to treat serious infections (risk difference = 0.6%, 95% CI 0.1–1.2) [2]. This result has been confirmed by a study that associated the increased risk mortality with resistant pathogens, hospital-acquired pneumonia, and increased age of patients [11]. However the type of serious infections didn't include BSI. We used the same effect metric to assess our results, and noted that the risk difference of all-cause mortality was not significant (−3.5%, 95% CI −13 to −6; $I^2 = 85.4\%$, P = 0.001).

Although the overall mortality did not differ between tigecycline and the control groups, subgroup analysis found the mortality was significantly lower in the tigecycline combination group than in the tigecycline monotherapy therapy group. Tigecycline in combination with colistin, carbapenem in combination with colistin, and tigecycline in combination with gentamicin were the commonly administered antibiotic treatment regimens among the included studies and might result in lower mortality than other combinations of antibiotics. The most common combination was tigecycline with colistin in tigecycline combination therapy group, yet this data did not necessarily predict tigecycline plus polymyxins based therapy was significantly better than other antibiotics combination therapy. For the patients with KPC-Kp BSI, antibiotic therapy with tigecycline was associated with lower mortality.

With regard to clinical response, the evidence that we could compile from studies was that tigecycline therapy may have no clinical advantage over comparator therapy, but may result in better clinical cure in treatment of CAP presenting with bacteremia.

Tigecycline had good eradication ability for most pathogens recorded at baseline, as a novel glycylcycline antibiotic, it has a broad spectrum of antimicrobial activity, ranging from aerobic to anaerobic bacteria, and gram-positive, gram-negative (exceptions of *Pseudomonas aeruginosa* and *Proteus mirabilis*), and atypical organisms [12]. Eradication was better than with control regimens in all cases, although no significant difference was found when tigecycline was compared with the comparators.

Previous studies have shown that the most common adverse effects of tigecycline had increased incidence in the tigecycline group, such as nausea, vomiting, and diarrhea [13, 14]. According to a recently published review, tigecycline induces acute pancreatitis, indicating that surveillance for adverse events from the digestive system is needed during treatment [15]. But lack of data from all trials results can not be obtained about adverse events outcomes in our meta-analysis.

Small non-comparative series have reported relatively poor clinical and microbiological outcomes with tigecycline for tigecycline-susceptible CR-Ab bacteremia [16–18]. The high severity of illness and the notable delays in initiation of effective antimicrobial therapy could also explain these results. In a pooled, retrospective data analysis of phase 3 clinical trials, 91 patients being treated with tigecycline had secondary bacteremia detected, tigecycline appeared safe and well tolerated in the treatment of secondary bacteremia associated with cSSSI, cIAI, and CAP; cure rates were similar to comparative standard therapies [19]. Recently, a high-dose regimen (loading dose 200 mg followed by 100 mg every 12 h) has been successfully and safely used in critically ill patients with severe infections due to multi drug resistant bacteria although the number of primary bacteremia was anecdotal [20].

Several potential limitations should be taken into consideration when interpreting the present results. Firstly, the number of subjects included was not large enough. We would have preferred to contact researchers directly for missing data, but this approach was not attempted because of time constraints. Secondly, in some subgroup analyses, the sample size was small, which may have reduced the power of the statistical analysis. Another important issue is that the administrations of the antibiotics differed among the studies with regard to the duration of infusion or the total daily dose. Thirdly, due to the included studies did not provide relevant data, we were unable to assess the impact of tigecycline on adverse drug reactions. Accordingly, these differences might influence the clinical outcomes. Last, the matter of the emergence of resistance during therapy was not raised by any of the included studies.

In conclusion, based on a review of published cases, tigecycline appears to have produced some favourable clinical and microbiological outcomes in patients with BSI, even when used as monotherapy. This research was needed to clarify whether tigecycline was suitable for treatment such infections when other antibiotics fail, especially because indications for increased risk of all-cause mortality have been reported in patients treated with this drug. The FDA has recently reported an increased risk of death when intravenous tigecycline is used for FDA approved purposes [21], which may be explained by a worsening infection or potential complications [11].

The available evidence suggests that combination antibiotic treatment may offer a comparative advantage over monotherapy with regard to the mortality of critically ill patients with severe infections due to BSI. The number of currently available appropriate antimicrobial agents is limited, combination therapy with tigecycline, it could be a fine option for the treatment of BSI, especially in patients with KPC-Kp BSI.

Abbreviations

BSI: bloodstream infection; cIAI: complicated intra-abdominal infections; cSSSI: complicated skin and skin-structure infections; CAP: community-acquired pneumonia; CR-Kp: carbapenem-resistant *K. pneumoniae*; CVC-CoNS: central venous catheter-related coagulase-negative staphylococcal; KPC-Kp: *Klebsiella pneumoniae* carbapenemase-producing *K. pneumoniae*; MRSA: methicillin-resistant *Staphylococcus aureus*; VAP: ventilator-associated pneumonia; VRE: vancomycin-resistant enterococci; XDR-Ab: extensively drug-resistant *Acinetobacter baumannii*.

Authors' contributions

WJ and PYP designed the study, performed the articles search and screen. WJ wrote the paper. WJ, PYP and XYH performed the Statistical analysis. SJL reviewed the manuscript. All authors read and approved the final manuscript.

Acknowledgements

Not applicable.

Competing interests

The authors declare that they have no competing interests.

Consent for publication

Informed consent was obtained from all individual participants included in the review.

References

1. Muralidharan G, Micalizzi M, Speth J, Raible D, Troy S. Pharmacokinetics of tigecycline after single and multiple doses in healthy subjects. Antimicrob Agents Chemother. 2004;49(1):220–9.
2. FDA drug safety communication: increased risk of death with Tygacil (tigecycline) compared to other antibiotics used to treat similar infections. http://www.fda.gov/drugs/drugsafety/ucm224370.htm.
3. Stein GE, Babinchak T. Tigecycline: an update. Diagn Microbiol Infect Dis. 2013;75(4):331–6.
4. Prasad P, Sun J, Danner RL, Natanson C. Excess deaths associated with tigecycline after approval based on noninferiority trials. Clin Infect Dis. 2012;54(12):1699–709.
5. Yahav D, Lador A, Paul M, Leibovici L. Efficacy and safety of tigecycline: a systematic review and meta-analysis. J Antimicrob Chemother. 2011;66(9):1963–71.
6. Food and Drug Administration: Tygacil (tigecycline): drug safety communication-increased risk of death. http://www.fda.gov/Safety/MedWatch/SafetyInformation/SafetyAlertsforHumanMedicalProducts/ucm370170.htm.
7. Vardakas KZRP, Falagas ME. Effectiveness and safety of tigecycline: focus on use for approved indications. Clin Infect Dis. 2012;54(11):1672–4.
8. Jean SS, Hsieh TC, Hsu CW, Lee WS, Bai KJ, Lam C. Comparison of the clinical efficacy between tigecycline plus extended-infusion imipenem and sulbactam plus imipenem against ventilator-associated pneumonia with pneumonic extensively drug-resistant *Acinetobacter baumannii* bacteremia, and correlation of clinical efficacy with in vitro synergy tests. J Microbiol Immunol Infect. 2016;49(6):924–33.
9. Roberts FJ, Geere IW, Coldman A. A three-year study of positive blood cultures, with emphasis on prognosis. Rev Infect Dis. 1991;13(1):34–46.
10. Weinstein MP, Towns ML, Quartey SM, Mirrett S, Reimer LG, Parmigiani G, Reller LB. The clinical significance of positive blood cultures in the 1990s: a prospective comprehensive evaluation of the microbiology, epidemiology, and outcome of bacteremia and fungemia in adults. Clin Infect Dis. 1997;24(4):584–602.
11. McGovern PC, Wible M, El-Tahtawy A, Biswas P, Meyer RD. All-cause mortality imbalance in the tigecycline phase 3 and 4 clinical trials. Int J Antimicrob Agents. 2013;41(5):463–7.
12. Nicolau DP. Management of complicated infections in the era of antimicrobial resistance: the role of tigecycline. Expert Opin Pharmacother. 2009;10(7):1213–22.
13. Tasina E, Haidich AB, Kokkali S, Arvanitidou M. Efficacy and safety of tigecycline for the treatment of infectious diseases: a meta-analysis. Lancet Infect Dis. 2011;11(11):834–44.
14. McGovern P, Leister N, Zito E, Tucker N, Mansfield D, Babinchak T. Efficacy of tigecycline versus ceftriaxone and metronidazole for complicated intra-abdominal infections-analysis of pooled clinical trial data. Clin Microbiol Infect. 2010;16(suppl 2):S448.
15. Hung WY, Kogelman L, Volpe G, Iafrati M, Davidson L. Tigecycline-induced acute pancreatitis: case report and literature review. Int J Antimicrob Agents. 2009;34(5):486–9.
16. Kim NH, Hwang JH, Song KH, Choe PG, Kim ES, Park SW, Kim HB, Kim NJ, Park WB, Oh MD. Tigecycline in carbapenem-resistant *Acinetobacter baumannii* bacteraemia: susceptibility and clinical outcome. Scand J Infect Dis. 2013;45(4):315–9.
17. Guner R, Hasanoglu I, Keske S, Kalem AK, Tasyaran MA. Outcomes in patients infected with carbapenem-resistant *Acinetobacter baumannii* and treated with tigecycline alone or in combination therapy. Infection. 2011;39(6):515–8.
18. Gordon NC, Wareham DW. A review of clinical and microbiological outcomes following treatment of infections involving multidrug-resistant *Acinetobacter baumannii* with tigecycline. J Antimicrob Chemother. 2009;63(4):775–80.
19. Gardiner D, Dukart G, Cooper A, Babinchak T. Safety and efficacy of intravenous tigecycline in subjects with secondary bacteremia: pooled results from 8 phase III clinical trials. Clin Infect Dis. 2010;50(2):229–38.
20. De Pascale G, Montini L, Pennisi M, Bernini V, Maviglia R, Bello G, Spanu T, Tumbarello M, Antonelli M. High dose tigecycline in critically ill patients with severe infections due to multidrug-resistant bacteria. Crit Care. 2014;18(3):R90.
21. FDA drug safety communication: FDA warns of increased risk of death with IV antibacterial Tygacil (tigecycline) and approves new Boxed Warning. http://www.fda.gov/Drugs/DrugSafety/ucm369580.htm.
22. Oliva ME, Rekha A, Yellin A, Pasternak J, Campos M, Rose GM, Babinchak T, Ellis-Grosse EJ, Loh E. A multicenter trial of the efficacy and safety of tigecycline versus imipenem/cilastatin in patients with complicated intra-abdominal infections [Study ID Numbers: 3074A1-301-WW; ClinicalTrials.gov Identifier: NCT00081744]. BMC Infect Dis. 2005;5:88.
23. Daikos GL, Tsaousi S, Tzouvelekis LS, Anyfantis I, Psichogiou M, Argyropoulou A, Stefanou I, Sypsa V, Miriagou V, Nepka M, et al. Carbapenemase-producing *Klebsiella pneumoniae* bloodstream infections: lowering mortality by antibiotic combination schemes and the role of carbapenems. Antimicrob Agents Chemother. 2014;58(4):2322–8.

24. Florescu I, Beuran M, Dimov R, Razbadauskas A, Bochan M, Fichev G, Dukart G, Babinchak T, Cooper CA, Ellis-Grosse EJ, et al. Efficacy and safety of tigecycline compared with vancomycin or linezolid for treatment of serious infections with methicillin-resistant *Staphylococcus aureus* or vancomycin-resistant enterococci: a phase 3, multicentre, double-blind, randomized study. J Antimicrob Chemother. 2008;62(Suppl 1):i17–28.
25. Sacchidanand S, Penn RL, Embil JM, Campos ME, Curcio D, Ellis-Grosse E, Loh E, Rose G. Efficacy and safety of tigecycline monotherapy compared with vancomycin plus aztreonam in patients with complicated skin and skin structure infections: results from a phase 3, randomized, double-blind trial. Int J Infect Dis. 2005;9(5):251–61.
26. Liou BH, Lee YT, Kuo SC, Liu PY, Fung CP. Efficacy of tigecycline for secondary Acinetobacter bacteremia and factors associated with treatment failure. Antimicrob Agents Chemother. 2015;59(6):3637–40.
27. Cheng A, Chuang YC, Sun HY, Sheng WH, Yang CJ, Liao CH, Hsueh PR, Yang JL, Shen NJ, Wang JT, et al. Excess mortality associated with colistin-tigecycline compared with colistin-carbapenem combination therapy for extensively drug-resistant *Acinetobacter baumannii* bacteremia: a multicenter prospective observational study. Crit Care Med. 2015;43(6):1194–204.
28. Tanaseanu C, Bergallo C, Teglia O, Jasovich A, Oliva ME, Dukart G, Dartois N, Cooper CA, Gandjini H, Mallick R, et al. Integrated results of 2 phase 3 studies comparing tigecycline and levofloxacin in community-acquired pneumonia. Diagn Microbiol Infect Dis. 2008;61(3):329–38.
29. Tumbarello M, Viale P, Viscoli C, Trecarichi EM, Tumietto F, Marchese A, Spanu T, Ambretti S, Ginocchio F, Cristini F, et al. Predictors of mortality in bloodstream infections caused by *Klebsiella pneumoniae* carbapenemase-producing *K. pneumoniae*: importance of combination therapy. Clin Infect Dis. 2012;55(7):943–50.
30. Zarkotou O, Pournaras S, Tselioti P, Dragoumanos V, Pitiriga V, Ranellou K, Prekates A, Themeli-Digalaki K, Tsakris A. Predictors of mortality in patients with bloodstream infections caused by KPC-producing *Klebsiella pneumoniae* and impact of appropriate antimicrobial treatment. Clin Microbiol Infect. 2011;17(12):1798–803.
31. Bucaneve G, Micozzi A, Picardi M, Ballanti S, Cascavilla N, Salutari P, Specchia G, Fanci R, Luppi M, Cudillo L, et al. Results of a multicenter, controlled, randomized clinical trial evaluating the combination of piperacillin/tazobactam and tigecycline in high-risk hematologic patients with cancer with febrile neutropenia. J Clin Oncol. 2014;32(14):1463–71.
32. Papadimitriou-Olivgeris M, Marangos M, Christofidou M, Fligou F, Bartzavali C, Panteli ES, Vamvakopoulou S, Filos KS, Anastassiou ED. Risk factors for infection and predictors of mortality among patients with KPC-producing *Klebsiella pneumoniae* bloodstream infections in the intensive care unit. Scand J Infect Dis. 2014;46(9):642–8.
33. Breedt J, Teras J, Gardovskis J, Maritz FJ, Vaasna T, Ross DP, Gioud-Paquet M, Dartois N, Ellis-Grosse EJ, Loh E, et al. Safety and efficacy of tigecycline in treatment of skin and skin structure infections: results of a double-blind phase 3 comparison study with vancomycin-aztreonam. Antimicrob Agents Chemother. 2005;49(11):4658–66.
34. Babinchak T, Ellis-Grosse E, Dartois N, Rose GM, Loh E. The efficacy and safety of tigecycline for the treatment of complicated intra-abdominal infections: analysis of pooled clinical trial data. Clin Infect Dis. 2005;41(Suppl 5):S354–67.
35. Ellis-Grosse EJ, Babinchak T, Dartois N, Rose G, Loh E. The efficacy and safety of tigecycline in the treatment of skin and skin-structure infections: results of 2 double-blind phase 3 comparison studies with vancomycin-aztreonam. Clin Infect Dis. 2005;41(Suppl 5):S341–53.
36. Fomin P, Beuran M, Gradauskas A, Barauskas G, Datsenko A, Dartois N, Ellis-Grosse E, Loh E, Three Hundred Six Study G. Tigecycline is efficacious in the treatment of complicated intra-abdominal infections. Int J Surg. 2005;3(1):35–47.
37. Dartois N, Cooper CA, Castaing N, Gandjini H, Sarkozy D. Tigecycline versus levofloxacin in hospitalized patients with community-acquired pneumonia: an analysis of risk factors. Open Respir Med J. 2013;7:13–20.
38. Qureshi ZA, Paterson DL, Potoski BA, Kilayko MC, Sandovsky G, Sordillo E, Polsky B, Adams-Haduch JM, Doi Y. Treatment outcome of bacteremia due to KPC-producing *Klebsiella pneumoniae*: superiority of combination antimicrobial regimens. Antimicrob Agents Chemother. 2012;56(4):2108–13.
39. Lauf L, Ozsvar Z, Mitha I, Regoly-Merei J, Embil JM, Cooper A, Sabol MB, Castaing N, Dartois N, Yan J, et al. Phase 3 study comparing tigecycline and ertapenem in patients with diabetic foot infections with and without osteomyelitis. Diagn Microbiol Infect Dis. 2014;78(4):469–80.
40. Gomez-Simmonds A, Nelson B, Eiras DP, Loo A, Jenkins SG, Whittier S, Calfee DP, Satlin MJ, Kubin CJ, Furuya EY. Combination regimens for treatment of carbapenem-resistant *Klebsiella pneumoniae* bloodstream infections. Antimicrob Agents Chemother. 2016;60(6):3601–7.
41. Maki D, Lentnek A, Sheftel T, Paladino J, Feuerstein S, Jagodzinski L, Schentag J. P284 Prospective multicenter trial of tigecycline for treatment of central venous catheter (CVC)-related coagulase-negative staphylococcal (CoNS) bacteremia. Int J Antimicrob Agents. 2009;34(09):S115.
42. de Oliveira MS, de Assis DB, Freire MP, do Prado GB, Machado AS, Abdala E, Pierrotti LC, Mangini C, Campos L, Caiaffa Filho HH, et al. Treatment of KPC-producing Enterobacteriaceae: suboptimal efficacy of polymyxins. Clin Microbiol Infect. 2015;21(2):179.

20

Dose-dependent artificial prolongation of prothrombin time by interaction between daptomycin and test reagents in patients receiving warfarin: a prospective in vivo clinical study

Makoto Saito[1], Shuji Hatakeyama[1,2*], Hideki Hashimoto[1], Takumitsu Suzuki[1], Daisuke Jubishi[1], Makoto Kaneko[3], Yukio Kume[3], Takehito Yamamoto[4], Hiroshi Suzuki[4] and Hiroshi Yotsuyanagi[1]

Abstract

Background: Daptomycin has been reported to cause artificial prolongation of prothrombin time (PT) by interacting with some test reagents of PT. This prolongation was particularly prominent with high concentrations of daptomycin in vitro. However, whether this prolongation is important in clinical settings and the optimal timing to assess PT remain unclear.

Methods: A prospective clinical study was conducted with patients who received daptomycin for confirmed or suspected drug-resistant, gram-positive bacterial infection at a university hospital in Japan. PT at the peak and trough of daptomycin was tested using nine PT reagents. Linear regression analyses were used to examine the difference in daptomycin concentration and the relative change of PT-international normalized ratios (PT-INR).

Results: Thirty-five patients received daptomycin (6 mg/kg). The mean ± standard deviation of the trough and peak concentrations of daptomycin were 13.5 ± 6.3 and 55.1 ± 16.9 μg/mL, respectively. Twelve patients (34%) received warfarin. With five PT reagents, a significant proportion of participants experienced prolongation of PT-INR at the daptomycin peak concentration compared to the PT-INR at the trough, although the mean relative change was less than 10%. None of the participants clinically showed any signs of bleeding. A linear, dose-dependent prolongation of PT was observed for one reagent [unadjusted coefficient β 3.1 × 10^{-3}/μg/mL; 95% confidence interval (CI) 2.3 × 10^{-5}–6.3 × 10^{-3}; $p = 0.048$]. When patients were stratified based on warfarin use, this significant linear relationship was observed in warfarin users for two PT reagents (adjusted coefficient β, 6.4 × 10^{-3}/μg/mL; 95% CI 3.5 × 10^{-3}–9.3 × 10^{-3}; $p < 0.001$; and adjusted coefficient β, 8.3 × 10^{-3}/μg/mL; 95% CI 4.4 × 10^{-3}–1.2 × 10^{-2}; $p < 0.001$). In non-warfarin users, this linear relationship was not observed for any PT reagents.

Conclusions: We found that a higher concentration of daptomycin could lead to artificial prolongation of PT-INR by interacting with some PT reagents. This change may not be clinically negligible, especially in warfarin users receiving a high dose of daptomycin. It may be better to measure PT at the trough rather than at the peak daptomycin concentration.

Keywords: Daptomycin, Prothrombin time, Warfarin, Drug resistance, Gram-positive infections, High dose

*Correspondence: shatake-tky@umin.ac.jp
[2] Division of General Internal Medicine, Division of Infectious Diseases, Jichi Medical University Hospital, 3311-1 Yakushiji, Shimotsuke-shi, Tochigi 329-0498, Japan
Full list of author information is available at the end of the article

Background

Daptomycin is a cyclic lipopeptide antimicrobial agent, which exerts its bactericidal effects against gram-positive bacteria by decreasing the integrity of bacterial phospholipid cell membranes in the presence of Ca^{2+} [1]. It is licensed for use against skin and soft tissue infections and bloodstream infection by gram-positive pathogens. Since its use was first approved in the USA in 2003, several reports have shown that prothrombin time (PT) was prolonged in daptomycin users, especially those who were on warfarin [2, 3]. This prolongation was considered artificial because those patients did not show evidence of bleeding [3]. In addition, daptomycin does not interfere with cytochrome P450 and thus it is unlikely to interact with warfarin in vivo [4]. It is possible that some PT reagents may interfere with daptomycin, resulting in an artificial increase in PT. Indeed, this prolongation was confirmed for some PT reagents in vitro by adding daptomycin to the blood samples, and this effect was particularly prominent in samples with elevated baseline PT due to warfarin use [3, 5, 6]. This finding is critical as a finer control of PT is needed for those treated with warfarin to prevent bleeding and intravascular clotting. In addition, patients who require warfarin and patients who need daptomycin frequently overlap. For example, anticoagulants are used in patients with intravascular devices, who are also at risk for bloodstream infection by gram-positive bacteria. The prolongation effect by daptomycin has been reported to depend on the daptomycin concentration [3, 5, 6], and some have suggested that PT should be measured at the trough rather than at the peak of the daptomycin concentration [3]. However, this suggestion has not been assessed in clinical settings. In addition, the effect of some PT reagents used in Japan on daptomycin has not been evaluated.

In this study, we compared for the first time PT at the trough and the peak concentrations of daptomycin using clinical samples prospectively collected from patients treated with daptomycin. The objective of this study was to assess whether there were any PT reagents affected by daptomycin and whether there was any difference in this effect depending on concomitant use of warfarin.

Methods

This prospective study was conducted at the University of Tokyo Hospital, Japan between February 2013 and October 2014. Participants were patients treated with daptomycin for confirmed or suspected drug-resistant, gram-positive bacterial infections (i.e. infections caused by methicillin-resistant *Staphylococcus aureus* and vancomycin-resistant enterococci) after they gave full written consents. Children younger than 12 years and anaemic patients with a haemoglobin concentration <9.0 mg/dL were excluded.

We examined the impact of daptomycin on PT measurement by comparing PT-international normalised ratio (PT-INR) at the trough and peak blood concentrations of daptomycin. Daptomycin was administered intravenously at a 6 mg/kg/dose over 30 min every 24 h (clearance of creatinine ≥30 mL/min) or 48 h (<30 mL/min) [4]. Blood samples (one 4.5 mL 3.2% sodium citrate tube for PT and one 2.0 mL ethylenediamine tetraacetic acid anticoagulant tube for daptomycin concentration) were taken at ≤30 min before (trough) and 30–60 min after (peak) the ≥3rd daptomycin administration. Blood samples were also taken for PT measurement at enrolment before the initiation of daptomycin. Within 1 h after collection, plasma was isolated by centrifugation (3000 rpm, room temperature, 10 min; 1500*g*, 4 °C, 15 min) and stored at −80 or −70 °C until assay of PT and daptomycin, respectively. We measured PTs using nine commercial reagents that are commonly used in Japan (Table 1). Samples were examined up to three times for each sample using each reagent, and median values were used for the statistical analyses. Plasma concentrations of daptomycin were measured using ultra-performance liquid chromatography with tandem mass spectrometric detection (UPLC-MS/MS) according to a previous report with some modifications [7]. Briefly, 50 µL of plasma specimens spiked with an internal standard (4-hydroxychalcone, 10 mg/L) was deproteinated by addition of 200 µL of methanol and centrifuged for 15 min at 15,000 rpm, 4 °C. Then, the clear supernatant was diluted 10 times with 80% methanol, and 5 µL aliquots were analysed with a UPLC-MS/MS system consisting of an ACQUITY UPLC® instrument coupled with a Quattro Premier XE triple-quadrupole MS/MS system (Waters Corp., Milford, MA, USA) operated under electrospray ionization (ESI) mode. Chromatographic separation was performed on ACUITY UPLC® BEH C18 column (1.7 µm, 2.1 × 100 mm, Waters Corp.) in isocratic separation mode. The mobile phase was 50/50 (v/v) milliQ water/acetonitrile containing 0.1% formic acid, and the flow rate was set at 0.3 mL/min. Analytes were monitored in multiple reaction monitoring (MRM) mode, and the m/z of precursor and product ions was 811.33 > 313.26 and 223.15 > 117.00 (ESI-) for daptomycin and 4-hydroxychalcone, respectively. The calibration ranges were 0.25–100 mg/L. Samples were anonymised with unique patient identifiers, and laboratories were blinded to the patients' information.

Statistical tests were conducted using STATA/MP 14.2 (Stata Corp, College Station, TX, USA). The binomial test and Fisher's exact test were used for binary and

Table 1 Characteristics of prothrombin time test reagents used in the study

No	Brand name	Manufacturer	Laboratory	ISI	Thromboplastin	Phospholipid
1	HemosIL Recombi PlasTin 2G	Instrumental Laboratories	University of Tokyo Hospital	1.01	Recombinant human tissue factor	Synthetic phospholipid
2	Neoplastin plus	Roche Diagnostics	Roche Diagnostics	1.33	Rabbit brain	Confidential
3	STA Neoplastin R	Roche Diagnostics	Roche Diagnostics	0.96	Recombinant human tissue factor	Confidential
4	Dade Innovin	Dade Behring (Sysmex)	Sysmex	1.0	Recombinant human tissue factor	No data
5	Thromborel S	Dade Behring (Sysmex)	Sysmex	1.0	Human placenta	No data
6	Thrombocheck PT	Sysmex	Sysmex	1.6	Rabbit brain	No data
7	Simplastin Excel S	BioMerieux	Kyowa Medex	1.22	Rabbit brain	No PG
8	Simplastin HTF	BioMerieux	Kyowa Medex	1.26	Cultured human lung cell	No PG
9	Coagupia PT–N	Sekisui Medical	Sekisui Medical	1.09	Rabbit brain	Confidential

ISI international sensitivity index, *PG* phosphatidylglycerol

categorical variables, respectively. For continuous variables, t test and linear regression model were used. The Huber-White sandwich estimator was used to measure the standard errors for linear regression analyses. Outliers that lay outside the 95% confidence interval (95% CI) based on the standard error of forecast were excluded from the linear regression model. Effect modification by warfarin use was our a priori interest. More than 10% relative change of PT-INR was regarded as clinically significant [8].

This study was approved by the Ethics Committee of the University of Tokyo Hospital (10026).

Results

Patient characteristics

Of the 36 participants recruited for this study, one withdrew because of the cessation of daptomycin before the third administration. Among the remaining 35 patients, 25 (71%) were men, and the median age was 61 years (Table 2). Twelve patients received warfarin. The median baseline PT-INR at trough was 2.62 [interquartile range (IQR) 1.63–3.29] in warfarin users and 1.19 (IQR 1.06–1.42) in non-warfarin users using our routine reagent (Reagent 1). The median time interval between trough and peak blood sample collections was 105 min (IQR

Table 2 Patient characteristics stratified by warfarin use

Characteristic	All (n = 35)	Warfarin user (n = 12)	Non-warfarin user (n = 23)
Age (years)	61 (51–77)	65.5 (52.5–79)	59 (51–74)
Male	25 (71%)	8 (67%)	17 (74%)
PT-INR at trough	1.39 (1.12–2.38)	2.62 (1.63–3.29)	1.19 (1.06–1.42)
Time interval between trough and peak (min)	105 (95–120)	95 (95–110)	112.5 (90–120)
Daptomycin dose (mg/kg/dose)	6.0 (5.9–6.1)	6.0 (5.9–6.4)	6.0 (5.8–6.0)
Number of daptomycin administered before peak	4 (3–5)	4.5 (4–5.5)	4 (3–5)
Creatinine clearance (mL/min)	84.8 ± 54.1	74.2 ± 40.4	89.9 ± 59.7
Source of infection			
Skin/joint infection	19 (54%)	7 (58%)	12 (52%)
Bacteraemia	12 (34%)	5 (42%)	7 (30%)
Other infections	4 (11%)	0 (0%)	4 (17%)
Comorbidity			
Autoimmune disease	5 (14%)	2 (17%)	3 (13%)
Cancer	6 (17%)	2 (17%)	4 (17%)
Cardiovascular disease	13 (37%)	8 (67%)	5 (22%)
Others	11 (31%)	0 (0%)	11 (48%)
Concomitant antibiotic use	17 (49%)	7 (58%)	10 (43%)

Data are shown as a number (%), mean ± standard deviation or median (interquartile range)

PT-INR prothrombin time-international normalised ratio. PT-INR by Reagent 1 is shown

95–120 min). Daptomycin treatment (results determined according to administered dose per body weight and number of administrations before the PT measurement) was comparable between the two groups. Most of the patients were receiving treatment for skin/joint infection (19/35; 54%) or bloodstream infection (12/35; 34%). There were more patients with cardiovascular disease in the warfarin group (8/12; 67%) than in the non-warfarin group (5/23; 22%). A total of 49% (17/35) patients were given concomitant antibiotics in addition to daptomycin. None of the patients showed any signs of bleeding during this study.

Comparison of PT-INRs between the trough and the peak concentrations of daptomycin

The average ± standard deviation of the trough and peak concentrations of daptomycin were 13.5 ± 6.3 and 55.1 ± 16.9 μg/mL, respectively. Both trough and peak concentrations were slightly higher in the warfarin group (16.6 ± 6.1, 57.6 ± 16.3) than in the non-warfarin group (11.9 ± 5.9, 53.8 ± 17.5), which could be due to the slightly impaired renal function in the warfarin group. The differences between the trough and peak concentrations were roughly equal (41.0 ± 14.0 in warfarin group and 41.9 ± 14.9 in non-warfarin group). The maximum peak concentration observed in this study cohort was 96.4 μg/mL.

PT-INRs at the trough and the peak daptomycin concentration were compared. Regarding Reagent 1, 2, 3, 7, and 8, more than 70% of patients had higher PT-INR at the peak than at the trough level (Table 3). This trend was not different between warfarin users and non-users for the same PT reagent (data not shown). Based on the PT-INR values, however, no reagents showed a clinically important relative change of >10%. The highest relative change of PT-INR was observed in the warfarin group with Reagent 3 at 1.13 (95% CI 1.03–1.22). The absolute difference of PT-INRs was biggest in warfarin users at 0.26 (95% CI 0.02–0.50) with Reagent 3 and in non-warfarin users at 0.06 (95% CI 0.01–0.12) with Reagent 1.

Linear relationship between the relative change of PT-INR and the difference in daptomycin concentrations between the trough and peak

The difference in daptomycin concentrations (Δ-daptomycin) between trough and peak was assessed as an explanatory variable for the relative change of PT-INR (Fig. 1). For Reagent 3, a significant linear association was observed between Δ-daptomycin and relative change of PT-INR: unadjusted coefficient β, 3.1×10^{-3}/μg/mL; 95% CI 2.3×10^{-5}–6.3×10^{-3}; $p = 0.048$; $r^2 = 0.19$ (Table 4). This relationship was unchanged after adjusting for warfarin use: adjusted coefficient β, 3.3×10^{-3}/μg/mL; 95% CI 5.2×10^{-4}–6.0×10^{-3}; $p = 0.02$; $r^2 = 0.34$.

For Reagent 2 and 3, effect modification by warfarin use was indicated (p value for effect modification, 0.0003 and 0.001, respectively). When taking this effect modification into account, only warfarin users showed a linear association for both Reagent 2 (adjusted coefficient β, 6.4×10^{-3}/μg/mL; 95% CI 3.5×10^{-3}–9.3×10^{-3}; $p < 0.001$; $r^2 = 0.57$) and Reagent 3 (adjusted coefficient β, 8.3×10^{-3}/μg/mL; 95% CI 4.4×10^{-3}–1.2×10^{-2}; $p < 0.001$; $r^2 = 0.56$). No linear association between Δ-daptomycin and relative change of PT-INR was observed for other reagents (Table 5).

Discussion

PT-INR at the peak concentration increased compared to that at the trough concentration of daptomycin in 56% (5/9) of the reagents, although the difference was not clinically meaningful (<10%). The magnitude of PT

Table 3 Proportion of patients with prolonged PT-INR at peak daptomycin concentration and the relative change of PT-INR between trough and peak

Reagent	$PT\text{-}INR_{peak} > PT\text{-}INR_{trough}$ (%)	p value[a]	$PT\text{-}INR_{peak}/PT\text{-}INR_{trough}$ (95% CI)	p value[b]
1	26/35 (74%)	0.006	1.05 (1.02–1.07)	1.00
2	27/35 (77%)	0.002	1.04 (1.01–1.07)	1.00
3	31/35 (89%)	<0.001	1.07 (1.03–1.11)	0.94
4	20/35 (57%)	0.50	1.00 (0.98–1.02)	1.00
5	20/35 (57%)	0.50	1.01 (0.98–1.03)	1.00
6	20/35 (57%)	0.50	1.02 (0.97–1.07)	1.00
7	25/35 (71%)	0.02	1.04 (1.01–1.08)	1.00
8	25/35 (71%)	0.02	1.05 (1.01–1.09)	0.99
9	19/35 (54%)	0.74	1.00 (0.98–1.02)	1.00

PT-INR prothrombin time-international normalised ratio, *CI* confidence interval

[a] p values by binomial test compared to 0.50

[b] One-sided p value by t test to test whether the ratio is more than 1.10

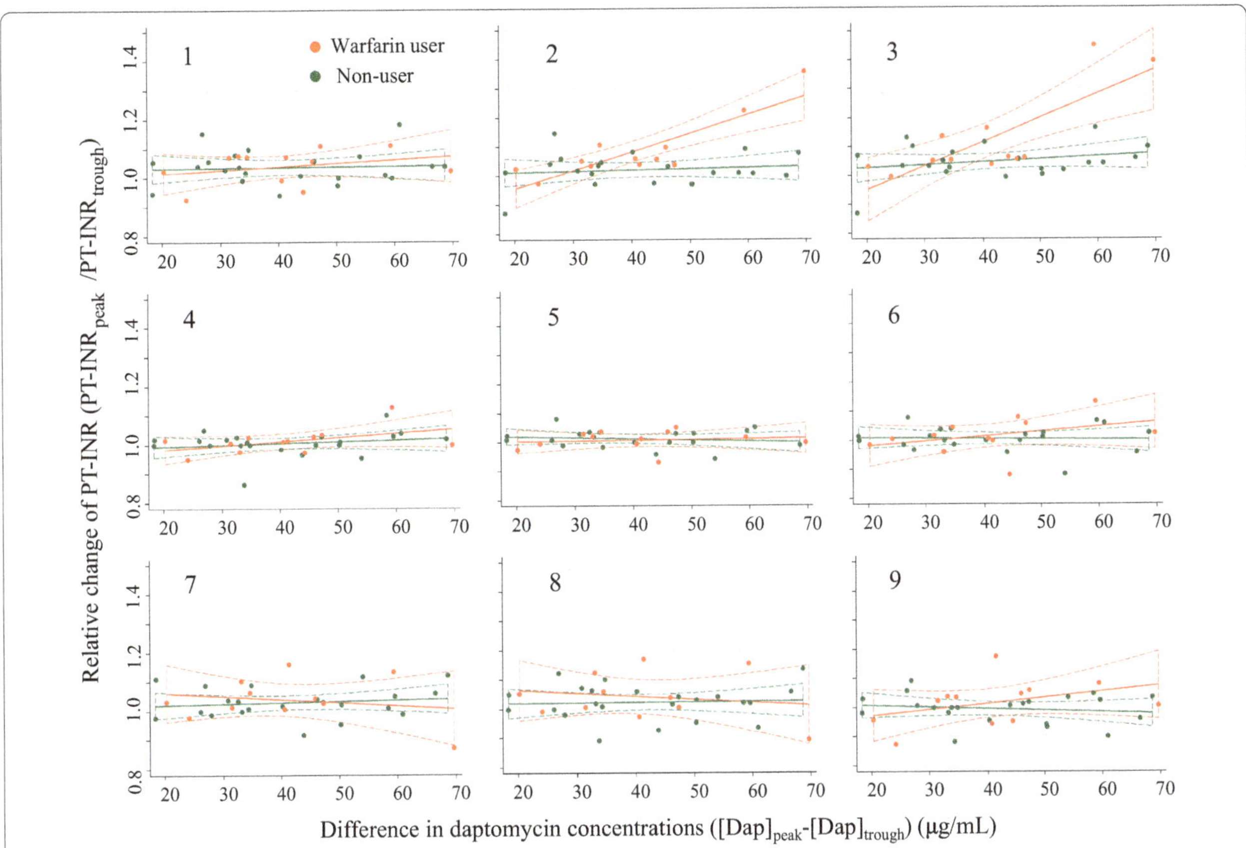

Fig. 1 The relative change of PT-INR and the difference in daptomycin concentrations [Dap] between trough and peak. Linear regression lines with a 95% confidence interval for the predicted mean are shown separately for warfarin users and non-users. The *reagent numbers* are shown in the *top left*. *PT-INR* prothrombin time international normalised ratio

Table 4 Linear relationship between the relative change of PT-INR and the difference in daptomycin concentrations between the trough and peak

Reagent	n	Unadjusted β (95% CI) (/μg/mL)	p value $H_0: \beta = 0$	r^2
1	34	5.1×10^{-4} (-9.2×10^{-4}–1.9×10^{-3})	0.48	0.02
2	34	2.2×10^{-3} (-5.6×10^{-4}–4.9×10^{-3})	0.12	0.15
3	34	3.1×10^{-3} (2.3×10^{-5}–6.3×10^{-3})	0.048	0.19
4	34	8.5×10^{-4} (-2.2×10^{-4}–1.9×10^{-3})	0.12	0.08
5	32	-1.8×10^{-4} (-9.2×10^{-4}–5.6×10^{-4})	0.62	0.006
6	33	4.3×10^{-4} (-7.3×10^{-4}–1.6×10^{-3})	0.45	0.02
7	33	-5.0×10^{-5} (-2.0×10^{-3}–1.9×10^{-3})	0.96	<0.001
8	34	-2.3×10^{-4} (-2.1×10^{-3}–1.6×10^{-3})	0.80	0.003
9	34	2.3×10^{-4} (-1.1×10^{-3}–1.6×10^{-3})	0.73	0.003

prolongation, however, could depend on the concentration of daptomycin. Based on the linear regression results in warfarin users, the PT-INR at a daptomycin peak concentration of 70 μg/mL is predicted to be 1.15 times (Reagent 2) and 1.20 times (Reagent 3) higher than the PT-INR at a trough concentration of 20 μg/mL. These estimates are in the similar range of effects previously reported by in vitro studies (ranging from 1.15 to more than three times higher at 100 μg/mL than at 0 μg/mL) [3, 5, 6, 9]. These magnitudes of elevation are clinically relevant, especially considering that higher daptomycin dosing (>6 mg/kg) was recently suggested and used for certain clinical situations [10, 11].

Susceptibility of PT reagents to the interaction with daptomycin has been reported to depend on two factors: the type of thromboplastin reagents used and the condition of phospholipids [3, 5]. One common feature among the affected reagents was that they were derived from recombinant human or rabbit tissue factors [3, 5, 6]. Phosphatidylglycerol (PG) concentration is considered to be the other key factor for this interaction [5]. When PG was added, reagents containing recombinant rabbit or

Table 5 Adjusted linear relationship between the relative change of PT-INR and the difference in daptomycin concentrations between the trough and peak

Reagent	Adjusted β (95% CI) (/μg/mL)	p value $H_0: \beta = 0$	p value for interaction	r^2
1	5.1×10^{-4} (-9.5×10^{-4}–2.0×10^{-3})	0.48		0.02
Warfarin (+)	1.2×10^{-3} (-1.3×10^{-3}–3.7×10^{-3})	0.34	0.79	0.03
Warfarin (−)	2.0×10^{-4} (-1.7×10^{-3}–2.1×10^{-3})	0.83		
2	2.3×10^{-3} (-1.1×10^{-4}–5.0×10^{-3})	0.06		0.33
Warfarin (+)	6.4×10^{-3} (3.5×10^{-3}–9.3×10^{-3})	<0.001	0.0003	0.57
Warfarin (−)	4.2×10^{-4} (-1.6×10^{-3}–2.5×10^{-3})	0.68		
3	3.3×10^{-3} (5.2×10^{-4}–6.0×10^{-3})	0.02		0.34
Warfarin (+)	8.3×10^{-3} (4.4×10^{-3}–1.2×10^{-2})	<0.001	0.001	0.56
Warfarin (−)	9.8×10^{-4} (-1.2×10^{-3}–3.2×10^{-3})	0.36		
4	8.5×10^{-4} (-2.5×10^{-4}–2.0×10^{-3})	0.13		0.08
Warfarin (+)	1.4×10^{-3} (-1.1×10^{-3}–3.9×10^{-3})	0.26	0.52	0.10
Warfarin (−)	5.6×10^{-4} (-6.1×10^{-4}–1.7×10^{-3})	0.33		
5	-1.8×10^{-4} (-9.2×10^{-4}–5.7×10^{-4})	0.63		0.009
Warfarin (+)	2.3×10^{-4} (-7.1×10^{-4}–1.2×10^{-3})	0.63	0.78	0.03
Warfarin (−)	-4.0×10^{-4} (-1.4×10^{-3}–6.5×10^{-4})	0.44		
6	4.4×10^{-4} (-7.3×10^{-4}–1.6×10^{-3})	0.45		0.03
Warfarin (+)	1.7×10^{-3} (-4.7×10^{-4}–3.8×10^{-3})	0.12	0.45	0.09
Warfarin (−)	-1.4×10^{-4} (-1.5×10^{-3}–1.2×10^{-3})	0.84		
7	-3.3×10^{-5} (-2.1×10^{-3}–2.0×10^{-3})	0.97		0.006
Warfarin (+)	-1.1×10^{-3} (-5.9×10^{-3}–3.8×10^{-3})	0.65	0.81	0.03
Warfarin (−)	4.4×10^{-4} (-1.3×10^{-3}–2.2×10^{-3})	0.61		
8	-2.1×10^{-4} (-2.2×10^{-3}–1.8×10^{-3})	0.83		0.02
Warfarin (+)	-1.0×10^{-3} (-5.6×10^{-3}–3.5×10^{-3})	0.65	0.72	0.04
Warfarin (−)	1.5×10^{-4} (-1.7×10^{-3}–2.0×10^{-3})	0.87		
9	2.6×10^{-4} (-1.1×10^{-3}–1.7×10^{-3})	0.71		0.03
Warfarin (+)	2.1×10^{-3} (-7.9×10^{-4}–4.9×10^{-3})	0.15	0.32	0.12
Warfarin (−)	-5.6×10^{-4} (-2.1×10^{-3}–9.6×10^{-4})	0.46		

For each PT reagent, the first row is based on the linear regression model adjusted for warfarin use, and the second and the third rows are strata-specific values based on the linear regression model with interaction by warfarin use

recombinant human tissue factor showed concentration-dependent prolongation of PT by daptomycin, whereas a reagent containing human placenta was less affected [5]. One of the two affected reagents in our study contained recombinant human tissue factor, whereas the other contained rabbit brain. All samples were centrifuged within 1 h after collection and then kept at −80 °C; therefore, the time between collection and measurement, and transportation were not likely to considerably affect our results [12].

Our comparison between trough and peak concentrations was based on the assumption that PT was otherwise unchanged between trough time and peak time, which were 1–3 h apart on the same day. Although factors other than increased daptomycin concentration might have caused true prolongation of PT between the trough and peak concentrations, such factors were not likely, and even if they played a role in the effect, they would not explain why this prolongation was only observed for the two PT reagents. First, this trend was not attributable to increased warfarin concentration, as only one patient took warfarin between the two sample collections, and all others took warfarin after blood collection at peak of daptomycin. Second, the circadian rhythm of PT, which is approximately 5–10% [13–15], did not likely to affect our results. If this circadian rhythm was affecting our results, all reagents should have shown the same pattern. Furthermore, although the PT seems to vary in a day, it is still controversial whether there is a certain circadian pattern of PT that is the same across patients on warfarin [13–15]. Third, the impact of the concomitant use of other antibiotics on the change of PT between the two time points could be limited. There are mainly three mechanisms by which antibiotics can affect PT: interaction between warfarin and antibiotics; reduced vitamin K production resulting from interference by the

N-methylthiotetrazole side chain of certain antibiotics; and the effect of antibiotics on normal gut flora producing vitamin K. Only one patient took both warfarin and a concomitant antibiotic that was known to interact with warfarin. This patient took sulphamethoxazole-trimethoprim (ST) and he was the only person in the warfarin group who showed more than a 5% relative increase in PT-INR with all PT reagents. Nonetheless, Reagent 2 and 3 showed a greater relative increase in PT-INR (1.23 and 1.45, respectively) than the rest of the PT reagents (mean 1.11, 95% CI 1.07–1.15). Interaction between ST and test reagents was also unlikely, as this prolongation of PT by Reagent 2 and 3 was not observed in the other three patients who used ST. There was only one patient who took warfarin and an antibiotic with a N-methylthiotetrazole side chain (i.e. cefmetazole). Similar to the previous patient, only Reagents 2 and 3 showed an increase in PT-INR in this patient (relative increase of 1.36 and 1.40, respectively), and the mean value for the rest of the PT reagents did not increase (mean 0.98, 95% CI 0.92–1.03). Thus, true prolongation of PT by the N-methylthiotetrazole side chain of cefmetazole was unlikely. Additionally, artificial prolongation of PT resulting from the interaction between cefmetazole and the two PT test reagents was unlikely. This was because the blood level of cefmetazole was considered to decrease between the two time points of blood sample collection, as cefmetazole was administered 3 h before the first blood sample collection. The effect on normal gut flora was not likely to change PT dramatically in 1–3 h. Lastly, the prolongation of PT was not likely due to regression to the mean, as this trend of PT prolongation was unchanged even when patients with a lower initial PT-INR of <1.0 were excluded from the analyses (data not shown).

There were some differences between warfarin users and non-users. Both the absolute and relative increases in PT-INR between trough and peak were smaller in non-warfarin users compared to those in warfarin users. Similarly, the dose-dependent effect of daptomycin on PT prolongation was only observed in warfarin users in our study. In previous in vitro studies, normal plasma samples were less reactive to daptomycin than samples from patients with anti-vitamin K therapy [5], or with prolonged baseline PT (PT-INR > 2.0) [6]. Another study revealed that samples with normal PT were slightly less affected by daptomycin than that those obtained from warfarin users, whereas warfarin users with different PT levels showed a similar increase rate [3]. Another possibility is that the apparent discrepancy between the response in warfarin users and the non-response in non-users in our study might be due to the relatively low peak concentration of daptomycin in our patients rather than the warfarin effect. In all in vitro studies, changes of PT in normal PT samples were small, particularly if the daptomycin concentration was low.

This study has some limitations. As we used clinical samples, we could not finely control the daptomycin concentration, which led to a relatively small difference between trough and peak daptomycin concentrations. Samples with a high peak concentration (e.g. >70 μg/mL) were also scarce in our study. Therefore, care is required when interpreting our results showing an increasing trend in the relative change of PT-INR caused by increased difference in the daptomycin concentrations for Reagents 2 and 3 because the prediction relied on a small number of samples with a high peak concentration. It is also possible that other tested agents are affected by daptomycin under a higher peak concentration. We cannot conclude whether the effect of daptomycin occurred in warfarin users or patients with high PT-INR for any reason because these patients largely overlapped in this study. Therefore, in the future, it is necessary to assess whether the measurement of PT from patients with elevated PT due to coagulopathy but not on warfarin will be affected by daptomycin.

Conclusion

In summary, we found that a higher concentration of daptomycin could lead to artificial prolongation of PT-INR by interacting with some PT reagents, particularly in patients on warfarin. Because we used clinical samples, the results of this study relied on a relatively small number of samples, especially those with a high peak daptomycin concentration, which could have been influenced by many time-varying confounding factors in addition daptomycin concentration. Therefore, in vitro studies assessing the impact of daptomycin on some reagents may be warranted. In the meantime, we suggest that it may be better to measure PT near the trough concentration of daptomycin, especially when PT is elevated or warfarin is used.

Abbreviations

CI: confidence interval; ESI: electrospray ionization; IQR: interquartile range; MRM: multiple reaction monitoring; PG: phosphatidylglycerol; PT: prothrombin time; PT-INR: prothrombin time international normalised ratios; UPLC-MS/MS: ultra-performance liquid chromatography with tandem mass spectrometric detection; USA: United States of America.

Authors' contributions

SH and HY conceived and conducted this study; MS, HH, DJ, and TS performed the clinical assessment and data collection; TS, MK, YK, TY and HS conducted laboratory work; MS and SH conducted statistical analysis and interpreted the data. MS, SH and TY drafted the manuscript; all the authors critically revised the manuscript for intellectual content. All authors read and approved the final manuscript.

Author details
[1] Department of Infectious Diseases, University of Tokyo Hospital, 7-3-1 Hongo, Bunkyo-ku, Tokyo 113-8655, Japan. [2] Division of General Internal Medicine, Division of Infectious Diseases, Jichi Medical University Hospital, 3311-1 Yakushiji, Shimotsuke-shi, Tochigi 329-0498, Japan. [3] Department of Clinical Laboratory, University of Tokyo Hospital, 7-3-1 Hongo, Bunkyo-ku, Tokyo 113-8655, Japan. [4] Department of Pharmacy, University of Tokyo Hospital, 7-3-1 Hongo, Bunkyo-ku, Tokyo 113-8655, Japan.

Acknowledgements
We would like to thank the patients who participated in this study and the staff who took care of them. We acknowledge the following diagnostics companies for technical support on PT reagents: Kyowa Medex Co., Ltd. (Tokyo, Japan), Roche Diagnostics K.K. (Tokyo, Japan), Sekisui Medical Co., Ltd. (Tokyo, Japan) and Sysmex Corporation (Hyogo, Japan).

Competing interests
MS received a scholarship from the GlaxoSmithKline International Scholarship Charitable Trust Fund and is receiving another scholarship from the University of Oxford Clarendon Fund. These funding sources had no roles in this study. All other authors declare that they have no competing interests.

Consent for publication
Not applicable: all data are fully anonymised and do not include any identifiable information.

Funding
The authors declare that they did not have any funding source or grant to support their research work.

References

1. Steenbergen JN, Alder J, Thorne GM, Tally FP. Daptomycin: a lipopeptide antibiotic for the treatment of serious Gram-positive infections. J Antimicrob Chemother. 2005;55(3):283–8.
2. Drug information: CUBICIN® (daptomycin for injection). 2016. https://www.merck.com/product/usa/pi_circulars/c/cubicin/cubicin_pi.pdf. Accessed 25 Oct 2016.
3. Webster PS, Oleson FB Jr, Paterson DL, Arkin CF, Mangili A, Craven DE, Adcock DM, Lindfield KC, Knapp AG, Martone WJ. Interaction of daptomycin with two recombinant thromboplastin reagents leads to falsely prolonged patient prothrombin time/International Normalized Ratio results. Blood Coagul Fibrinolysis. 2008;19(1):32–8.
4. Kosmidis C, Levine DP. Daptomycin: pharmacology and clinical use. Expert Opin Pharmacother. 2010;11(4):615–25.
5. van den Besselaar AM, Breukink E, Koorengevel MC. Phosphatidylglycerol and daptomycin synergistically inhibit tissue factor-induced coagulation in the prothrombin time test. J Thromb Haemost. 2010;8(6):1429–30.
6. Yamada T, Kato R, Oda K, Tanaka H, Suzuki K, Ijiri Y, Ikemoto T, Nishihara M, Hayashi T, Tanaka K, et al. False prolongation of prothrombin time in the presence of a high blood concentration of daptomycin. Basic Clin Pharmacol Toxicol. 2016;119(4):353–9.
7. Verdier MC, Bentue-Ferrer D, Tribut O, Collet N, Revest M, Bellissant E. Determination of daptomycin in human plasma by liquid chromatography-tandem mass spectrometry. Clinical application. Clin Chem Lab Med. 2011;49(1):69–75.
8. Poller L. Screening INR deviation of local prothrombin time systems. J Clin Pathol. 1998;51(5):356–9.
9. van den Besselaar AM, Tripodi A. Effect of daptomycin on prothrombin time and the requirement for outlier exclusion in International Sensitivity Index calibration of thromboplastin. J Thromb Haemost. 2007;5(9):1975–6.
10. Baddour LM, Wilson WR, Bayer AS, Fowler VG Jr, Tleyjeh IM, Rybak MJ, Barsic B, Lockhart PB, Gewitz MH, Levison ME, et al. Infective endocarditis in adults: diagnosis, antimicrobial therapy, and management of complications: a Scientific Statement for Healthcare Professionals From the American Heart Association. Circulation. 2015;132(15):1435–86.
11. Seaton RA, Gonzalez-Ruiz A, Cleveland KO, Couch KA, Pathan R, Hamed K. Real-world daptomycin use across wide geographical regions: results from a pooled analysis of CORE and EU-CORE. Ann Clin Microbiol Antimicrob. 2016;15:18.
12. van Geest-Daalderop JH, Mulder AB. Boonman-de Winter LJ, Hoekstra MM, van den Besselaar AM: Preanalytical variables and off-site blood collection: influences on the results of the prothrombin time/international normalized ratio test and implications for monitoring of oral anticoagulant therapy. Clin Chem. 2005;51(3):561–8.
13. Bleske BE, Welage LS, Warren EW, Brown MB, Shea MJ. Variations in prothrombin time and international normalized ratio over 24 hours in warfarin-treated patients. Pharmacotherapy. 1995;15(6):709–12.
14. García A, Marín F, Sánchez B, Roldán V, Marco P. Diurnal variation in the intensity of anticoagulation in atrial fibrillation. Stroke. 2002;33(1):322–4.
15. Ho C-H, Lin M-W, You J-Y, Chen C-C, Yu T-J. Variations of prothrombin time and international normalized ratio in patients treated with warfarin. Thromb Res. 2002;107(5):277–80.

21

The emergence of a novel sequence type of MDR *Acinetobacter baumannii* from the intensive care unit of an Egyptian tertiary care hospital

Doaa Mohammad Ghaith[1], Mai Mahmoud Zafer[2], Mohamed Hamed Al-Agamy[3,4*], Essam J. Alyamani[5], Rayan Y. Booq[5] and Omar Almoazzamy[6]

Abstract

Background and aim of work: *Acinetobacter baumannii* is known for nosocomial outbreaks worldwide. In this study, we aimed to investigate the antibiotic susceptibility patterns and the clonal relationship of *A. baumannii* isolates from the intensive care unit (ICU) of an Egyptian hospital.

Methods: In the present study, 50 clinical isolates of multidrug resistant (MDR)-*A. baumannii* were obtained from patients admitted into the ICU from June to December 2015. All isolates were analyzed for antimicrobial susceptibilities. Multiplex PCR was performed to detect genes encoding oxacillinase genes (bla_{OXA-51}-like, bla_{OXA-23}-like, bla_{OXA-24}-like, and bla_{OXA-58}-like). Multilocus sequence typing (MLST) based on the seven-gene scheme (*gltA, gyrB, gdhB, recA, cpn60, gpi, rpoD*) was used to examine these isolates.

Results: All *A. baumannii* clinical isolates showed the same resistance pattern, characterized by resistance to most common antibiotics including imipenem (MIC $\geq$ 8μ/mL), with the only exception being colistin. Most isolates were positive for bla_{OXA-51}-like and bla_{OXA-23}-like (100 and 96%, respectively); however, bla_{OXA-24}-like and bla_{OXA-58}-like were not detected. MLST analysis identified different sequence types (ST195, ST208, ST231, ST441, ST499, and ST723) and a new sequence type (ST13929) with other sporadic strains.

Conclusions: MDR *A. baumannii* strains harboring bla_{OXA-23}-like genes were widely circulating in this ICU. MLST was a powerful tool for identifying and epidemiologically typing our strains. Strict infection control measures must be implemented to contain the worldwide spread of MDR *A. baumannii* in ICUs.

Keywords: MDR-*A. baumannii*, bla_{OXA-23}-like, MLST

Background

The clinical care of intensive care unit (ICU) patients with infections has been complicated by the emergence and spread of extremely drug-resistant (XDR) *Acinetobacter baumannii* strains [1]. Due to scarce current therapeutic options; higher infection rates; poor patient outcomes because of life-threatening infections, including ventilator-related pneumonia, sepsis, urinary tract infections, and skin and soft tissue disorders may occur [1, 2].

Extensively drug-resistant (XDR) *A. baumannii* strains exhibiting resistance to three or more antibiotic classes, except for polymyxins, have been recently described in nosocomial outbreaks [2, 3]. The essential role of *A. baumannii* resistance to carbapenems, is mediated by oxacillinases (OXA-class D) and, less frequently, by metallo-β-lactamases (MBL-class B) [4, 5]. The class D carbapenemases are the most predominant carbapenemases in *A. baumannii.* They are categorized into six subclasses:

*Correspondence: malagamy@KSU.EDU.SA; elagamy71@yahoo.com
[3] Department of Pharmaceutics, College of Pharmacy, King Saud University, PO box 2457, Riyadh 11451, Saudi Arabia
Full list of author information is available at the end of the article

intrinsic chromosomal OXA-51-like, the acquired OXA-23-like, OXA-24/40-like, OXA-58-like, OXA-143-like, and OXA-235-like β-lactamases [6]. In this study, we aimed to investigate the antimicrobial susceptibility, class D carbapenemases and clonal relationship of *A. baumannii* strains isolated from a tertiary care hospital ICU in Egypt.

Methods

The study was carried out in EL Sheikh Zayed hospital which provides tertiary care from specialists and consultants after referral (in orthopedic, trauma, neuro/spine surgeries) from primary care and secondary care hospitals in Egypt. A lab-based surveillance was performed over a period of 6 months (June–December 2015) after the isolation of five MDR *A. baumannii* strains in a period of 1 week showing the same phenotypic characteristics.

Bacterial strains

All clinical samples of the patients admitted during the above-mentioned period were processed at the microbiology unit. All samples were cultured on blood agar and MacConkey agar (Oxoid Co. England). All culture plates were incubated aerobically at 35 °C for 24–48 h. Identification of isolated organisms was performed by conventional biochemical reactions. During the experimental period, 50 *A. baumannii* non-duplicate strains were isolated.

Antimicrobial susceptibility testing

Susceptibility testing was performed by the disc diffusion method (Modified Kirby-Bauer technique) using Mueller–Hinton agar and aerobic incubation at 35 °C for 16–18 h. Antimicrobial discs containing imipenem (10 μg), meropenem (10 μg), gentamicin (10 μg), ciprofloxacin (5 μg), amikacin (30 μg), cotrimoxazole (25 μg), cefepime (30 μg), cefotaxime (30 μg), cefotaxime/clavulanic acid (30/10 μg), aztreonam (30 μg), ceftazidime (30 μg), ceftazidime/clavulanic acid (30/10 μg), amoxicillin/clavulanic acid (20/10 μg), and cefoxitin (30 μg) were obtained from Oxoid Co. (Oxoid Limited, Basingstoke, Hampshire, England) [7].

Multidrug resistance was defined in this analysis as resistance to three or more representatives of the following classes of antibiotics: fluoroquinolones, extended-spectrum cephalosporins, aminoglycosides, and carbapenems [8].

Escherichia coli ATCC 25922, *Pseudomonas aeruginosa* ATCC 27853, and *Staphylococcus aureus* ATCC 29213 were used as reference strains for susceptibility testing per Clinical and Laboratory Standards Institute (CLSI, 2015) guidelines and interpretations [7].

Minimum inhibitory concentrations (MICs) were determined by broth microdilution and interpreted using CLSI, 2015 guidelines [7].

The presence of *A. baumannii* genes encoding oxacillinases (bla_{OXA-23}-like, bla_{OXA-24}-like, bla_{OXA-51}-like, and bla_{OXA-58}-like) was assessed in all 50 isolates using multiplex PCR.

Multiplex PCR assay

The sequences of bla_{OXA} alleles encoding carbapenemases were aligned and group-specific regions were identified using BioEdit software (http://www.mbio.ncsu.edu/BioEdit/bioedit.html). The primers: 5′-TAA TGC TTT GATCGG CCT TG and 5′-TGG ATT GCA CTT CAT CTT GG were used to amplify a 353 bp fragment of genes encoding the intrinsic OXA-51-like enzymes of *A. baumannii* [9].

A set of primers were designed to amplify OXA-23-like genes (501 bp: 5′-GAT CGG ATT GGA GAA CCAGA and 5′-ATT TCT GAC CGC ATT TCC AT), OXA-24-like genes (246 bp: 5′-GGT TAG TTG GCC CCC TTA AA and 5′-AGT TGA GCG AAA AGG GGA TT), and OXA-58-like genes (599 bp: 5′-AAG TAT TGG GGC TTG TGC TG and 5′-CCCCTCTGCGCTCTACATAC) [9]. The primers were evaluated separately against control strains and then in a multiplex format. The amplification conditions were: initial denaturation at 94 °C for 5 min, 30 cycles of 94 °C for 25 s, 52 °C for 40 s, and 72 °C for 50 s, and a final elongation at 72 °C for 6 min [9].

Multilocus sequence typing

MLST analysis was performed per the protocol of the Pasteur Institute. Fragments of seven internal housekeeping genes (*gltA, gyrB, gdhB, recA, cpn60, gpi,* and *rpoD*) were amplified and sequenced as previously described [10]. Briefly, PCR amplifications were performed with a MasterCycler Nexus (Eppendorf, Hamburg, Germany) with an initial denaturation at 94 °C for 5 min, followed by 35 cycles of denaturation at 94 °C for 1 min, annealing at 55 °C for 1 min, and extension at 72 °C for 2 min, and a 4-min final extension at 72 °C. The amplicons were verified by agarose gel electrophoresis and were subsequently purified for bidirectional Sanger sequencing reactions. Multiple allele sequences were assigned for each locus with an arbitrary allele number to obtain characterization of sequence types (STs) for each *A. baumannii* isolate. Each sequence was compared with sequences deposited in the Institute of Pasteur MLST schema (http://pubmlst.org/perl/bigsdb/bigsdb.pl?db=pubmlst_abaumannii_pasteur_seqdef).

Results

Out of 358 patients admitted to ICU from June to December 2015, 56 (15.6%) patients were diagnosed with various types of hospital-acquired infections (HAI) as shown in Table 1. A total of 50 non-duplicate *A. baumannii* strains

Table 1 Patient's data

	Age (mean ± SD)	Sex %		APACHE %		Length of stay (mean ± SD)	More than one device inserted %
		Male	Female	<15%	>15%		
VAP	(42.62 ± 17.63)	72%	28%	40%	60%	(48.96 ± 77.3)	(100%)
CLABSI	(41 ± 23.4)	88.8%	11.1%	33.3%	66.6%	(22.33 ± 11.4)	(55.55%)
CAUTI	(44.53 ± 22.1)	76.9%	23.0%	38.4%	61.5%	(82.307 ± 67.8)	(100%)
P value	0.900	0.535		0.880		0.131	0.00

VAP ventilator associated pneumonia, *CLABSI* central line associated blood stream infection, *CAUTI* catheter associated urinary tract infection, *APACHI* acute physiology and chronic health evaluation

were isolated from different patient samples. Phenotypic antibiotic susceptibility testing for all *A. baumannii* isolates showed the same drug resistance pattern, characterized by resistance to all antibiotics used including imipenem, except for colistin. Genotypic analysis of bla_{OXA-51}-like, bla_{OXA-23}-like, bla_{OXA-24}-like, and bla_{OXA-58}-like genes by multiplex PCR (Fig. 1) showed that bla_{OXA-51}-like and bla_{OXA-23}-like were the most prevalent genes with 100 and 96% prevalence, respectively. However, bla_{OXA-24}-like and bla_{OXA-58}-like were not detected in the current study. Multilocus sequence typing (MLST) of the 50 clinical isolates of *A. baumannii* has yielded different sequence types; ST195, ST208, ST231, ST441, ST499, and ST723. Interestingly, a new sequence type ST13929 was identified among *A. baumannii* clinical isolates as shown in Table 2 and Fig. 2. *A. baumannii* ST13929 has been isolated from a young male (21 years old) patient who had no history of overseas travel. He was admitted to ICU at El Sheikh Zayed Specialized Hospital, Giza, Egypt on 5th of December 2014. The patient had multiple traumas due to motor car accident. After 7 days of ventilation the patient diagnosed to have ventilator associated pneumonia (VAP). Empirical antibiotic therapy of intravenous ceftriaxone/cefotaxime had been initiated. Endotracheal aspiration has been cultured on blood, chocolate and MacConkey agars. The recovered colonies had been identified as *A. baumannii.* Further genotypic identification was done by restriction analysis of 16S–23S rRNA spacer sequences using *Alu*I and *Nde*II. The isolate exhibited XDR towards imipenem (MIC > 32 mg/L), meropenem (MIC > 32 mg/L), ceftazidime (>256 mg/L), cefepime (MICs > 256 mg/L), gentamicin (MICs > 256 mg/L), amikacin (MICs > 256 mg/L), and ciprofloxacin (MICs > 32 mg/L). Tigecycline susceptibility was observed at MIC of 1 mg/L. The antimicrobial therapy was changed to tigecycline on day 11. The patient had spent 107 days in the hospital. The patient was alive after the hospitalization period. There was an ongoing XDR- *A. baumannii* outbreak in the institution in the same period and multiple isolates had been investigated.

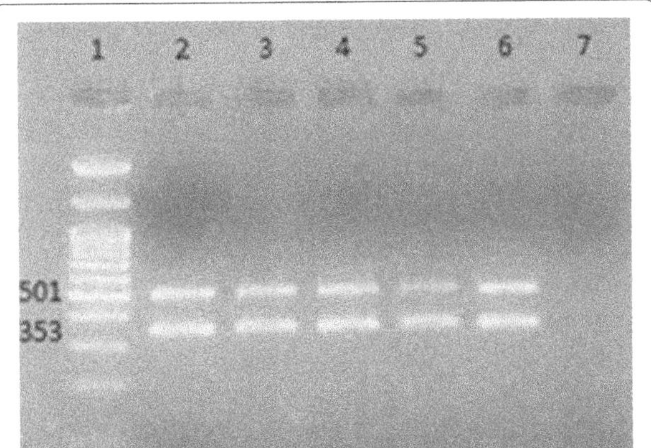

Fig. 1 Results of multiplex PCR for detection of bla_{OXA-51}-like, bla_{OXA-23}-like, bla_{OXA-24}-like, and bla_{OXA-58}-like genes. *Lane 1* 100 bp DNA Ladder, *Lane 2* positive control, *Lanes 3–6 A. baumannii* clinical isolates showing bla_{OXA-51}-like and bla_{OXA-23}-like positivity (353 and 501 bp, respectively). bla_{OXA-24}-like and bla_{OXA-58}-like were not detected at (246 and 599 bp) respectively. *Lane 7* negative control

Discussion

MDR *A. baumannii* is a problematic, multidrug-resistant pathogen identified in healthcare settings worldwide, especially in ICUs [12]. *A. baumannii* has a notable ability to capture and express resistance genes. All resistance mechanisms including target modification, efflux pump expression, and enzymatic inactivation have been described in *A. baumannii* [13].

In the current study, five MDR *A. baumannii* strains were isolated over 1 week from the same ICU. All isolates showed the same phenotypic characteristics which prompted us to start a survey study of the antimicrobial susceptibility and clonal relationship of *A. baumannii* strains isolated from this ICU.

All our isolates were resistant to imipenem. The main role of the *A. baumannii* resistance to carbapenems is mediated by oxacillinases and, less frequently, by metallo-β-lactamases [4, 5].

bla_{OXA-23}-like, $bla_{OXA-24/40}$-like, and bla_{OXA-58}-like genes have been repetitively reported in *A. baumannii* outbreaks from diverse parts of the world. The

Table 2 Sequence types (STs), allele profiles of 50 carbapenem-resistant *A. baumannii* isolates, carbapenem-hydrolyzing class D β-lactamase genes, minimum inhibitory concentration (MIC), site of isolation and patient outcome

	Sample ID	Site of isolation	Allele profile							ST	Carbapenem-hydrolyzing class D β-lactamase genes				MIC R ≥ 8 (mg/L)	Patient outcome
			gltA	*gyrB*	*gdhB*	*recA*	*cpn60*	*gpi*	*rpoD*		bla_{OXA-51}	bla_{OXA-23}	bla_{OXA-24}	bla_{OXA-58}	IMI	
A. baumannii	21	ETA	1	3	3	2	2	96	3	195	+	+	–	–	25	Deceased
A. baumannii	22	ETA	1	3	3	2	2	96	3	195	+	+	–	–	20	Deceased
A. baumannii	30	ETA	1	3	3	2	2	97	3	208	+	+	–	–	25	Deceased
A. baumannii	33	ETA	1	3	No gene	2	2	97	3	NA	+	+	–	–	25	Deceased
A. baumannii	34	ETA	1	3	3	2	2	97	3	208	+	–	–	–	35	Deceased
A. baumannii	36	ETA	1	3	3	2	2	97	3	208	+	+	–	–	20	Deceased
A. baumannii	37	ETA	1	3	3	2	2	97	3	208	+	+	–	–	30	Deceased
A. baumannii	44	Blood	1	3	3	2	2	97	3	208	+	+	–	–	25	Deceased
A. baumannii	46	Urine	1	3	3	2	2	97	3	208	+	+	–	–	25	Deceased
A. baumannii	47	Urine	1	3	No gene	2	2	97	3	NA	+	+	–	–	30	Discharged
A. baumannii	49	Urine	1	3	3	2	2	96	3	195	+	+	–	–	25	Deceased
A. baumannii	5	ETA	1	12	3	2	2	79	3	1114	+	+	–	–	20	Deceased
A. baumannii	29	ETA	1	87	3	2	2	96	3	13929[a]	+	+	–	–	20	Discharged
A. baumannii	24	ETA	1	107	12	10	23	195	26	723	+	+	–	–	25	Deceased
A. baumannii	25	ETA	1	107	12	10	23	195	26	723	+	+	–	–	25	Deceased
A. baumannii	38	ETA	1	107	12	10	23	195	26	723	+	+	–	–	30	Deceased
A. baumannii	48	urine	1	107	12	10	23	195	26	723	+	+	–	–	25	Deceased
A. baumannii	1	ETA	10	12	4	11	4	100	5	441	+	+	–	–	30	Deceased
A. baumannii	3	ETA	10	12	4	11	4	79	5	945	+	+	–	–	15	Deceased
A. baumannii	4	ETA	10	12	4	11	4	100	5	441	+	+	–	–	35	Discharged
A. baumannii	8	ETA	10	12	4	11	4	100	5	441	+	+	–	–	35	Deceased
A. baumannii	11	ETA	10	12	4	11	4	100	5	441	+	+	–	–	20	Deceased
A. baumannii	14	ETA	10	12	4	11	4	100	5	441	+	+	–	–	20	Deceased
A. baumannii	16	ETA	10	12	4	11	4	100	5	441	+	+	–	–	25	Discharged
A. baumanii	18	ETA	10	12	No gene	11	4	98	5	NA	+	+	–	–	20	Deceased
A. baumanii	19	ETA	10	12	4	11	4	98	5	231	+	+	–	–	20	Deceased
A. baumannii	20	ETA	10	12	4	11	4	98	5	231	+	+	–	–	20	Deceased
A. baumannii	23	ETA	10	12	4	11	4	98	5	231	+	+	–	–	15	Deceased
A. baumannii	26	ETA	10	12	4	11	4	98	5	231	+	+	–	–	25	Deceased
A. baumannii	27	ETA	10	12	4	11	4	98	5	231	+	+	–	–	20	Deceased
A. baumannii	28	ETA	10	12	4	11	4	98	5	231	+	+	–	–	20	Deceased
A. baumannii	31	ETA	10	12	4	11	4	100	5	441	+	+	–	–	25	Deceased

Table 2 continued

	Sample ID	Site of isolation	Allele profile							ST	Carbapenem-hydrolyzing class D β-lactamase genes				MIC R ≥ 8 (mg/L)	Patient outcome
			gltA	*gyrB*	*gdhB*	*recA*	*cpn60*	*gpi*	*rpoD*		bla_{OXA-51}	bla_{OXA-23}	bla_{OXA-24}	bla_{OXA-58}	IMI	
A. baumannii	32	ETA	10	12	4	11	4	98	5	231	+	+	–	–	20	Deceased
A. baumannii	35	ETA	10	12	4	11	4	98	5	231	+	+	–	–	25	Deceased
A. baumannii	40	ETA	10	12	4	11	4	100	5	441	+	+	–	–	25	Deceased
A. baumannii	41	Blood	10	12	4	11	4	100	5	441	+	+	–	–	25	Discharged
A. baumannii	45	ETA	10	12	4	11	4	98	5	231	+	+	–	–	20	Deceased
A. baumannii	12	ETA	12	17	12	1	29	102	39	236	+	+	–	–	35	Deceased
A. baumannii	17	ETA	12	17	12	1	29	102	39	236	+	+	–	–	35	Deceased
A. baumannii	2	ETA	24	92	96	11	49	162	26	499	+	+	–	–	20	Discharged
A. baumannii	6	ETA	24	92	96	11	49	162	26	499	+	+	–	–	25	Deceased
A. baumannii	7	ETA	24	92	96	11	49	162	26	499	+	+	–	–	20	Deceased
A. baumannii	13	ETA	24	92	96	11	49	162	26	499	+	+	–	–	15	Deceased
A. baumannii	15	ETA	24	92	96	11	49	162	26	499	+	+	–	–	15	Deceased
A. baumannii	39	ETA	24	92	96	11	49	162	26	499	+	+	–	–	35	Deceased
A. baumannii	42	Blood	24	92	96	11	49	162	26	499	+	+	–	–	25	Deceased
A. baumannii	50	Swab	24	92	96	11	49	162	26	499	+	+	–	–	20	Deceased
A. baumannii	43	Blood	28	38	45	1	16	66	2	1089	+	–	–	–	25	Deceased
A. baumannii	9	ETA	44	73	No gene	11	44	‡	4	NA	+	+	–	–	40	Deceased
A. baumannii	10	ETA	44	73	No gene	11	44	‡	4	NA	+	+	–	–	20	Discharged

ETA endotracheal aspirate, + positive, – negative

[a] New sequence type (ST13929)

‡ *gpi* 173, 1 difference found. 33T → 33C

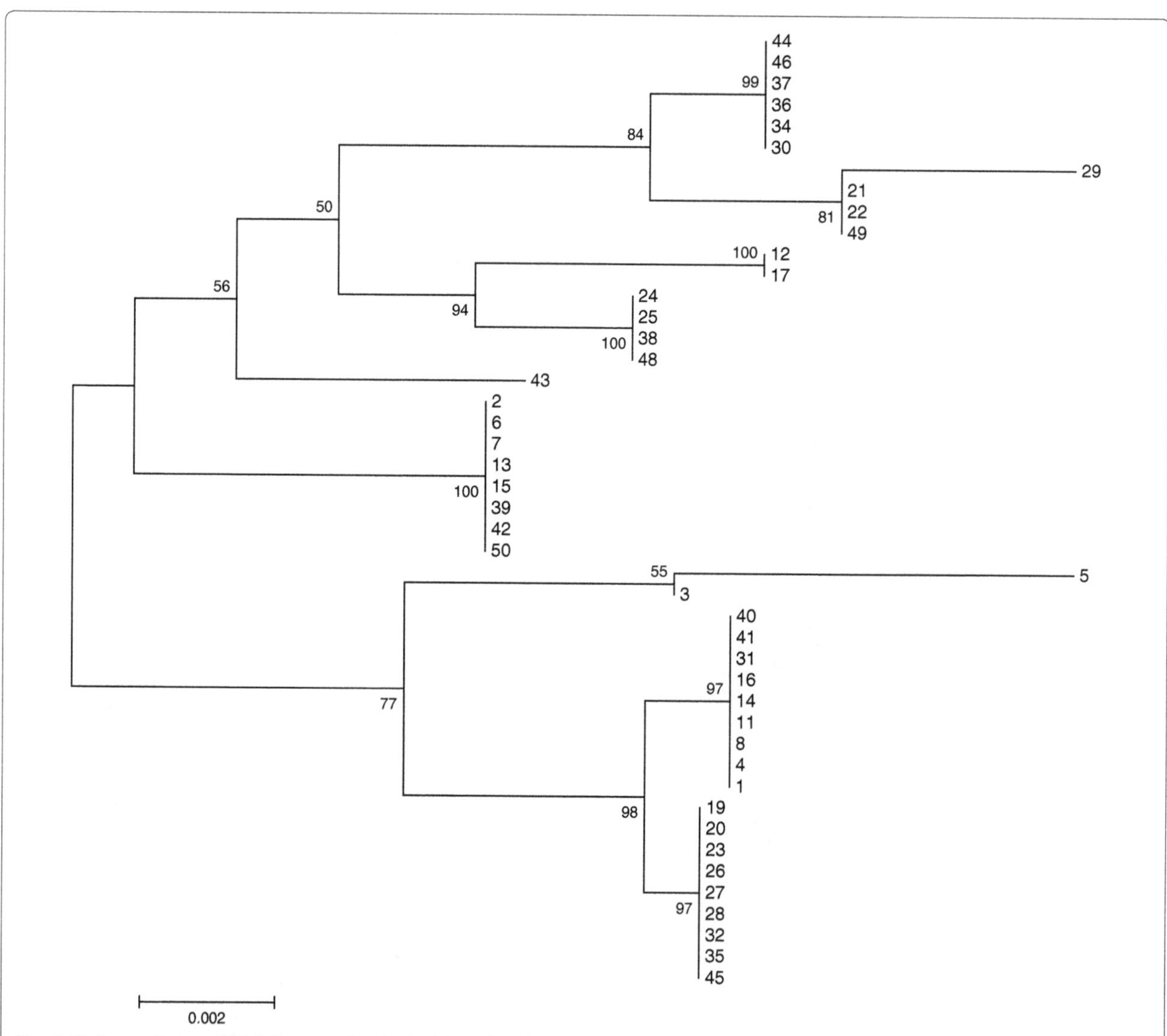

Fig. 2 Phylogenetic tree of 50 *A. baumannii* strains built based on the maximum likelihood algorithm in the MEGA6 software [11] and the concatenated alleles of seven housekeeping genes with bootstrap values. The phylogenetic analysis identified ST195, ST208, ST231, ST441, ST499, and ST723 and the new sequence type ST13929. The numbers in the branches depict the sample ID of *A. baumannii*

localization of numerous β-lactamase genes on plasmids facilitates their horizontal mobilization from one bacterium to another [13, 14].

All our isolates harbored the *bla*$_{OXA-51}$-like gene, which is ubiquitous in *A. baumannii* [15]. *bla*$_{OXA-23}$ was the most universally identified gene, while *bla*$_{OXA-24}$-like and *bla*$_{OXA-58}$-like genes were not detected in any strain. *bla*$_{OXA-23}$ is the most prevalent carbapenemase-encoding gene in the Mediterranean region. This might be explained by the higher carbapenemase activity of *bla*$_{OXA-23}$ and/or acquisition of carbapenem resistance through horizontal gene transfer [16–18]. The *bla*$_{OXA-23}$ gene was either encoded on the chromosome or on plasmids and was associated with four dissimilar genetic structures, with the most common being transposons Tn2006. *bla*$_{OXA-23}$ has been reported in different regions of the Middle East, The United Arab Emirates, Algeria, Libya, Bahrain, and recently, Qatar [16, 19].

Mugnier et al. found an isolate from Egypt harboring plasmid containing *bla*$_{OXA-23}$. This finding might indicate the prevalence of the genetic environment of *bla*$_{OXA-23}$ in Egyptian isolates [16]. Moreover, a recent study including three Egyptian hospitals revealed the emergence and spread of *bla*$_{NDM-1}$ and *bla*$_{OXA-23}$ in addition to the co-occurrence of 16S rRNA methylase *armA* with *bla*$_{NDM-1}$ and *bla*$_{OXA-23}$ in 27 distinct sequence types, 11 of which were novel among *A. baumannii* clinical isolates [20].

Per MLST results, ST195, ST208, ST231, ST441, ST499, and ST723 were the most prevalent isolates. Another Egyptian study illustrated the large diversity found within the strains where ten distinct sequence types (STs) were identified, ST408–ST414, ST331, ST108, and ST208 [21]. However, a study showed that the most prevalent sequence types in the gulf area were ST195, ST208, ST229, ST436, ST450, ST452, and ST499 [22].

Taking into consideration that ST208 is the ancestor strain of several STs including ST89, ST88, ST190, ST225, and ST75, it has been identified in different parts of the world such as Japan, China, Thailand, Korea, Italy, Australia, Portugal, and the Czech Republic [23].

In conclusion, MDR *A. baumannii* strains harboring the $bla_{OXA\ 23}$-like gene were widely circulating in our ICU. MLST provided us with a powerful tool for identifying and epidemiologically typing our strains. Studying the epidemiology of HAIs is urgent to prevent the clonal dissemination of antibiotic-resistant pathogens, not only in hospital settings, but in the community, as well. Strict infection control measures and antimicrobial stewardship programs are necessary to contain the worldwide spread of MDR *A. baumannii.* Proving the clonal relation between clinical isolates emphasizes the importance of surveillance programs and strict IC measures that would influence decision-making and health policy.

Authors' contributions

DG, and MA conceived and designed the study, carried out the collection of the bacterial strains, participated in antibiotic sensitivity and molecular genetic studies. DG drafted the manuscript. MZ participated in antibiotic sensitivity, and MHA. EA and RB carried out the MLST and participated in the design of the study. OA participated in the antimicrobial sensitivity testing and multiplex PCR. All authors read and approved the final manuscript.

Author details

[1] Department of Clinical and Chemical Pathology, Faculty of Medicine, Cairo University, Cairo, Egypt. [2] Department of Microbiology and Immunology, Faculty of Pharmacy, Ahram Canadian University, Giza, Egypt. [3] Department of Pharmaceutics, College of Pharmacy, King Saud University, PO box 2457, Riyadh 11451, Saudi Arabia. [4] Department of Microbiology and Immunology, Faculty of Pharmacy, Al-Azhar University, Cairo, Egypt. [5] National Center for Biotechnology, King Abdulaziz City for Science and Technology, Riyadh, Saudi Arabia. [6] Department of Microbiology, Faculty of Science, Zagazig University, Zagazig, Egypt.

Acknowledgements

The authors extend their appreciation to the Deanship of Scientific Research at King Saud University for funding the study through research group project no. RGP-038.

Competing interests

The authors declare that they have no competing interests.

Ethics approval

Ethical Committee of faculty of medicine, Cairo University approved the study and a written informed consent was not obtained from patients because the bacterial isolates studied were collected from the routine work of microbiology laboratory for patient care and no additional clinical specimens were collected for the study. It is a standard practice not to get written informed consent for use of bacterial isolates unlinked to patient identity from the routine clinical laboratory.

References

1. Ghaith DM, Hassan RM, Hasanin AM. Rapid identification of nosocomial *A. baumannii* isolated from a surgical intensive care unit in Egypt. Ann Saudi Med. 2015;36(5):440–4.
2. Hasanin A, Mukhtar A, El-Adawy A, Elazizi H, Lotfyn A, Nassar H, Ghaith D. Ventilator associated pneumonia caused by extensive-drug resistant *Acinetobacter* species: colistin is the remaining choice. Egypt J Anaesth. 2016. doi:10.1016/j.egja.2016.03.004.
3. Helal S, El Anany M, Ghaith D, Rabeea S. The role of MDR- *A. baumannii* in orthopedic surgical site infections. Surg Infect. 2015. doi:10.1089/sur.2014.187.
4. Poirel L, Nordmann P. Carbapenem resistance in *A. baumannii*: mechanisms and epidemiology. Clin Microbiol Infect. 2006;12:826–36.
5. Higgins PG, Dammhayn C, Hackel M, Seifert H. Global spread of carbapenem resistant *A. baumannii*. J Antimicrob Chemother. 2010;65:233–8.
6. Turton JF, Woodford N, Glover J, Yarde S, Kaufmann ME, Pitt TL. Identification of *A. baumannii* by detection of the bla_{OXA-51}-like carbapenemase gene intrinsic to this species. J Clin Microbiol. 2006;44:2974–6.
7. Clinical and Laboratory Standards Institute. Performance standards for antimicrobial susceptibility testing; twenty-fifth informational supplement. Document M100-S25. Wayne: CLSI; 2015.
8. Magiorakos AP, Srinivasan A, Carey RB, Carmeli Y, Falagas ME, Giske CG, et al. Multidrug-resistant, extensively drug-resistant and pandrug-resistant bacteria: an international expert proposal for interim standard definitions for acquired resistance. Clin Microbiol Infect. 2012;18:268–81.
9. Woodford N, Ellington M, Coelho J, Turton J, Ward M, Brown S, Amyes S, Livermore D. Multiplex PCR for genes encoding prevalent OXA Carbapenemases in *Acinetobacter* spp. Int J Antimicrob Agents. 2006. doi:10.1016/j.ijantimicag.2006.01.004.
10. Alyamani EJ, Khiyami MA, Booq RY, Alnafjan BM, Altammami MA, Bahwerth FS. Molecular characterization of extended-spectrum beta-lactamases (ESBLs) produced by clinical isolates of *Acinetobacter baumannii* in Saudi Arabia. Ann Clin Microbiol Antimicrob. 2015. doi:10.1186/s12941-015-0098-9.
11. Tamura K, Stecher G, Peterson D, Filipski A, Kumar S. MEGA6: molecular evolutionary genetics analysis version 6.0. Mol Biol Evol. 2013. doi:10.1093/molbev/mst197.
12. Hasanin A, Eladawy A, Mohamed H, Salah Y, Lotfy A, Mostafa H, Ghaith D, Mukhtar A. Prevalence of extensively drug-resistant gram negative bacilli in surgical intensive care in Egypt. Pan Afr Med J. 2014. doi:10.11604/pamj.2014.19.177.4307.
13. Higgins PG, Dammhayn C, Hackel M, Seifert H. Global spread of carbapenem-resistant *A. baumannii*. Br Soc Antimicrob Chemother. 2010. doi:10.1093/jac/dkp428.
14. Djahmi N, Dunyach-Remy C, Pantel A, Dekhil M, Sotto A, Lavigne JP. Epidemiology of carbapenemase-producing *Enterobacteriaceae* and *A. baumannii* in Mediterranean countries. Biomed Res Int. 2014. doi:10.1155/2014/305784.

15. Hamouda A, Evans BA, Towner KJ. Amyes SBG. Characterization of epidemiologically unrelated *A. baumannii* isolates from four continents by use of multilocus sequence typing, pulsed-field gel electrophoresis, and sequence-based typing of blaOXA-51-like genes. J Clin Microbiol. 2010;48:2476–83.
16. Mugnier PD, Poirel L, Naas T, Nordmann P. Worldwide dissemination of the blaOXA-23 carbapenemase gene of *Acinetobacter Baumannii*. Emerg Infect Dis. 2009. doi:10.3201/eid1601.090852.
17. Minandri F, D'Arezzo S, Antunes LCS, Pourcel C, Principe L, Petrosillo N, Visca P. Evidence of diversity among epidemiologically related carbapenemase-producing *Acinetobacter Baumannii* strains belonging to international clonal lineage II. J Clin Microbiol. 2011. doi:10.1128/jcm.05555-11.
18. Grosso F, Quinteira S, Peixe L. Understanding the dynamics of imipenem-resistant *A. baumannii* lineages within Portugal. Clin Microbiol Infect Dis. 2011. doi:10.1111/j.1469-0691.2011.03469.x.
19. Rolain JM, Loucif L, Al-Maslamani M, Elmagboul E, Al-Ansari N, Taj-Aldeen S, et al. Emergence of multidrug-resistant *A. baumannii* producing OXA-23 carbapenemase in qatar. New Microbes New Infect. 2016. doi:10.1016/j.nmni.2016.02.006.
20. El-Sayed MAEG, Amin MA, Tawakol WM, Loucif L, Bakour S, Rolain JM. High prevalence of blaNDM-1 carbapenemase-encoding gene and 16S rRNA *armA* methyltransferase gene among *Acinetobacter baumannii* clinical isolates in Egypt. Antimicrob Agents Chemother. 2015. doi:10.1128/AAC.04412-14.
21. Al-Hassan L, El Mehallawy H, Amyes SG. Diversity in *Acinetobacter baumannii* isolates from paediatric cancer patients in Egypt. Clin Microbiol Infect. 2013. doi:10.1111/1469-0691.12143.
22. Zowawi HM, Sartor AL, Sidjabat HE, Balkhy HH, Walsh TR, Al Johani SM, et al. Molecular epidemiology of carbapenem-resistant *Acinetobacter baumannii* isolates in the Gulf Cooperation Council states: dominance of OXA-23-type producers. J Clin Microbiol. 2015. doi:10.1128/JCM.02784-14.
23. Liu F, Zhu Y, Yi Y, Lu N, Zhu B, Hu Y. Comparative genomic analysis of *Acinetobacter baumannii* clinical isolates reveals extensive genomic variation and diverse antibiotic resistance determinants. BMC Genomics. 2014. doi:10.1186/1471-2164-15-1163.

22

Babesiosis in Long Island: review of 62 cases focusing on treatment with azithromycin and atovaquone

Ekaterina A. Kletsova[1*], Eric D. Spitzer[2], Bettina C. Fries[1] and Luis A. Marcos[1,3*]

Abstract

Background: Babesiosis is a potentially life-threatening, tick-borne infection endemic in New York. The purpose of this study was to review recent trends in babesiosis management and outcomes focusing on patients, who were treated with combination of azithromycin and atovaquone.

Methods: A retrospective chart review of patients seen at Stony Brook University Hospital between 2008 and 2014 with peripheral blood smears positive for *Babesia* was performed. Clinical and epidemiological information was recorded and analyzed.

Results: 62 patients had confirmed babesiosis (presence of parasitemia). Forty six patients (74%) were treated exclusively with combination of azithromycin and atovaquone; 40 (87%) of these patients were hospitalized, 11 (28%) were admitted to Intensive Care Unit (ICU), 1 (2%) died. Majority of patients presented febrile with median temperature 38.5 °C. Median peak parasitemia among all patients was 1.3%, and median parasitemia among patients admitted to ICU was 5.0%. Six patients (15%) required exchange transfusion. Majority of patients (98%) improved and were discharged from hospital or clinic.

Conclusion: Symptomatic babesiosis is still rare even in endemic regions. Recommended treatment regimen is well tolerated and effective. Compared to historical controls we observed a lower overall mortality.

Keywords: Babesiosis, Tick-borne, Babesia, Azithromycin, Atovaquone

Background

Tick-bone infections are common in some geographic areas of the United States—mainly northeastern regions particularly in New York, Massachusetts, Rhode Island, and Connecticut [1–5]. Babesiosis is an emerging, usually tick-mediated infection caused by intra-erythrocytic parasites that may also be transmitted by blood transfusions [6].

The severity of Babesiosis ranges from asymptomatic or mild, self-limited febrile illness [5, 7] to potentially life threatening infection and may have a complicated clinical course especially in people with certain risk factors such as those with splenectomy, cancer, human immunodeficiency virus infection (HIV), chronic heart, lung, or live disease, or patients receiving immunosuppressive therapy [8]. A trend of increasing frequency of transfusion mediated babesiosis since the early 2000s was noted in recent studies [6, 9].

The combination of clindamycin and quinine was the first regimen of choice for the treatment of *Babesia microti* infection [8]. A combination of atovaquone and azithromycin is now recommended for mild to moderate disease [10] since it was shown that this combination is as effective as the combination of clindamycin and quinine but is associated with fewer adverse reactions. Clindamycin plus quinine is still recommended for patients with severe babesiosis, including those who require an

*Correspondence: katklevtsova@gmail.com; Luis.marcos@stonybrookmedicine.edu
[1] Department of Medicine, Division of Infectious Diseases, Stony Brook University, Stony Brook, USA
[3] Global Health Institute, Stony Brook University, Stony Brook, NY, USA
Full list of author information is available at the end of the article

exchange transfusion, as these patients were excluded from the azithromycin/atovaquone trial [11].

The purpose of this study was to review demographic, clinical characteristics, and outcomes of patients with proven babesiosis, who were treated with the combination of azithromycin and atovaquone.

Methods

Case definition

Laboratory records were reviewed to identify all adult patients who had a positive peripheral blood smear at Stony Brook University Hospital (SBUH) between 2008 and 2014. All initial positive smears were confirmed to be positive for *B. microti* by PCR analysis performed at the NY State Department of Health. Only symptomatic patients who had at least one positive smear were included in the study. These criteria met the definition of active babesiosis used in the current IDSA guidelines [10].

Study design

A retrospective chart review was performed to gather descriptive clinical and epidemiological information. Only patients who were treated with combination of azithromycin and atovaquone were included into the analysis. Patients' demographic information, past medical history, laboratory values, and outcomes were recorded and analyzed. SAPS II scores were calculated as previously described [12].

Statistical analysis

Microsoft EXCEL was used to record and analyze the data. Proportions were calculated for all categorical variables and medians with interquartile ranges (IQR) were calculated for continuous variables.

Results

Number of cases

Between 2008 and 2014 a total of 62 patients presented to SBUH with active babesiosis confirmed by the presence of parasitemia on a peripheral blood smear. The incidence of babesiosis had trended up over the years from 1 case of an active babesiosis diagnosed in 2008 to 16 cases diagnosed in 2014 (Fig. 1). Fifty-three of the patients (85%) who presented with active babesiosis were admitted to the hospital. Twenty-seven of these patients (44%) were transferred from other hospitals in eastern Long Island with severe babesiosis for potential exchange transfusion; however, only 10 of these patients (38%) ultimately required exchange transfusion based on percent parasitemia and clinical findings.

Treatment and ICU stay

Forty six patients (74%), who presented with active babesiosis, were treated exclusively with combination of atovaquone and azithromycin and were included into the analysis. Forty of the included patients (87%) were admitted to the hospital and 11 of the hospitalized patients (28%) required the intensive care unit (ICU) admission. The decision regarding ICU admission and management at the highest level of care was made based on clinical presentation as well as severity and number of comorbidities that increase risk for potential complication of babesiosis.

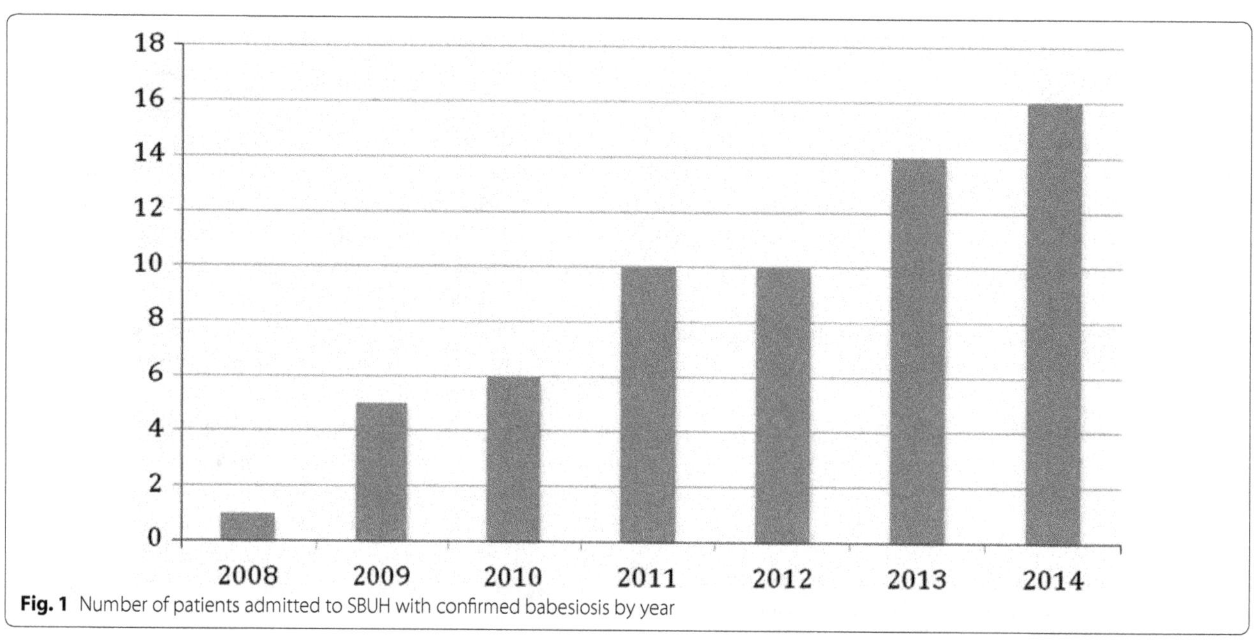

Fig. 1 Number of patients admitted to SBUH with confirmed babesiosis by year

Demographics and comorbidities

The median age of all admitted patients was 64 years (IQR 47–81 years). Twenty six patients (65%) were males (Table 1). Only 5 patients (13%) had a prior splenectomy but 4 (10%) had a history of malignancy, 17 (43%) had hypertension, 9 (23%) had a history of heart disease and some had multiple comorbidities (Table 1).

Table 1 Demographic and clinical characteristics of the patients treated with the combination of azithromycin and atovaquone

Characteristic	All (N = 40)	Admitted to ICU (n = 11)	Not admitted to ICU (n = 29)	P value
Age	64 (47–81)	60 (47–73)	66 (52–80)	0.44
Gender				
Male	26 (65)	8 (73)	18 (62)	0.58
Female	14 (35)	3 (27)	11 (38)	0.72
Race				
White	24 (60)	8 (73)	16 (55)	0.39
African American	0	0	0	
Hispanic	8 (20)	3 (27)	5 (17)	0.74
Asian	1 (3)	0 (0)	1 (3)	
Declined	2 (5)	0 (0)	2 (7)	
Other	5 (13)	0 (0)	5 (17)	
Comorbidities				
Hypertension	17 (43)	6 (55)	11 (38)	0.49
Diabetes mellitus	7 (18)	6 (55)	1 (3)	0.33
Heart disease (CHF/CAD/Arrhythmias)	9 (23)	3 (27)	6 (21)	0.84
Blood disease	2 (5)	0	2 (7)	
Cancer	4 (10)	0	4 (14)	
CKD	3 (8)	1 (9)	2 (7)	
COPD/asthma	6 (15)	2 (18)	4 (14)	0.89
Liver disease	2 (5)	2 (18)	0	
Autoimmune disease	3 (8)	0	3 (10)	
HIV	1 (3)	0	1 (3)	
Splenectomy	5 (13)	1 (9)	4 (14)	
Days in hospital	5 (1–9)	6 (2–11)	5 (1–11)	0.55
Clinical/lab characteristics				
SAPS II score (points)	20 (14–26)	21 (10–32)	20 (14–26)	0.69
Temperature on admission (C)	38.5 (37.2–39.8)	37.2 (35.6–38.8)	38.6 (37.6–39.8)	0.03
Peak parasitemia (%)	1.3 (2.5–5.1)	5.0 (1.5–11.5)	1.1 (1.1–3.3)	0.003
Days of parasitemia (number)	4 (1.75–6.25)	4.5 (1.5–7.5)	4 (1.2–6.8)	0.70
Hemoglobin (g/dL)	10.7 (8.4–13.0)	10.0 (7.9–12.2)	11.1 (8.7–13.5)	0.33
Platelets ($\times 10^3/\mu L$)	74 (8.3–138.8)	64 (1.8–128.8)	74 (8.0–139.0)	0.66
AST (U/L)	79 (13–146)	87 (29–146)	72 (2–142)	0.52
ALT (U/L)	59 (4–114)	63 (1–125)	46 (4–96)	0.33
Total bilirubin (mg/dL)	1.3 (0.8–1.8)	1.5 (0.4–2.6)	1.3 (0.8–1.8)	0.40
LDH (U/L)	605 (231–979)	719 (282–1157)	535 (208–862)	0.12
Haptoglobin (mg/dL)	7.4 (6.7–8.1)	7.2 (1.5–15.9)	7.4 (7.1–7.7)	0.66
Exchange transfusions				
No	34 (85)	6 (55)	28 (97)	0.002
Yes (one)	6 (15)	5 (45)	1 (3)	0.42
Outcome				
Improved and discharged	39 (98)	11 (100)	28 (97)	
Died	1 (2)	0	1 (3)	

Data are presented as median (IQR) or No. (%)

Fever and parasitemia

The median temperature on admission among all patients was 38.5 °C (IQR 37.2–39.8 °C). Interestingly, the median temperature of patient, admitted to the ICU was lower than median body temperature of those, admitted to regular medical floor (Table 1). The median recorded peak parasitemia among all patients was 1.3% and the maximum parasitemia observed was 11%. The median peak parasitemia tended to be significantly higher in patients admitted to the ICU (Table 1). Calculated median SAPS II score for all admitted patient was 20 points (IQR 14–26 points) indicating that patients had an average 4% hospital mortality risk during their admission. The score was not significantly different among the groups.

Laboratory findings

The majority of patients in our sample exhibited anemia (median hemoglobin 10.7 g/dL), thrombocytopenia (median platelets 74 × 10^3/μL), and elevated liver function tests (median alanine aminotransferase (ALT) 59 U/L, median aspartate aminotransferase (AST) 79 U/L, median total bilirubin 1.3 mg/dL). Also, laboratory evidence of hemolysis (median lactate dehydrogenase 605 units/L and median haptoglobin 7.4 mg/dL) was common. Generally, laboratory parameters were more abnormal in patients admitted to the ICU.

Exchange transfusion

Six patients (15%) required an exchange transfusion in addition to antibiotic therapy. Five of these patients were admitted to the ICU. One patient, who had an exchange transfusion started on the floor prior to being admitted to the ICU, developed pulmonary edema followed by cardiac arrest and died on day two of hospitalization.

In general, the combination of atovaquone and azithromycin was well tolerated and effective. All except one patient improved and were discharged from the hospital in stable condition.

Discussion

Our data suggested that incidence of babesiosis is trending up over the years (Fig. 1) in Suffolk county that is consistent with previous studies [5]. We cannot exclude that increased awareness of the infection leading to the increased overall number of tested patients confound these numbers.

This study was performed at a referral center in Long Island, NY, where babesiosis is endemic. Compared to historical controls ([13, 14]; Table 2), fewer patients were transferred to SBUH from other facilities suggesting better understanding of the disease in the medical community. Most of the patients diagnosed with acute symptomatic babesiosis were older adults. This may reflect under-recognition of this infection in younger adults and/or the presence of comorbidities in older adults. Babesiosis may be missed on a routine CBC (complete blood count) and requires a specific order for blood smear examination or other diagnostic tests. In their prospective case-finding and serosurvey study of babesiosis on Block Island, Rhode Island, Krause et al. [5] observed that the number and duration of symptoms due to Babesia infection were similar in people 20–49 years of age versus those older than 50 years of age; however, the latter group was more likely to be hospitalized.

The combination of atovaquone and azithromycin is now widely used for the treatment of patients presenting with babesiosis. The randomized study by Krause et al. [11] that demonstrated the effectiveness of atovaquone plus azithromycin specifically excluded patients with evidence of life-threatening babesiosis (e.g. encephalopathy, shock, congestive heart failure, pulmonary edema, DIC, or renal) or those who required exchange transfusion or assisted ventilation [11]. The current IDSA Guidelines contain an AIII recommendation for quinine plus clindamycin along with red blood cells (RBC) exchange transfusion for patients with severe babesiosis, defined as high grade parasitemia (≥10%), significant hemolysis, or renal, hepatic, or pulmonary compromise. All patients in our report had a disease severe enough to be hospitalized and to be admitted to the ICU, therefore our retrospective study suggests that atovaquone plus azithromycin is often effective for patients with moderate to severe babesiosis, many of whom may be admitted to ICUs because of associated comorbidities. Perhaps good supportive care and exchange transfusions, when indicated, together with antibiotics play more crucial role in patients' outcomes than antiparasitic medications alone.

Compared to historical controls we observed a lower mortality—2 vs. 6.5% from the study of 139 hospitalized patients with babesiosis ([13]; Table 2) and 2 vs. 8.8% from the study of 34 hospitalized patients with babesiosis ([14]; Table 2).

Even though our report is focused on babesiosis patients treated with combination of azithromycin and atovaquone, it is noteworthy to discuss those patients, who were treated otherwise. Two pregnant patients

Table 2 Comparison to other studies

	SBUH, 62 cases review	UAlbany 139 cases review	SBUH 34 cases review
Methods	Chart review of patients with positive smears from 2008 to 2014	Hospital records of babesiosis in NYS for 11 years (1982–1993) Classified to have mild or severe (death, >2 weeks in hospital, ICU admission)	Records of SBUH and VA[a] hospitalized patients for 13 years with positive blood smears Controls with FUO[b], negative blood smears, matched by age and sex
Transferred from other hospital	27 (44%)	NA	30 (88%)
Median age (years)	64	66	46
Mean hospital stay (days)	9.6	11.7	12.7
ICU admission	20 (38%)	35 (25.2%)	–
Splenectomy	9 (15%)	16 (11.5%)	11 (32%)
Mean hemoglobin (g/dL)	10.6	11.3	10
Mean platelets ($\times 10^3/\mu L$)	86	102	92
Mean LDH (U/L)	742	572	–
Mean ALT (U/L)	66	–	99
Mean AST (U/L)	85	–	121
Mean parasitemia (%)	3.4%	–	7.4%
Mean peak parasitemia (%)	4.4%	–	7.6%
Max parasitemia	25%	–	30%
Mean days of parasitemia	6	–	8.5
Treatment	Clindamycin 15 (24%) Quinine 13 (21%) Azithromycin 59 (95%) Atovaquone 59 (95%)	Clindamycin 110 (79%) Quinine 106 (76%)	Clindamycin 33 (97.1%) Quinine 28 (82.3%) Azithromycin 2 (5.9%) Atovaquone 15 (44%)
Exchange transfusions	12 (19%)	6 (4.3%)	7 (20.6%)
Died	1 (2%)	9 (6.5%)	3 (8.8%)
Associations	High-grade parasitemia and: Malignancy Splenectomy LDH AST Total bilirubin	Severe disease and: Cardiac disease/murmur Splenectomy Alkaline phosphatase WBC Higher parasitemia	Complicated babesiosis and: Hemoglobin <10 g/dL Higher parasitemia

For the purpose of a comparison, all patients from SBUH with positive blood smear were included in this table regardless of antimicrobials that were used for babesiosis therapy (n = 62)

[a] VA–Veteran Affairs Hospital

[b] FUO–Fever of Unknown Origin

were treated solely with clindamycin and quinine and 11 patients received all four antibiotics (clindamycin, quinine, azithromycin, and atovaquone), however not simultaneously (Table 3). Only 2 out of 62 patients with confirmed babesiosis did not respond to azithromycin/atovaquone combination (patient 1 and patient 5 in Table 1) suggesting that this regimen may be a reasonable initial therapy even in patients with a severe babesiosis. Even though two more patient were switched from azithromycin atovaquone to quinine/clindamycin (patients 2 and 3 in Table 3), the decision was made based on percent parasitemia on admission, but not on clinical failure of initial regimen.

Potential limitations

First, as the infection is rare and sample size is small, some associations may remain undetected. Second, due to retrospective nature of the study, patients' past medical history may be not complete and additional risk factors for severe babesiosis may be overlooked. Third, effectiveness of azithromycin/atovaquone therapy was also retrospectively assessed and there was no control group in our study. However, no clinical trials are available at this time to compare azithromycin/atovaquone regimen to clindamycin/quinine regimen in patients with severe babesiosis.

Table 3 Patients treated with clindamycin and quinine in addition to azithromycin and atovaquone

Patient	Initial therapy	Changes	Admitted to ICU	ID involved
1	Azithromycin/atovaquone	Changed to clindamycin/quinine on day #5 due to poor clinical response	Yes	Yes
2	Azithromycin/atovaquone	Changed to clindamycin/quinine on day #2 due to high % parasitemia on admission → changed back to azithromycin/atovaquone on day #4 due to QT prolongation	Yes	Yes
3	Azithromycin/atovaquone	Initial therapy at outside hospital; started on clindamycin/quinine on admission to SBUH	No	No
4	Clindamycin/quinine	Changed to azithromycin/atovaquone on day #2 per ID recommendations	Yes	Yes
5	Azithromycin/atovaquone	Initial therapy started at the outside hospital → patient developed respiratory failure, intubated, changed to clindamycin/quinine, and transferred to SBUH	Yes	No
6	Clindamycin/quinine	Initial therapy was changed to azithromycin/atovaquone on day #1 per ID recommendations	Yes	Yes
7	Clindamycin/quinine	ID recommended to change regimen to azithromycin/atovaquone on day #2, however antibiotics were changed to azithromycin/clindamycin per primary team due to lack of IV formulation of atovaquone → therapy changed to azithromycin/atovaquone on day #7	Yes	Yes
8	Clindamycin/quinine	Therapy changed to azithromycin/atovaquone on day #6	No	No
9	Clindamycin/quinine	Therapy changed to azithromycin/atovaquone on day #3	No	Yes
10	Clindamycin/quinine/azithromycin	Azithromycin discontinued on day #5 → changed to azithromycin/atovaquone on day #17 due to hypoglycemia. Patient with prolonged parasitemia	Yes	Yes
11	Clindamycin/Quinine/Atovaquone	Atovaquone discontinued on day #2 → regimen changed to azithromycin/atovaquone on day #3	Yes	Yes

ID infectious diseases

Conclusion

In conclusion, our data indicate that symptomatic babesiosis is uncommon even in endemic regions. Furthermore, these data suggest that recommended treatment regimens for babesia infections are well tolerated and effective even in patients with severe babesiosis.

Authors' contributions

EAK, EDS, BCF and LAM designed the study. EAK wrote the first draft of the manuscript. EAK and LAM perform statistical analysis. EAK, BCF, EDS and LAM reviewed and edited the final manuscript. All authors read and approved the final manuscript.

Authors' information

LAM is a Clinical Professor of Medicine in the Division of Infectious Diseases at Stony Brook University whose research interest is in tick-borne diseases.

Author details

[1] Department of Medicine, Division of Infectious Diseases, Stony Brook University, Stony Brook, USA. [2] Department of Pathology, Stony Brook University, Stony Brook, NY, USA. [3] Global Health Institute, Stony Brook University, Stony Brook, NY, USA.

Acknowledgements

Not applicable.

Competing interests

The authors declare that they have no competing interests.

Funding

Dr. Fries is supported by the NIH R21 AI114259.

References

1. Rodgers SE, Mather TN. Human *Babesia microti* incidence and ixodes scapularis distribution, Rhode Island, 1998–2004. Emerg Infect Dis. 2007;13:633–5.
2. Kogut SJ, Thill CD, Prusinski MA, Lee J-H, Backenson PB, Coleman JL, et al. *Babesia microti* upstate New York. Emerg Infect Dis. 2005;11:476–8.
3. Krause PJ, Telford SR III, Ryan R, Hurta AB, Kwasnik I, Luger S, et al. Geographical and temporal distribution of babesial infection in connecticut. J Clin Microbiol. 1991;29:1–4.
4. Smith RP Jr, Elias SP, Borelli TJ, Missaghi B, York BJ, Kessler RA, et al. Human Babesiosis, Maine, USA, 1995–2011. Emerg Infect Dise. 2014;20:1727–30.
5. Krause PJ, McKay K, Gadbaw J, Christianson D, Closter L, Lepore T, et al. Increasing health burden of human babesiosis in endemic sites. Am J Trop Med Hyg. 2003;68:431–6.
6. Gubernot DM, Lucey CT, Lee KC, Conley GB, Holness LG, Wise RP. Babesia infection through blood transfusions: reports received by the US Food and Drug Administration, 1997–2007. Clin Infect Dis. 2009;48:25–30.

7. Ruebush TK II, Juranek DD, Chisholm ES, Snow PC, Healy R, Sulzer AJ. Human babesiosis on Nantucket Island: evidence for self-limited and subclinical infections. New Engl J Med. 1977;297:825–7.
8. Vannier E, Krause PJ. Human babesiosis. New Engl J Med. 2012;366:2397–407.
9. Herwaldt BL, Linden JV, Bosserman E, et al. Transfusion-associated babesiosis in the United States: a description of cases. Ann Intern Med. 2011;155:509–20.
10. Wormser GP, Dattwyler RJ, Shapiro ED, Halperin JJ, Steere AC, Klempner MS, et al. The clinical assessment, treatment, and prevention of Lyme disease, human granulocytic anaplasmosis, and babesiosis: clinical practice guidelines by the infectious diseases society of America. Clin Infect Dis. 2006;43:1089–134.
11. Krause PJ, Lepore T, Sikand VK, Gadbaw J Jr, Burke G, Telford SR III, et al. Atovaquone and azithromycin for the treatment of babesiosis. New Engl J Med. 2000;343:1454–8.
12. Le Gall JR, Lemeshow S, Saulnier F. A new simplified acute physiology score (SAPS II) based on a European/North American multicenter study. JAMA. 1993;270:2957–63.
13. White DJ, Talarico J, Chang H-G, Birkhead GS, Heimberger T, Morse DL. Human babesiosis in New York State: review of 139 hospitalized cases and analysis of prognostic factors. Arc Intern Med. 1998;158:2149–54.
14. Hatcher JC, Greenberg PD, Antique J, Jimenez-Lucho VE. Severe babesiosis in Long Island: review of 34 cases and their complications. Clin Infect Dis. 2001;32:1117–25.

23

Prevalence of *Chlamydia trachomatis*, *Neisseria gonorrhoeae*, *Mycoplasma genitalium* and *Ureaplasma urealyticum* infections using a novel isothermal simultaneous RNA amplification testing method in infertile males

Ling Qing[1], Qi-Xiang Song[2], Jian-Li Feng[3], Hai-Yan Li[1], Guiming Liu[4] and Hai-Hong Jiang[1*]

Abstract

Background: The purpose of this study was to evaluate the prevalence of *Chlamydia trachomatis*, *Neisseria gonorrhoeae*, *Mycoplasma genitalium* and *Ureaplasma urealyticum* infections in infertile men that consulted our outpatient departments using a novel simultaneous amplification testing (SAT) that is RNA-detection based. The possible impact of *C. trachomatis*, *N. gonorrhoeae*, *M. genitalium* and *U. urealyticum* infections on semen parameters was also noted in the present study.

Methods: A total of 2607 males that were diagnosed with infertility were included in this study. *C. trachomatis*, *N. gonorrhoeae*, *M. genitalium* and *U. urealyticum* infections were detected in the urine samples using SAT method. Related data, including semen parameters and age as well as *C. trachomatis*, *N. gonorrhoeae*, *M. genitalium* and *U. urealyticum* infections were collected and analyzed.

Results: A total of 51 and 1418 urine samples were found positive for *M. genitalium* RNA and *U. urealyticum* RNA, respectively, while the prevalence of *C. trachomatis* and *N. gonorrhoeae* was relatively lower. Men with positive *M. genitalium* RNA and *U. urealyticum* RNA had higher sperm DNA fragmentation index (DFI) while the comparisons of other semen parameters yielded nonsignificant results between the RNA positive and negative group. A multivariate linear regression analysis revealed that *U. urealyticum* and *M. genitalium* infections posed significant factors of DFI (adjusted $R^2 = 46.2\%$).

Conclusions: Our study suggested a relative high prevalence of *U. urealyticum* and *M. genitalium* infection based on this novel SAT detection method. *U. urealyticum* and *M. genitalium* infection could possibly impair male fertility potential through promoting sperm DNA damage.

Keywords: Simultaneous amplification testing, *Chlamydia trachomatis*, *Neisseria gonorrhoeae*, *Mycoplasma genitalium*, *Ureaplasma urealyticum*, Male infertility, Sperm DNA fragmentation index

Background

Male infertility is a world health problem affecting about 10–15% of couples, which accounts for half of the infertile cases [1]. The cause of male infertility has been multidimensional, in which the role of genitourinary tract infections has been the focus in contemporary medicine. The major genitourinary tract infections include *Chlamydia trachomatis*, *Neisseria gonorrhoeae*, mycoplasma species (*Mycoplasma genitalium* and *Mycoplasma hominis*), ureaplasma species (*Ureaplasma urealyticum* and *Ureaplasma parvum*) and *Treponema pallidum*. The

*Correspondence: jianghh.md@foxmail.com
[1] Departments of Reproductive Medicine, Urology, and Nursing, The First Affiliated Hospital of Wenzhou Medical University, #2-4P07 Nan Bai Xiang, Ouhai, Wenzhou 325000, Zhejiang, China
Full list of author information is available at the end of the article

exact mechanisms that genitourinary pathogens affecting male fertility potential remains unknown. The inflammatory processes triggered by genitourinary pathogens can lead to deterioration of spermatogenesis and seminal tract obstruction. The apoptosis process associated with inflammatory conditions could possibly result in the impaired semen parameters, although the relationship between the infections and semen parameters are still under debate [2].

The diagnosis of genitourinary pathogens have been based on bacterial culture, which are time consuming and fail to show adequate sensitivity. Recently, the diagnosis methods based on nucleic acid amplification methods have been widely applied in clinic, being feasible and having relative high sensitivity and specificity [3]. The first voided urine specimen has been proven be just as accurate as a urethral swab in the detection of *C. trachomatis* and *N. gonorrhoeae* [4]. Notably, a novel simultaneous amplification testing method (SAT) based on isothermal amplification of pathogens RNA has been reported providing accurate and rapid detection of several pathogens [5, 6]. To the best of our knowledge, there is no data available published regarding the prevalence of *C. trachomatis, N. gonorrhoeae, M. genitalium* and *U. urealyticum* in infertile men using this novel SAT method. Therefore, in the present study, we aimed to observe the prevalence of *C. trachomatis, N. gonorrhoeae, M. genitalium* and *U. urealyticum* in 2607 urine samples based on SAT methods of infertile men included, and to investigate the association between genitourinary infections and semen parameters. This study helps to define the diagnostic role of genitourinary infections in the assessment of male fertility potential.

Methods

Study population

The present multicentre study involved following medical centers: the First Affiliated Hospital of Wenzhou Medical University, Changhai Hospital, the 324 Hospital of PLA while the data was summarized and analyzed in the Case Western Reserve University and the First Affiliated Hospital of Wenzhou Medical University. From February 2016 to June 2016, we recruited males complained of infertility diagnosed with having had no pregnancies in the past of unprotected intercourse with their partners for more than 1 year that attended the outpatient department of the participated centers. All patients underwent semen analysis, semen chromatin structure assay (SCSA) analysis and *C. trachomatis, N. gonorrhoeae, M. genitalium* and *U. urealyticum* test using urine samples with SAT method. The exclusion criteria were male with reproductive system abnormalities, hormonal abnormalities, varicocele, heavy use of smoking or alcohol, exposure to physical or chemical agents with known negative reproductive effects, other causes of infertility that has been medical proven, advanced female partner age $\geq$38 years, detected female causes of infertility with medical evidence. Participants were also asked to confirm that they did not have any genitourinary symptoms such as pain, micturition, urethral discharge or dysuria.

Semen analyses

Routine semen analyses were conducted by one examer according to the 4th edition of World Health Organization (WHO) laboratory manual for the examination and processing of human semen. Sperm parameters including seminal value, concentration, progressive (PR%) motility (a + b%) and normal sperm morphology were collected for further analyses. Azoospermia was defined as the absence of spermatozoa, oligospermia as the sperm concentration <20 $\times$ 10^6/ml, asthenospermia as PR% <40%, teratospermia as normal morphology of spermatozoa <15%.

Semen chromatin structure assay (SCSA)

Semen chromatin structure assay was performed by one examer using flow cytometry SCSA methods described previously [7]. Briefly, the acid induced sperm nuclear DNA denaturation, the semen samples were processed with acridine orange staining. Acridine orange binds to the fragmented sperm DNA that fluoresces red while the double-strand DNA fluoresces green. The SCSA parameters are calculated based on the red/(red + green) fluorescence intensity. The SCSA parameters included DFI as the percentage of the denatured sperm DNA that fluoresces red and high DNA stainability (HDS) as the percentage of sperm with abnormally high DNA statinability.

C. trachomatis, N. gonorrhoeae, M. genitalium and *U. urealyticum* detection in urine samples in infertile men using SAT methods

The presence of genitourinary pathogen was carried out in urine specimens. The presence of *C. trachomatis, N. gonorrhoeae, M. genitalium* and *U. urealyticum* 16S rRNA in urine samples of infertile males, which has highly conserved sequence, were detected using SAT methods, according to the methods of the manufacture (Shanghai Rendu biotechnology Co., Ltd). Briefly, the genitourinary pathogen 16S rRNA were isolated from the sample and reverse transcribed to generate cDNA fragment. The specific 16S rRNA sense primer and anti-sense primer contains T7 promoter sequence, and is used for RNA fragment amplification. The probe sequence was labeled with 6-carboxyfluorescein (FAM) at the 5′ end and with quencher 4-[4-(dimethylamino) phenylazo] benzoic acid *N*-succinimidylester (DABCYL) at the 3′ end. Real-time PCR was performed in a real-time PCR system (Applied Biosystems Inc., Foster City, CA, USA).

Statistical analyses

One-way Kolmogorov–Smirnov was used to test the normal distribution. Continuous variables were presented as mean ± standard deviation (SD) and compared by independent sample t test. The Chi square test or Fisher's exact Chi square was used to for categorical variables; quantitative data non-normally distributed were presented as median (interquartile range) and compared using non-parametric test. Multivariate linear regression with likelihood ratio test was used to observe the significant predictors of DFI.

Results

Prevalence of *C. trachomatis, N. gonorrhoeae, M. genitalium* and *U. urealyticum* infection in infertile males

A total of 2607 urine samples of infertile males were collected and analyzed in the present study. A relative high prevalence of *U. urealyticum* was found in the detected urine samples (1418/2607, 54.5%). A total of 27 patients were positive for *C. trachomatis* (27/2607, 1.0%), 51 patients were positive for *M. genitalium* (51/2607, 2.0%), 6 patients were positive for *N. gonorrhoeae* (6/2607, 0.2%). Mix infection, defined as more than one pathogen infection, was also common in the detected samples (148/2607, 5.9%). A total of 957 samples were found negative for *C. trachomatis, N. gonorrhoeae, M. genitalium* or *U. urealyticum* infections (Table 1).

C. trachomatis, N. gonorrhoeae, M. genitalium and *U. urealyticum* infection and semen parameters

The comparisons in terms of semen concentration, seminal volume, PR%, normal morphology, DFI, HDS were conducted between the pathogens positive and negative group, which were demonstrated in Table 2. The patients in *M. genitalium* positive group tended to have higher DFI% than that in *M. genitalium* negative cases (25.29 ± 15.70 versus 19.01 ± 12.80, $p = 0.03$). *U. urealyticum* positive subjects had about 10% higher DFI than *U. urealyticum* negative subjects (30.30 ± 16.90 versus 20.09 ± 10.56, $p = 0.02$). However, we failed to identify this significant differences between *C. trachomatis* positive and *C. trachomatis negative* groups, either between *N. gonorrhoeae* positive and *N. gonorrhoeae* negative groups. The mean values of seminal volume, sperm concentration, PR%, normal morphology and HDS were neither related to the detection of *C. trachomatis* RNA nor to those of *N. gonorrhoeae* or *U. urealyticum* and *M. genitalium* RNA in the detected specimens.

The distribution of *C. trachomatis, N. gonorrhoeae, M. genitalium* and *U. urealyticum* positive cases in azoospermia versus non-azoospermia cases, oligospermia versus non-oligospermia, asthenospermia versus asthenospermia and teratospermia versus teratospermia cases were also analyzed. 2 semen specimens (2/27, 7.4%) were azoospermic in the 27 cases that were *C. trachomatis* positive while it was 11 (11/27, 40.7%), 17/27 (63.0%), 15/27 (55.6%) for oligospermia, asthenospermia and teratospermia cases, respectively. Neither *C. trachomatis* nor *N. gonorrhoeae, M. genitalium* or *U. urealyticum* positive was found to be related with azoospermia, oligospermia, asthenospermia or teratospermia in the current study (Table 3).

C. trachomatis, N. gonorrhoeae, M. genitalium and *U. urealyticum* infection and DFI elevation

DFI was the only semen parameter that correlated with pathogen infection in the current study. Hence, all parameters were introduced into multivariate linear regression analysis in the prediction of DFI. The results indicated that *U. urealyticum* and *M. genitalium* infections accounted for 46.2% of the variability in the prediction of DFI: *U. urealyticum* positive, $p = 0.023$; *M. genitalium* positive, $p = 0.030$ (Table 4).

Table 1 Prevalence of CT/MG/NG/UU *C. trachomatis, N. gonorrhoeae, M. genitalium* and *U. urealyticum* in detected urine samples

	n	%
Uninfected	957	36.7
CT *C. trachomatis* only	27	1.0
MG *M. genitalium* only	51	2.0
NG *N. gonorrhoeae* only	6	0.23
UU *U. urealyticum* only	1418	54.5
Mixed infection	148	5.68

Discussion

Male genitourinary tract infections has always been the focus of debate in the era of male infertility. It is also estimated that approximately 15% of male infertility is related to genital tract infection [8]. *C. trachomatis, N. gonorrhoeae, M. genitalium* and *U. urealyticum* are common genitourinary tract pathogens and are widely studied in the current literature. It is also difficult to identify these infections due to their being clinically silent nature, the possibility of contamination with other organisms and the culture difficulty [9].

In our study, *C. trachomatis, N. gonorrhoeae, M. genitalium* and *U. urealyticum* infection was detected in 1.0, 2.0, 0.2 and 54.5% of infertile men, respectively. Huang et al. found that *U. urealyticum* and *M. genitalium*

Table 2 Comparisons of semen parameters between *C. trachomatis*, *N. gonorrhoeae*, *M. genitalium* and *U. urealyticum* CT, NG, MG, UU positive and negative subjects

	Sperm concentration ($\times 10^6$/ml)	Semen volume (ml)	PR (%)	Normal morphology (%)	DFI (%)	HDS (%)
CT *C. trachomatis*						
Positive	55.70 ± 30.80	3.18 ± 1.40	29.00 ± 19.10	9.13 ± 4.58	25.90 ± 14.45	10.15 ± 8.70
Negative	61.08 ± 40.67	3.42 ± 1.41	29.67 ± 18.78	11.45 ± 5.90	21.61 ± 10.50	12.19 ± 7.10
MG *M. genitalium*						
Positive	57.10 ± 41.40	3.51 ± 1.30	30.08 ± 18.01	12.10 ± 4.48	25.29 ± 15.70	11.65 ± 5.79
Negative	59.65 ± 41.90	3.09 ± 1.60	25.89 ± 19.01	10.10 ± 5.45	17.01 ± 12.80	15.57 ± 4.40
NG *N. gonorrhoeae*						
Positive	67.80 ± 30.90	3.78 ± 1.60	30.53 ± 17.20	15.67 ± 5.78	20.19 ± 15.67	15.00 ± 9.00
Negative	55.08 ± 30.61	3.50 ± 1.39	28.54 ± 18.34	11.45 ± 6.89	20.10 ± 15.09	13.43 ± 9.61
UU *U. urealyticum*						
Positive	50.50 ± 34.89	3.89 ± 1.21	21.90 ± 21.43	12.78 ± 6.89	30.30 ± 16.90	17.68 ± 6.05
Negative	56.90 ± 34.54	3.80 ± 1.30	21.29 ± 21.45	13.45 ± 6.89	20.09 ± 10.56	14.46 ± 5.01

Table 3 The distribution of CT, NG, MG, UU positive cases in semen specimens

	Azoospermia		Oligospermia		Asthenospermia		Teratospermia	
	Yes (106)	No (2445)	Yes (1230)	No (1377)	Yes (1507)	No (1100)	Yes (1310)	No (1297)
C. trachomatis CT-positive (n = 27)	2 (1.88%)	25 (1.02%)	11 (0.89%)	16 (1.16%)	17 (1.13%)	10 (0.91%)	15 (1.15%)	12 (0.93%)
M. genitalium MG-positive (n = 51)	2 (1.88%)	49 (2.00%)	24 (1.95%)	27 (1.96%)	31 (2.06%)	20 (1.82%)	27 (2.06%)	24 (1.85%)
N. gonorrhoeae NG-positive (n = 51)	0 (0%)	6 (0.24%)	3 (0.24%)	3 (0.22%)	3 (0.20%)	3 (0.27%)	3 (0.23%)	3 (0.23%)
U. urealyticum UU-positive (n = 1418)	56 (52.8%)	1362 (55.7%)	679 (50.7%)	816 (54.1%)	816 (54.1%)	602 (54.7%)	702 (53.6%)	716 (55.2%)

Table 4 Multivariate linear regression analysis of DFI and HDS prediction

DFI%	Partial regression coefficient	SE	p	HDS%	Partial regression coefficient	SE	p
Constant	20.50	9.60	0.100		18.29	8.23	0.340
Age	0.15	2.30	0.850		0.10	0.56	0.340
UU *U. urealyticum*							
U. urealyticum UU-negative	Reference						
U. urealyticum UU-positive	8.56	5.18	0.023		−6.23	10.35	0.42
MG *M. genitalium*							
M. genitalium MG-negative	Reference						
M. genitalium MG-positive	6.26	2.45	0.030		2.20	9.35	0.59

infections were found in 19.6 and 2.5% in infertile males, respectively [10]. *C. trachomatis* prevalence showed a wide variance, with reported rates of 0.4–42.3% in asymptomatic males in infertile couples [11]. *N. gonorrhoeae* was less evaluated in the current literature when compared to *C. trachomatis*, *M. genitalium* and *U. urealyticum*. In another study, *N. gonorrhoeae* was detected in 6.5% of infertile men, compared with 0% of fertile men [12]. These ambiguous results on the prevalence of detected pathogens can, at least partly, be the effect of differential diagnostic criteria and detection methods applied in different studies.

The consequences of genitourinary infections in the era of male fertility are still underdetermined, as well as the impact on semen parameters and sperm fertilizing capacity in the field of assisted reproductive medicine. Some studies failed to find any correlation between *C. trachomatis* infection and semen alternations [13, 14], while others reported a decrease in seminal volume, sperm concentration, motility and morphology [15–17] with *C. trachomatis* infections. Additionally, The semen quality impairments induced by *N. gonorrhoeae* and *M. genitalium* were not fully clarified in the field, with some studies reported a detrimental effect of genital pathogens on male fertility potential, while others reported altered alternation in semen parameters [2]. The heterogeneity in the male infertility diagnostic criteria and genital pathogens detection methods in different studies can partially interpret these ambiguous results. On the other hand, the effect of the presence of genital pathogens in semen on assisted reproductive technology consequences was also not fully clarified. Barbeyrac et al. found in a prospective study with 277 couples involved that the clinical pregnancy rate was comparable between the presence and absence of *C. trachomatis* infection biomarker [18]. However, in another prospective observational study, patients with *C. trachomatis* serology positive results had significant lower cumulative pregnancy rate than that in patients with *C. trachomatis* serology negative results in non-IVF treatments [19].

In our study cohort, more than half of the infertile males (54.5%) was found to have *U. urealyticum* infection. *U. urealyticum* is a natural inhabitant of the male urethra [20], while the role of *U. urealyticum* infections in male infertility pathogenesis are not fully determined. *U. urealyticum* infections has been implicated as the causative pathogen of urethritis, prostatitis and epididymitis [20]. Some researches failed to identify any correlation between *U. urealyticum* presence and semen alternations [11, 21], while others have reported a impairment on semen concentration [22], motility and morphology [11, 23]. *U. urealyticum* might have deleterious effect on sperm DNA integrity, leading to an impairment of embryo development. Sperm DNA integrity was assessed by DFI, known as sperm DNA fragmentation index, are now arising increasing attention for its diagnostic capabilities of male fertility potential and pregnancy outcome [24, 25]. *U. urealyticum* infections was found to induce sperm DNA damage and seminal reactive oxygen species and thus involved in male infertility pathogenesis in one study [26]. *U. urealyticum* was also found to cause sperm DNA denaturation both in vivo and in vitro, thus impairing embryonic development [27]. The rationality of *U. urealyticum* screening before ART cycles has also been fully acknowledged. Montagut et al. noted a significant reduction in the pregnancy rate in the *U. urealyticum* infected group [28], while there were another study reporting similar fertilization rate and pregnancy rate between the absence and presence of *U. urealyticum* in semen, although a higher abortion rate in the *U. urealyticum* positive was observed [29]. Notably, the possible influence of other detected genital pathogens infections on sperm DNA integrity had been noted in limited studies. Gallegos et al. found patients with *C. trachomatis* and *M. genitalium* infections have increased DFI and have DFI decreased from antibiotic therapy that aiming to control *C. trachomatis* and *M. genitalium* infections [30]. In our male infertility cohort, we found the routine semen parameters, including semen concentration, PR% and morphology remained unaltered regardless of *C. trachomatis, N. gonorrhoeae, M. genitalium* and *U. urealyticum* infections. However, *U. urealyticum* and *M. genitalium* infections was associated with the increase of DFI in the present study, indicating the male infertility potential impairments caused by genitourinary pathogens could possibly be mediated by a hazard impact on sperm DNA integrity.

Nucleic acid amplification tests (NAATs) has proven to provide the sensitivity, specificity and ease of specimen transport than that of any other tests available in the diagnosis of chlamydial and gonococcal infections, which was noted in the recommendations for *C. trachomatis* and *N. gonorrhoeae* detection issued by US Centers for Disease Control (CDC) and prevention [31]. Additionally, the detection progress based on RNA detection, including transcription-mediated amplification (TMA) and SAT methods has gained arising attention. TMA assay in *C. trachomatis* detection had higher sensitivity observed compared to that in DNA-based PCR detection assay [32]. This advantage of this approach is the presence of multiple copies of 16S rRNA per cell, leading to a possible higher sensitivity in comparison of PCR assays that is DNA-based that target single-copy genes. This TMA assay has proven to be the optimal methods in *M. genitalium* detection, facilitating a sensitive, specific and throughput test for MG detection [33].

Traditional methods of screening for genitourinary pathogens, like urethral swabs, are usually embarrassing and invasive, while noninvasive methods are clearly preferred by patients. Using RNA-based SAT testing method for *C. trachomatis* screening, the urine-based screening had a sensitivity and specificity 87.7 and 99.4%, respectively, which is nearly identical to those samples obtained from urethral swab (sensitivity 95.9%, specificity 99.4%) from a evidence-based medicine view [4], suggesting this urine-based noninvasive screening to be a potential alternative to invasive methods. On the other hand, the urine samples for and genitourinary pathogens detection, had been demonstrated a high concordance with semen specimens, with concordance 100% observed for *C. trachomatis, M. genitalium* and 85% for *U. urealyticum* detection [12]. The study of Gdoura et al. have also demonstrated a high concordance between semen and urine specimens for the detection of *C. trachomatis, U. urealyticum* and *M. genitalium* detection [11]. These data shed valuable light on the utility potential of urine specimens for the detection of genitourinary pathogens using SAT method, while offers a high concordance compared with semen specimens, thus facilitating the interpretation of the possible effect of these detected pathogens on semen quality and male infertility.

Several limitations should paid attention to our study. First, this is retrospective cohort study with no fertile males as "control" group included, which resulted in limited statistical power as well as provided limited information concerning the impact of *C. trachomatis, N. gonorrhoeae, M. genitalium* and *U. urealyticum* infections on male fertility potential. *U. urealyticum* and *M. genitalium* was found in 6.5 and 0.65% of the fertile males, respectively [10]. *U. urealyticum* and *M. genitalium* was found to cause sperm DFI elevation in the current study, this no "control" design makes the interpretation of the results less convincing for the prevalence of these pathogens in "control" fertile males was not detected. Second, the present study failed to compare the clinical performance in terms of prevalence, sensitivity and specificity of this novel SAT method and other existing detection method, such as bacterial culture and DNA-based assay, therefore more studies comparing this SAT and other assay are needed to uncover the advantage and disadvantage of this novel SAT method.

Despite these limitations, there are some advantages of our study that should take consideration. First, this was a cohort study with relatively large sample size (2607 cases) that evaluated *C. trachomatis, N. gonorrhoeae, M. genitalium* and *U. urealyticum* infections in infertile males and association with semen parameters. Second, to the best of our knowledge and belief, this was the first report regarding this novel SAT method using urine samples in the diagnose of genitourinary pathogens, thus providing the first hand evidence of the possible clinical utility of this SAT method. Third, the present study shed valuable light on the possibility that *M. genitalium* and *U. urealyticum* infections could cause sperm DNA damage other than impairing routine sperm parameters, thus providing the evidential proof that male genitourinary pathogens could impair male fertility potential, and this effect was possibly DFI mediated.

Conclusions

In conclusion, using this novel SAT method, we detected a relative high prevalence of *M. genitalium* and *U. urealyticum* infections in urine samples of a infertile men cohort. Our findings indicated that *M. genitalium* and *U. urealyticum* infections could impair sperm DNA integrity, thus was likely to cause male infertility.

Authors' contributions

LQ, QXS and JLF designed the project; HYL, GL and HHJ collected and analyzed the data; QL and HHJ wrote the manuscript. All authors read and approved the final manuscript.

Author details

[1] Departments of Reproductive Medicine, Urology, and Nursing, The First Affiliated Hospital of Wenzhou Medical University, #2-4P07 Nan Bai Xiang, Ouhai, Wenzhou 325000, Zhejiang, China. [2] Department of Urology, Changhai Hospital, Shanghai 200433, China. [3] Department of Urology, The 324 Hospital of PLA, Chongqing 400020, China. [4] Department of Surgery/Urology, MetroHealth Medical Center, Case Western Reserve University, Cleveland, OH 44109, USA.

Acknowledgements

Thanks are given to the patients enrolled in this study.

Competing interests

The authors declare that they have no competing interests.

Consent for publication

We have obtained consent to publish from the participant to report individual patient data.

Funding

The study was supported by the National Natural Science Foundation of China (Nos. 81670695 and 81500579) and cstc2012jjA10147 and China-America Promotion Society for Medical Doctor (CapsMD).

References

1. Gnoth C, Godehardt E, Frank-Herrmann P, Friol K, Tigges J, Freundl G. Definition and prevalence of subfertility and infertility. Hum Reprod (Oxford, England). 2005;20(5):1144–7.
2. Gimenes F, Souza RP, Bento JC, Teixeira JJ, Maria-Engler SS, Bonini MG, et al. Male infertility: a public health issue caused by sexually transmitted pathogens. Nat Rev Urol. 2014;11(12):672–87.
3. Lanjouw E, Ouburg S, de Vries HJ, Stary A, Radcliffe K, Unemo M. 2015 European guideline on the management of *Chlamydia trachomatis* infections. Int J STD AIDS. 2016;27(5):333–48.
4. Cook RL, Hutchison SL, Ostergaard L, Braithwaite RS, Ness RB. Systematic review: noninvasive testing for *Chlamydia trachomatis* and *Neisseria gonorrhoeae*. Ann Intern Med. 2005;142(11):914–25.
5. Fan L, Zhang Q, Cheng L, Liu Z, Ji X, Cui Z, et al. Clinical diagnostic performance of the simultaneous amplification and testing methods for detection of the *Mycobacterium tuberculosis* complex for smear-negative or sputum-scarce pulmonary tuberculosis in China. Chin Med J. 2014;127(10):1863–7.
6. Chen Q, Hu Z, Zhang Q, Yu M. Development and evaluation of a real-time method for testing human enteroviruses and coxsackievirus A16. Diagn Microbiol Infect Dis. 2016;85(1):36–41.
7. Evenson DP. Sperm chromatin structure assay (SCSA(R)). Methods Mol Biol (Clifton, NJ). 2013;927:147–64.
8. Keck C, Gerber-Schafer C, Clad A, Wilhelm C, Breckwoldt M. Seminal tract infections: impact on male fertility and treatment options. Hum Reprod Update. 1998;4(6):891–903.
9. Purvis K, Christiansen E. Male infertility: current concepts. Ann Med. 1992;24(4):259–72.

10. Huang C, Zhu HL, Xu KR, Wang SY, Fan LQ, Zhu WB. Mycoplasma and ureaplasma infection and male infertility: a systematic review and meta-analysis. Andrology. 2015;3(5):809–16.
11. Gdoura R, Kchaou W, Ammar-Keskes L, Chakroun N, Sellemi A, Znazen A, et al. Assessment of *Chlamydia trachomatis*, *Ureaplasma urealyticum*, *Ureaplasma parvum*, *Mycoplasma hominis*, and *Mycoplasma genitalium* in semen and first void urine specimens of asymptomatic male partners of infertile couples. J Androl. 2008;29(2):198–206.
12. Abusarah EA, Awwad ZM, Charvalos E, Shehabi AA. Molecular detection of potential sexually transmitted pathogens in semen and urine specimens of infertile and fertile males. Diagn Microbiol Infect Dis. 2013;77(4):283–6.
13. Vigil P, Morales P, Tapia A, Riquelme R, Salgado AM. Chlamydia trachomatis infection in male partners of infertile couples: incidence and sperm function. Andrologia. 2002;34(3):155–61.
14. Habermann B, Krause W. Altered sperm function or sperm antibodies are not associated with chlamydial antibodies in infertile men with leucocytospermia. J Eur Acad Dermatol Venereol JEADV. 1999;12(1):25–9.
15. Veznik Z, Pospisil L, Svecova D, Zajicova A, Unzeitig V. Chlamydiae in the ejaculate: their influence on the quality and morphology of sperm. Acta Obstet Gynecol Scand. 2004;83(7):656–60.
16. Senior K. Chlamydia: a much underestimated STI. Lancet Infect Dis. 2012;12(7):517–8.
17. Al-Mously N, Cross NA, Eley A, Pacey AA. Real-time polymerase chain reaction shows that density centrifugation does not always remove *Chlamydia trachomatis* from human semen. Fertil Steril. 2009;92(5):1606–15.
18. de Barbeyrac B, Papaxanthos-Roche A, Mathieu C, Germain C, Brun JL, Gachet M, et al. Chlamydia trachomatis in subfertile couples undergoing an in vitro fertilization program: a prospective study. Eur J Obstet Gynecol Reprod Biol. 2006;129(1):46–53.
19. Keltz MD, Sauerbrun-Cutler MT, Durante MS, Moshier E, Stein DE, Gonzales E. Positive *Chlamydia trachomatis* serology result in women seeking care for infertility is a negative prognosticator for intrauterine pregnancy. Sex Transm Dis. 2013;40(11):842–5.
20. Volgmann T, Ohlinger R, Panzig B. Ureaplasma urealyticum-harmless commensal or underestimated enemy of human reproduction? A review. Arch Gynecol Obstet. 2005;273(3):133–9.
21. Andrade-Rocha FT. *Ureaplasma urealyticum* and *Mycoplasma hominis* in men attending for routine semen analysis. Prevalence, incidence by age and clinical settings, influence on sperm characteristics, relationship with the leukocyte count and clinical value. Urol Int. 2003;71(4):377–81.
22. Zeighami H, Peerayeh SN, Yazdi RS, Sorouri R. Prevalence of *Ureaplasma urealyticum* and *Ureaplasma parvum* in semen of infertile and healthy men. Int J STD AIDS. 2009;20(6):387–90.
23. Xu C, Sun GF, Zhu YF, Wang YF. The correlation of *Ureaplasma urealyticum* infection with infertility. Andrologia. 1997;29(4):219–26.
24. Shamsi MB, Kumar R, Dada R. Evaluation of nuclear DNA damage in human spermatozoa in men opting for assisted reproduction. Indian J Med Res. 2008;127(2):115–23.
25. Agarwal A, Allamaneni SS. The effect of sperm DNA damage on assisted reproduction outcomes. A review. Minerva Ginecol. 2004;56(3):235–45.
26. Zhang Q, Xiao Y, Zhuang W, Cheng B, Zheng L, Cai Y, et al. Effects of biovar I and biovar II of *Ureaplasma urealyticum* on sperm parameters, lipid peroxidation, and deoxyribonucleic acid damage in male infertility. Urology. 2014;84(1):87–92.
27. Reichart M, Kahane I, Bartoov B. In vivo and in vitro impairment of human and ram sperm nuclear chromatin integrity by sexually transmitted *Ureaplasma urealyticum* infection. Biol Reprod. 2000;63(4):1041–8.
28. Montagut JM, Lepretre S, Degoy J, Rousseau M. Ureaplasma in semen and IVF. Hum Reprod (Oxford, England). 1991;6(5):727–9.
29. Kanakas N, Mantzavinos T, Boufidou F, Koumentakou I, Creatsas G. Ureaplasma urealyticum in semen: is there any effect on in vitro fertilization outcome? Fertil Steril. 1999;71(3):523–7.
30. Gallegos G, Ramos B, Santiso R, Goyanes V, Gosalvez J, Fernandez JL. Sperm DNA fragmentation in infertile men with genitourinary infection by *Chlamydia trachomatis* and *Mycoplasma*. Fertil Steril. 2008;90(2):328–34.
31. Papp JR, Schachter J, Gaydos CA, Van Der Pol B. Recommendations for the laboratory-based detection of *Chlamydia trachomatis* and *Neisseria gonorrhoeae*—2014. MMWR Recomm Rep. 2014;63(Rr-02):1–19.
32. Moller JK, Pedersen LN, Persson K. Comparison of Gen-probe transcription-mediated amplification, Abbott PCR, and Roche PCR assays for detection of wild-type and mutant plasmid strains of *Chlamydia trachomatis* in Sweden. J Clin Microbiol. 2008;46(12):3892–5.
33. Tabrizi SN, Costa AM, Su J, Lowe P, Bradshaw CS, Fairley CK, et al. Evaluation of the hologic panther transcription-mediated amplification assay for detection of *Mycoplasma genitalium*. J Clin Microbiol. 2016;54(8):2201–3.

24

Factors associated with *Staphylococcus aureus* nasal carriage and molecular characteristics among the general population at a Medical College Campus in Guangzhou, South China

B. J. Chen[1†], X. Y. Xie[1†], L. J. Ni[1†], X. L. Dai[1], Y. Lu[2], X. Q. Wu[1], H. Y. Li[1], Y. D. Yao[3*] and S. Y. Huang[1*]

Abstract

Background: The nasal cavity is the main colonization site of *Staphylococcus aureus* (*S. aureus*) in human body. Nasal carriage may be a strong risk factor for some serious infection. There was still limited information about the nasal carriage for *S. aureus* in south China.

Methods: Sought to determine the prevalence and molecular characteristics of *S. aureus* nasal carriage, 295 volunteers residing on a medicine campus were investigated and sampled the nasal cavity swab. Selected *S. aureus* isolates were carried through molecular analysis, including pulsed-field gel electrophoresis (PFGE), multilocus sequence analysis, staphylococcal cassette chromosome *mec* (SCC*mec*) and virulence gene detection.

Results: A total of 73 *S. aureus* isolates were recovered from separate subjects (24.7%, 73/295), with one methicillin-resistant *S. aureus* (MRSA) isolate (0.3%, 1/295). Among the 73 isolates, 71 isolates were successfully grouped into 13 pulsotypes by PFGE analysis, with profiles A and L the most prevalent; 12 sequence types (STs) were found among the 23 isolates which had similar drug resistant spectrum. ST59, ST188 and ST1 were the most prevalent, accounting for 17.4, 13.0 and 13.0% of all isolates, respectively. The MRSA isolate presented ST8-SCC*mec* III. 56.5% of isolates carried both the staphylococcal enterotoxin A (*sea*) and enterotoxin B (*seb*) genes. 83.6% of the *S. aureus* isolates were resistant to penicillin, all isolates were susceptible to quinupristin/dalfopristin, levofloxacin, teicoplanin and vancomycin. The most common risk factors for *S. aureus* carriage were being male, age ≤30 years, and nasal cavity cleaning habits.

Conclusions: Colonization by *S. aureus* was greater among male and young age (20–30 years) students and those with irregularity nasal cleaning. The *S. aureus* isolates selected were revealed into various sequence types and pulsotypes, indicating molecular heterogeneity among *S. aureus* isolates from the populations in the medical college in Guangzhou.

Keywords: *Staphylococcus aureus*, Nasal carriage, Antimicrobial susceptibility, Medical population, Molecular characteristics

*Correspondence: yaoyand@mail.sysu.edu.cn; hsongyin@126.com
†B. J. Chen, X. Y. Xie and L. J. Ni contributed equally to this work
[1] Department of Laboratory, Guangdong Provincial Key Laboratory of Malignant Tumor Epigenetics and Gene Regulation, Sun Yat-Sen Memorial Hospital, Sun Yat-Sen University, Guangzhou 510120, China
[3] Breast Tumor Center, Sun Yat-Sen Memorial Hospital, Sun Yat-Sen University, Guangzhou 510120, Guangdong, China
Full list of author information is available at the end of the article

Background

Staphylococcus aureus (*S. aureus*) can cause nosocomial and community-acquired infections in humans. As a medically pathogen, colonization is a strong risk factor and serious threat to human health. Multiple sites of the human body can be the ecological niche of *S. aureus*, but the main colonization site is the anterior nares [1]. The rates of infection in persistent carriers are higher than others [2]. Besides young age and being male, the main factors to colonize strains were the usage of antibiotics, chronic disease and hospitalization [3–5]. *S. aureus* could spread by contacting with a colonized individual [5]. That may be the reason why individuals without any healthcare-associated risk factors [6, 7] could have led to an increased awareness of community-associated methicillin-resistant *S. aureus* (CA-MRSA). Besides, the *S. aureus* that leads to an invasive infection were in distinguishable from carriage isolates previously isolated from the anterior nares by pulsed-field gel electrophoresis [8, 9] in a patient who gave pulmonary infection. The key to understand the transmission potential of *S. aureus* is to unravel the risk factors for carriage of *S. aureus*. Molecular typing of *S. aureus* is helpful for supporting infection control measures, investigating suspected outbreaks, and preventing nosocomial transmission [10, 11]. Nasal carriage rates were different among races. Moreover, the frequency with which *S. aureus* can be detected in the nose if human individuals, was shown to differ among people of different histocompatibility antigen types (HLA) [12, 13]. It still remains unclear whether carriage rates and risk factors among the Chinese populations that typically lived under crowded conditions are in the same range. And date on *S. aureus* nasal carriage among populations that typically gathered under crowded conditions in Guangzhou is very limited. The medical students need to carry through many experiments which relate to microorganism and go on a field trip to a hospital during their undergraduate career, so they are more likely to expose to the *S. aureus*. Therefore, we sought to determine the prevalence and risk factors of *S. aureus* nasal carriage from students, teachers, retirees among community residents at the campus of Zhongshan School of Medicine, Sun Yat-sen University (SYSU), Guangzhou, South China.

Methods

Population and study design

A cross-sectional study was conducted between October 2014 to May 2015, at the campus of Zhongshan School of Medicine, Sun Yat-sen University (SYSU), Guangzhou, South China. All the volunteers from 10 to 76 years old included middle school students, undergraduates, teachers, salesclerks and retirees. The pertinent demographic, medical information and potential factors that are related to *S. aureus* nasal carriage and transmission were collected through a standardized questionnaire. Eleven unqualified surveys whose responses were incomplete were eliminating, 295 nasal swabs were sampled. All volunteers, parents, or guardians signed informed consent documents approving the use of their samples for research purposes, and the study was approved by the Ethics Committee of Sun Yat-Sen Memorial Hospital. [Ethical Approval Number: 【2017】伦备第 (01) 号].

Bacterial strains

Both anterior nares were swabbed by rotating a sterile dry cotton swab 5 times inside the nostril. The samples were immediately stored in Copan eSwab Liquid Amies preservation medium (eSwab Collection and Preservation System, Copan Italia, Brescia, Italy). All swabs were kept at 4 °C, transported at room temperature to the department of bacteriology and processed in 4 h. The swabs were streaked on blood agar plates at 35 °C for 24 h. Gram-positive, β-hemolytic and coagulase positive isolates were confirmed as *S. aureus* using a Vitek® 2 microbial identification system (bioMérieux, Marcy l' Etoile, France) according to the manufacturer's instructions. All *S. aureus* were then cultured on MRSA select chromogenic agar. Presumptive MRSA strains, which grew as green colonies on the chromogenic medium, were confirmed by their resistance to cefoxitin and polymerase chain reaction (PCR) for the *mec*A gene [14].

Antibiotic susceptibility testing

All *S. aureus* isolates were tested for their susceptibility to the following antibiotics: penicillin, erythromycin, clindamycin, cefuroxime, ceftriaxone, cefotaxime, cefoxitin, gentamicin, rifampicin, imipenem, quinupristin/dalfopristin, tetracycline, teicoplanin, vancomycin, trimethoprim/sulfamethoxazole, ciprofloxacin, and levofloxacin. The sensitivity patterns of methicillin-susceptible *S. aureus* (MSSA) and MRSA strains were determined by disk diffusion method according to 25rd informational supplement (M100-S25) which recommended by the Clinical and Laboratory Standards Institute (CLSI; http://clsi.org). The inducible clindamycin resistance was determined by D-test. All disks were obtained from Oxoid Ltd (Oxoid, Basingstoke, England). American type culture collection (ATCC) 25923 *S. aureus* was used as the quality control strain.

Staphylococcal toxin genes detection

The Panton-Valentine leukocidin (*pvl*) and the staphylococcal enterotoxin A (*sea*) and enterotoxin B (*seb*) genes were detected by PCR as previously described [14, 15] (Fig. 1).

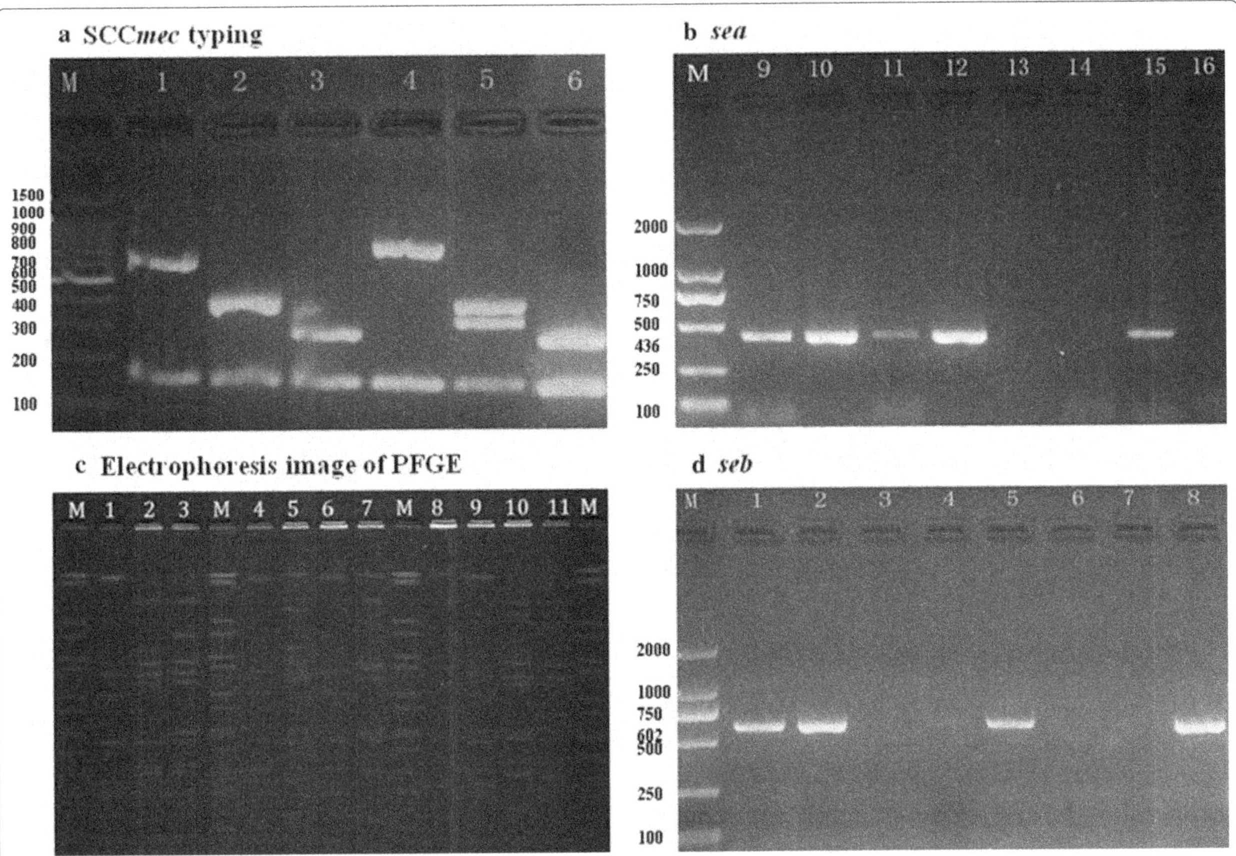

Fig. 1 Detection of SCC*mec* types and virulence factor genes. **a** Multiplex PCR assay identifies SCC*mec* types and subtypes I, II, III, IVa, and V. Simultaneously the *mecA* gene was detected. The following DNA templates were used for PCR (by lane): M, marker; 1–5, Control strains (SCC*mec* type I–V); 6, *S. aureus* strains isolated from the volunteers in the study. **b** PCR assay identifies *sea* gene. The following DNA templates were used for PCR (by lane): M, marker; 9, positive control; 10–16, *S. aureus* strains isolated from the volunteers in the study. **c** Electrophoresis image of Pulsed field gel electrophoresis. The following DNA templates were used for electrophoresis (by lane): M, The positive control strain *Salmonella ser. Braenderup standard strain H9812*; 1–11, *S. aureus* strains isolated from the volunteers in the study. **d** PCR assay identifies *seb* gene. The following DNA templates were used for PCR (by lane): M, marker; 1, positive control; 2–8, *S. aureus* strains isolated from the volunteers in the study

Staphyloccoccal cassette chromosome *mec* (SCC*mec*) typing

Multiplex PCR was performed for SCC*mec* typing of MRSA isolates by using eight unique pairs of primers for SCC*mec* types and subtypes I, II, III, IVa, IVb, IVc, IVd, and V, as described previously [16] (Fig. 1). Positive control strains for SCC*mec* types I (NCTC 10442), II (N315), III (85/2082), and IVa (JCSC 4744), were kindly provided by Dr. Fangyou Yu of the Department of Laboratory Medicine, the First Affiliated Hospital of Wenzhou Medical College.

Multilocus sequence typing (MLST)

MLST was performed using previously described primers and conditions [17], the sequence types (STs) was obtained through the website http://saureus.mlst.net and the clonal complexes (CCs) were defined by analyzing cluster related STs with the eBURST software (http://eburst.mlst.net/v3/enter_data/single). A neighbor-joining tree was constructed from the sequence data using MEGA version 6.06 [11]. STs that grouped together with ≥70% bootstrap support were considered part of the same CC.

Pulsed-field gel electrophoresis (PFGE)

PFGE was performed using *SmaI* as described previously [18] (Fig. 3). The relatedness of the strains were determined according to the criteria of Tenover et al. [19]. The isolates with >75% similarity were clustered in patterns. The dendrograms were generated by analyzing the electrophoretogram with BioNumerics version 5.01 statistical software, according to a simple matching coefficient and the unweighted pair group method with the arithmetic mean (UPGMA) algorithm. The same PFGE patterns were grouped as a pulsotype and assigned alphabetically (A, B, C etc.).

Statistical analysis

Frequencies were obtained and proportions were calculated for categorical variables. The only continuous variable, age, was transformed into a categorical variable using the quartiles of the frequency distribution (≤20, >20–30, >30–50, >50 years). Categorical variables were compared using the Chi square test or the Fisher exact test. Odds ratios (OR), 95% confidence intervals (CI), and *P* values were calculated. A *P* value of ≤0.05 was considered statistically significant. Univariable logistic regression models were applied to determine independent risk factors. Multiple logistic regression analysis was carried out by stepwise backward selection of variables with biological plausibility and a significance level <0.10 for entry into the model. Statistical comparisons were performed with SPSS (PASW Statistics 18) software (IBM, Armonk, NY). All susceptibility data were analyzed using WHONET software, version 5.6.

Results

Nasal colonization with *S. aureus*

A total of 295 volunteers were enrolled onto this study. The median age of the participating volunteers was 30.0 years (range 10–76 years), and 45.8% (135/295) were male. Distributions of *S. aureus* carriers and non-carriers stratified by population characteristics and variables associated with *S. aureus* carriage in the univariate analysis were shown in Table 1. The overall prevalence of *S. aureus* carriage was 24.7% (73/295). The nasal carriage of *S. aureus* was 32.6% (44/135) in males, which is higher than 18.1% (29/160) in females (OR 2.04, 95% CI 1.27–3.79). The difference between nasal carriage in male and female was statistically significant ($P < 0.05$). Highest nasal carriage, 33.1% (41/124) (OR 3.30; 95% CI 1.12–9.75) of *S. aureus* was recorded in the age group of

Table 1 Univariate and multivariate analysis of risk factors associated with *S. aureus* nasal carriage among 295 volunteers at the campus of Zhongshan School of Medicine, Sun Yat-sen University, Guangzhou

Characteristic	The healthy people (n = 295), n (%)		Univariate		Multivariate logistic	
	Carriers (n = 73) n (%)	Non-carriers (n = 222) n (%)	*P* value	OR (95% CI)	*P* value	OR (95% CI)
Sex						
Male	44 (32.6)	91 (67.4)	0.005	2.04 (1.27–3.79)	0.021	2.51 (1.29–3.91)
Female	29 (18.1)	131 (81.9)				
Age, years						
≤20	41 (33.1)	8 (66.9)	<0.001	0.25 (0.11–0.54)	0.01	3.30 (1.12–9.75)
>20–30	18 (26.5)	50 (73.5)	0.021	0.31 (0.11–0.84)	0.041	2.71 (1.15–7.51)
≥30–50	8 (17.0)	39 (83.0)	0.312	0.56 (0.18–1.74)	0.451	1.91 (0.44–4.91)
≥50	6 (10.7)	50 (89.3)		1		1
Antibiotic use in past 1 month						
Yes	4 (20.0)	16 (80.0)	0.612	0.75 (0.24–2.31)		
No	69 (25.1)	206 (74.9)				
Regular contact nasal cavity cleaning						
Yes	13 (13.0)	87 (87.0)	0.001	0.34 (0.17–0.65)	<0.001	0.29 (0.15–0.56)
No	59 (30.4)	135 (69.6)				
Hospitalization in past one year						
Yes	4 (36.4)	7 (63.6)	0.369	1.78 (0.51–6.27)		
No	69 (24.3)	215 (75.7)				
Underlying disease						
Yes	11 (36.7)	19 (63.3)	0.891	1.05 (0.50–2.21)		
No	62 (23.4)	203 (76.6)				
Household member working in Medical Institutions						
Yes	14 (26.4)	39 (73.6)	0.689	1.15 (0.58–2.27)		
No	59 (24.4)	183 (75.6)				

Underlying disease: hypertension, diabetes, chronic rhinitis, urticaria, hyperthyroidism

OR odds ratio, *CI* confidence interval

≤20 years, followed by 26.5% (18/68) (OR 2.71, 95% CI 1.15–7.51), 17.0% (8/47) (OR 1.91, 95% CI 0.44–4.91), and 10.7% (6/56) in the age groups of 20–30 years, 30–50 years and >50 years. There was statistical significant difference ($P < 0.05$) between ages <20 years and 20–30 years. The corresponding rates were 13.0% (13/100) and 30.4% (60/194) (OR 0.34, 95% CI 0.17–0.65) between those who clean their nasal frequently or occasionally, respectively, and there was statistical significant difference ($P < 0.05$). In multiple logistic regression analysis, nasal carriage of *S. aureus* was also significantly associated with male, age ≤20 years, and regular cleaning of the nasal cavity.

Antibiotic susceptibility

Susceptibility pattern of *S. aureus* to various antibiotics is shown in Fig. 2. Among the 73 *S. aureus* isolates, 61 (83.6%) were resistant to penicillin and 32 (43.8%) to erythromycin. The isolate resistant to tetracycline and clindamycin was found in 13 (17.8%) and 10 (13.7%) isolates respectively. Rates of resistance to cefuroxime, ceftriaxone, cefotaxime, cefoxitin, trimethoprim/sulfamethoxazole, gentamicin, rifampicin, and imipenem were <10%. All isolates were susceptible to levofloxacin, quinupristin/dalfopristin, teicoplanin, and vancomycin. Among 73 *S. aureus* isolates, only one isolate (1.4%, 1/73) was resistant to cefoxitin and further confirmed to be MRSA detecting *mec*A gene by PCR screening. It was resistant to penicillin, cefuroxime, ceftriaxone, cefotaxime, erythromycin, clindamycin, tetracycline, and gentamycin. The isolate was separated from a 17-year-old female middle school student, who had be in hospital for some days and taken antithyroid drugs because of thyroid problem in past half a year.

Detection of toxin genes and SCC*mec* typing

Detection of toxin genes and SCC*mec* typing were shown in Fig. 1. Only one isolate was clearly typed harbored SCC*mec* III. Among all the *S. aureus* isolates, 56.5% detected both *sea* and *seb*, 26.1% detected only *sea* and 13.0% detected only *seb*. And the MRSA isolate was only detected *seb*. Seven isolates that detected both *sea* and *seb* were found separated from the students who came from the same class. There was not statistical significant difference ($P > 0.05$) among age, gender and profession in detection of enterotoxin gene. Interestingly, the *pvl* gene was not detected among all the *S. aureus* isolates in this study.

MLST and PFGE typing

Twenty-three *S. aureus* isolates with similar drug-resistant spectrum were revealed 12 different sequence types. Among these, ST59, ST188 and ST1 were the most prevalent, accounting for 17.4% (4/23), 13.0% (3/23) and

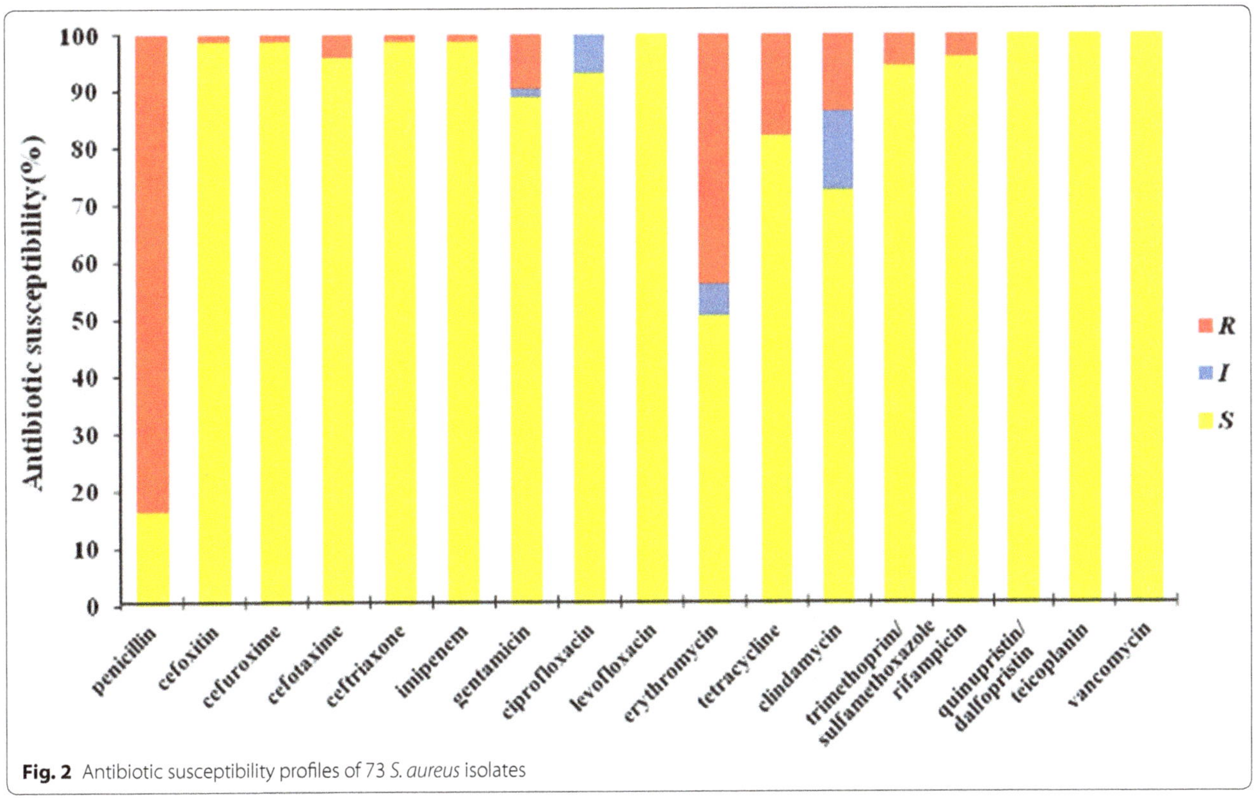

Fig. 2 Antibiotic susceptibility profiles of 73 *S. aureus* isolates

13.0% (3/23), respectively. Other ST types were ST965, ST30, ST6, ST7, ST5, ST8, ST72, ST537 and ST944. With the eBURST software, 10 CCs were identified. The main CC was CC59 (n = 5), followed by CC188 (n = 3), CC1 (n = 3), CC5 (n = 3), CC6 (n = 2), CC7 (n = 2), CC30 (n = 2), CC8 (n = 1), CC72 (n = 1) and CC182 (n = 1). The MRSA isolate was revealed ST8 (Table 2). Of the 73 *S. aureus* isolates collected, 71 isolates consisted of 13 different pulsotypes, while two isolates were untypable. Patterns were classified from A-M, each defining a clone in according with the previously reported interpretive criteria [19]. The most prevalent profiles were A (50.7%, 36/71) and L (18.3%, 13/71), the MRSA isolate belonged to pulsotype C. 69.4% (25/36) of the isolates separated from students were came from the same class in profiles A, and 84.6% (11/13) in profile L (Fig. 3).

Discussion

Staphylococcus aureus nasal carriage is not infrequent in China but few reports on the prevalence and the risk factors of *S. aureus* nasal carriage are found. The findings of this study are of significance to understand *S. aureus* nasal colonization dynamics within the special community, and to design strategies to prevent *S. aureus* infection and dissemination. *S. aureus* nasal carriage is a global phenomenon among healthy population. But detection rate of *S. aureus* nasal carriage is different in different area. The overall prevalence of *S. aureus* carriage was 24.7% in this study. Only one *S. aureus* was founded as MRSA (1.4%). Compared with the general population, this coincides with the recorded prevalence among 2448 healthy people from Beijing and Harbin in Northern China (16.5%), of which 0.3% were MRSA and in adults in community settings in Taiwan (22.1%) [20, 21]. Besides, previous studies revealed a similar nasal carriage rate (15.4–23.1%) and low prevalence of MRSA colonization (3.0–9.4%) in Chinese medical students from different regions. Another study also revealed a similar nasal carriage rate (20%) with no MRSA strains identified in military volunteers from Beijing [22]. In addition, it also coincides to multiple reports of CA-MRSA infections on college and high school campuses, with a concentration of cases occurring among student athletes [23]. But, in contrast, the nasal carriage rate of MRSA colonization

Table 2 Demographic characteristics and molecular features of 23 cases with *S. aureus* carried

Case	Age	Gender	Profession	Resistance profile	*pvl*	*sea/seb*	ST	CC	PFGE
1	20	Female	SCH	PEN, GEN, ERY, TCY, CLI, SXT	–	+/+	59	59	G
2	23	Male	SCH	PEN	–	±	6	6	A
3	22	Male	SCH	PEN, ERY, TCY, CLI	–	±	59	59	G
4	21	Male	SCH	NR.	–	–/+	188	188	A
5	20	Female	SCH	PEN, CTX	–	+/+	965	5	A
6	62	Female	SCH	PEN, ERY	–	+/+	30	30	C
7	23	Female	SOC	PEN	–	+/+	72	72	B
8	70	Female	SOC	PEN, CIP, CLI	–	+/+	1	1	A
9	17	Female	SOC	PEN, FOX, CXM, CTX, CRO, IPM, CIP,GEN, ERY, TCY, CLI	–	–/+	8	8	C
10	65	Female	SOC	PEN	–	–/+	188	188	A
11	62	Female	SOC	PEN	–	–/–	188	188	A
12	53	Male	SCH	PEN, CLI	–	+/+	1	1	A
13	24	Female	SCH	PEN, CLI	–	±	1	1	A
14	13	Female	SCH	GEN, ERY, CLI, SXT	–	+/+	5	5	A
15	14	Male	SCH	ERY	–	±	6	6	A
16	14	Male	SCH	PEN, GEN, ERY	–	±	30	30	C
17	14	Female	SCH	PEN, ERY, TCY, CLI	–	±	59	59	H
18	14	Male	SCH	PEN, GEN, ERY, TCY	–	+/+	965	5	A
19	13	Female	SCH	PEN, GEN, ERY, CLI, SXT	–	+/+	7	7	K
20	14	Male	SCH	NR.	–	+/+	59	59	G
21	13	Female	SCH	ERY	–	+/+	944	182	E
22	14	Male	SCH	NR.	–	+/+	7	7	A
23	14	Male	SCH	NR.	–	+/+	537	59	G

SCH the volunteers who work or study in the college, *SOC* the volunteers who work beside the college, *pvl* Panton-Valentine leukocidin gene, *sea* staphylococcal enterotoxin A gene, *seb* staphylococcal enterotoxin B gene, *ST* sequence type, *CC* clonal complexe, *PFGE* pulsed-field gelelectrophoresis, *PEN* penicillin, *FOX* cefoxitin, *CXM* cefuroxime, *CTX* cefotaxime, *CRO* ceftriaxone, *IPM* imipenem, *TCY* tetracycline, *CIP* ciprofloxacin, *CLI* clindamycin, *ERY* erythromycin, *GEN* gentamicin, *SXT* trimethoprim/sulfamethoxazole, *NR.* the isolate is sensitive to all the antibiotics, – negative, + positive

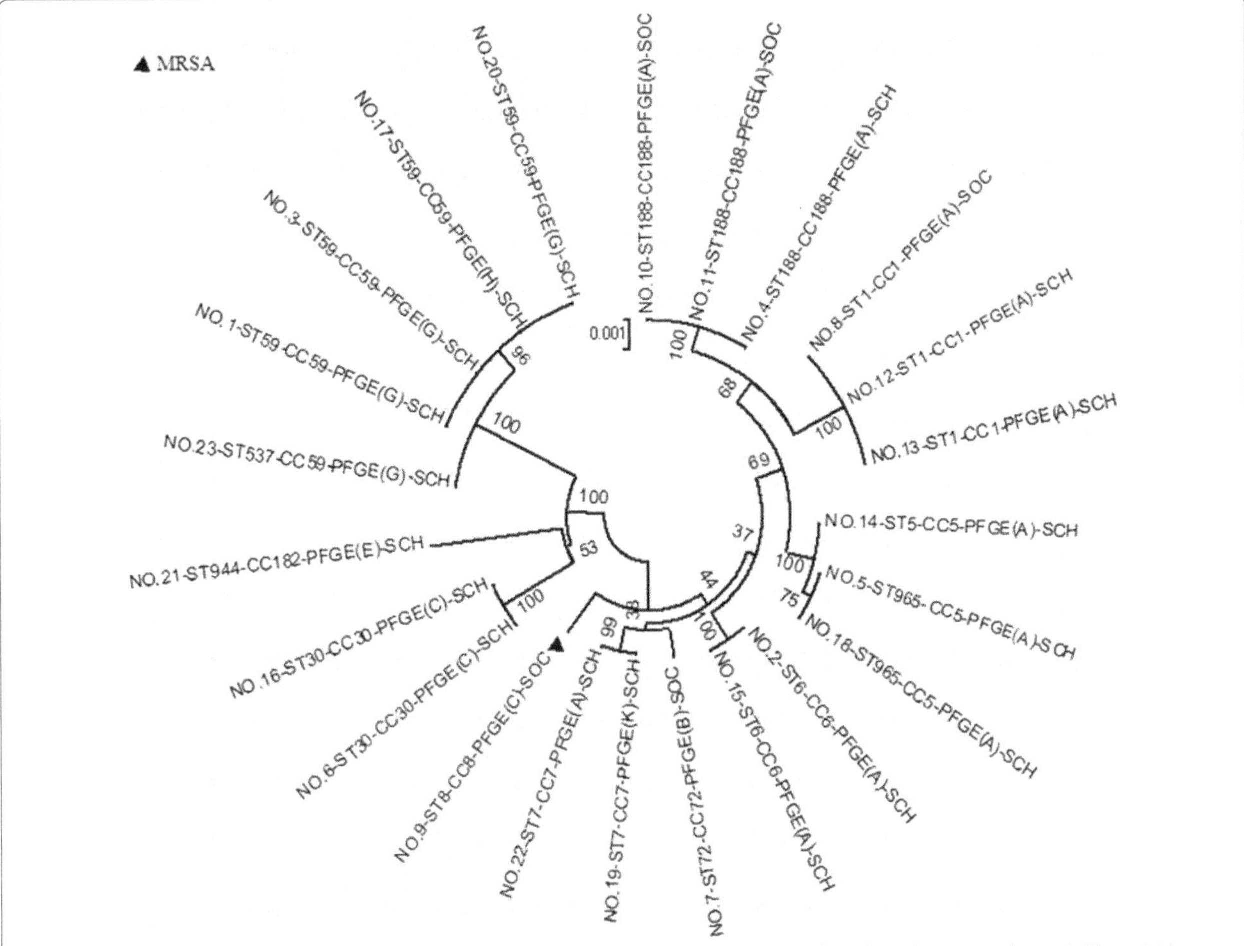

Fig. 3 A neighbour-joining tree reveals phylogenetic relationships of 23 *S. aureus* strains isolated from the volunteers in the study. The neighbor joining tree was based on the concatenated sequences of each of the 23 sequence types noted in the combined dataset, as determined using the *S. aureus* MLST database (http://saureus.mlst.net/) and implemented in MEGA v6.06 using Kimura-2-parameter distances. The relationships shown were based on 1000 re-samplings for bootstrapping. Each clonal complex (CC) is composed of STs that cluster with a ≥70% bootstrap confidence value. Bsides, Bayesian phylogram indicating the evolutionary relationships of *S. aureus* strains analyzed in this study. PFGE, pulsed-field gel electrophoresis; SCH, the volunteers who work or study in the college; SOC, the volunteers who work beside the college

was found to be 11.6% in a cohort of healthy children aged ≤14 years in community settings in Taiwan over a 5-year period [24], which was higher than that in this study. Compared with other nations, the detection rate of *S. aureus* nasal carriage is lower than that in America and Europe (20–30%) [25]. which coincides to the report that the detection rate of MRSA among adults is 1% in Thailand [26], 0.2% in Northern Europe and 3% in Northern America [27], but is lower than 8.6% in Mexico [28]. In addition, the analogous report that the detection rate of *S. aureus* at Wenzhou Medical College in Wenzhou was 15.4%, of which 3.0% were MRSA [29]. Besides, the study from Brasil reported that in a medical student community, the detection rate of *S. aureus* and MRSA were 20.6 and 3.4% [30]. In contrast, the detection rate of *S. aureus* in this study is higher than the analogous report, but the detection rate of MRSA is lower. In conclusion, though the special community living or working in crowded conditions are more likely to expose to *S. aureus* colonization and infection [29], but the nasal carriage detection rate of MRSA is not higher.

Previous studies have found that young age, male sex, chronic sinusitis, nonuse of antibiotics, the length of hospital stay, less education, and drug use were the risk factors associated with *S. aureus* colonization [31, 32]. Yan et al. [20] found that the populations that typically lived under crowded conditions would have higher opportunities for transmission and non-Han Chinese, youth male and chronic disease were the most possibly risk factors of nasal *S. aureus* carriage in healthy population. Higher *S. aureus* carriage rates were also found in men, individuals with obesity and children in Chinese medical college campus [29]. Another study reported that insufficient immunity, crowds or closed contacts, and inactivity was an ideal setting for *S. aureus* [22]. In Taiwan, a study also found that crowded environments, such as living with a greater number of children and attending day care, significantly increased the risk of MRSA colonization [24]. Our study also found that higher *S. aureus* carriage rates were associated with being male, young age and nonstandard nasal cleaning habits. Previous studies have reported that predisposes healthy individuals and transplant recipients to *S. aureus* nasal carriage with *S. aureus* will be affected by the human leukocyte antigen (HLA) DR3 antigen [13, 33]. Thus, gender specific frequencies of HLA haplotypes may lead to differential susceptibilities between male and female. However, HLA DR3 haplotype frequencies among the carriers have not been investigated. Cleaning the nasal cavity with regularity can protect against nasal colonization by *S. aureus* [34]. According to the standardized questionnaire we found that female volunteers were more likely to clean the nasal cavities with regularity, so it may be an important reason why the nasal carriage of *S. aureus* in males was higher than in females. So it was absolutely essential to clean the nasal cavity with regularity among those who were exposed to higher *S. aureus* carriage rates. Unfortunately, we could not find any difference between nasal carriage in the healthy people and the population under chronic disease was statistically significant because the number of the population under chronic disease was too small. It was observed that *pneumococcal* competition at the Youth of life would lead to a negative correlation for the cocolonization of *S. aureus* and *Streptococcus pneumonia* [35]. Besides, the volunteers whose ages ≤20 years were more likely to study together for more than 7 h per day, so they had more closely intimate contact with each other. What's more, compared with adults, they would not clean the nasal cavity with regularity. So it may be the explanation for the phenomenon that higher *S. aureus* carriage rates were associated with young age.

As known, the object of study to MLST was always MRSA but not MSSA. CC5, CC8, CC188, ST398 and CC59 [20, 21, 36, 37] were the major CCs among the *S. aureus* strains separated from both nasal and clinical according to those previous studies from China. But ST7 and CC188 occurred quite a lot in the recent Chinese studies, which indicated that the majority of the MSSA clones observed in China are globally distributed [36, 38]. In this study, 23 *S. aureus* isolates were separated into 12 STs, which belonged to 10 CCs, including 4 major CCs: CC59, CC188, CC1 and CC5, respectively. This coincides with the study to MLST of the *S. aureus* strains separated from nasal among healthy adults in China [20]. And ST59, which belonged to CC59, was the major ST of CA-MRSA in China [36], what's more, the major type of CA-MRSA in Taiwan was ST59-SCC*mec*V (*pvl*-positive), followed by ST59-SCC*mec*IV (*pvl*-negative), but 46–59% MRSA isolates that separated from the nasal of healthy adults belonged to ST59-SCC*mec*IV (*pvl*-negative). Interestingly, the MRSA isolate detected in this study belonged to ST8-SCC*mec*III (*pvl*-negative), which was the endemic genotype of hospital-acquired MRSA (HA-MRSA) but not CA-MRSA in China [39]. This finding lends further support to the notion that HA-MRSA was going to instead of CA-MRSA by nasal carriage transmission because the parasitifer of the MRSA isolates had a history of exposure to a hospital environment.

PFGE electrophoresis could separate large fragments of DNA, so it was recommended as the standard technique for *S. aureus* genotyping, using for pathogen traceability research and the investigation of hospital infection outbreak [40]. In this study, the *S. aureus* isolates separated from the population in the same class had the same PFGE pulsotype, which indicated that the *S. aureus* may spread from carrier to non carrier by nasal.

Panton-Valentine leukocidin [41, 42], encoded by *pvl* gene, was a toxin that lyses leukocytes in a receptor-dependent fashion and associated with skin and soft tissue infection. Previous study showed that the acquisition of a mobile genetic element carrying the genes coding for *pvl* gene was mainly based on the finding that most initially found CA-MRSA clones *pvl*-encoding genes, while HA-MRSA commonly do not [41]. But the role of *pvl* gene in the pathogenesis of CA-MRSA infections, in particular skin infection as the most common manifestation of CA-MRSA disease, is still controversial [43]. Interestingly, the *pvl* gene was not detected among all the *S. aureus* isolates in this study. It coincidesed with the study by Sanchini et al. [44], who collected 18 CA-MRSA strains from all over Italy but only found one of these tested positive for *pvl* gene.

Staphylococcus aureus enterotoxins (SE) are major causes of staphylococcal food poisoning [45]. Staphylococcal enterotoxin A and enterotoxin B genes, which were associated with severe disease such as necrotizing soft tissue infections, were confirmed as the most abundant toxin genes in clinical *S. aureus* isolates from patients and children in China [46, 47]. Previous reports have found that isolates from patients with bacteremia always detected *sea* and *seb* was identified in isolates from sputum samples, and the most abundant toxin genes in clinical *S. aureus* isolates from patients and children in China were *sea* and *seb* [46, 47]. Our recent study have shown that 56.5% CA-MRSA and 61.5% HA-MRSA carried the *sea* gene. However, *seb* gene was only detected in CA-MRSA isolates (52.2%) [48]. Another previous investigation has demonstrated that a significantly higher proportion of *sea* gene-positive isolates came from the community residents compared with the healthcare workers (26.1 vs. 5.6%, $P = 0.024$) [34]. The important finding of the current study was the high rate of detection of the enterotoxin genes in *S. aureus* (56.5% detected both *sea* and *seb*), which indicated that *S. aureus* carriers are at risk of autoinfection.

Broader concerns should be paid on the antimicrobial resistance problems in *S. aureus. S. aureus* strains can differ in their susceptibility profiles [49, 50]. In this study, we found that there was a high rate of resistance against penicillin and erythromycin. The reason might be the excessive use of penicillin and macrolides [49, 50]. Fortunately, most of the isolates remained sensitive to the majority of antibiotics, gentamicin, rifampicin, trimethoprim/sulfamethoxazole, quinupristin/dalfopristin and teicoplanin. Therefore, formulating more strategies for rational use of antibiotics are urgently required.

There are limitations to note about the current work. Most importantly, as a cross-sectional study, to detect variations in colonization patterns, e.g. persistent carriers, intermittent carriers, or non-carriers was unpractical. Secondly, because the number of volunteers is limit, recruitment of subjects from the college may mean that the results are not generalizable to the population of the medicos in Guangzhou as a whole, despite the good cross sections of age and occupation among the test subjects. Thirdly, sampling only the nostrils without including other body parts may underestimate the frequency of MRSA carriage overall [50].

Conclusions

This study showed that being male, young age (20–30 years) and irregularity nasal cleaning are more likely to be colonized by *S. aureus*. The finding lends further evidence of molecular heterogeneity among *S. aureus* isolates from the populations in the medical college in Guangzhou.

Authors' contributions

YDY, SYH and BJC contributed to the design of the study and the writing of the manuscript. XYX, LJN and XLD performed the experiments. YL, XQW and HYL assisted with quantitative data collection and volunteers follow up. All authors read and approved the final manuscript.

Author details

[1] Department of Laboratory, Guangdong Provincial Key Laboratory of Malignant Tumor Epigenetics and Gene Regulation, Sun Yat-Sen Memorial Hospital, Sun Yat-Sen University, Guangzhou 510120, China. [2] Cross Infection Control Office, Sun Yat-Sen Memorial Hospital, Sun Yat-Sen University, Guangzhou 510120, Guangdong, China. [3] Breast Tumor Center, Sun Yat-Sen Memorial Hospital, Sun Yat-Sen University, Guangzhou 510120, Guangdong, China.

Acknowledgements

This work was supported by Grant [2013]163 from Key Laboratory of Malignant Tumor Molecular Mechanism and Translational Medicine of Guangzhou Bureau of Science and Information Technology.

Competing interests

The authors declare that they have no competing interests.

Funding

This work was supported by grants from the National Natural Science Foundation of China (81272897), the Science and Technology Foundation of the Guangdong Province (2014A050503029), and the Sun Yat-sen Initiative Program for Scientific Research (YXQH201701). The funders played no role in the study design, data collection and analysis, decision to publish, or preparation of the manuscript.

References

1. Kluytmans J, van Belkum A, Verbrugh H. Nasal carriage of *Staphylococcus aureus*: epidemiology, underlying mechanisms, and associated risks. Clin Microbiol Rev. 1997;10:505–20.
2. Yu VL, Goetz A, Wagener M, Smith PB, Rihs JD, Hanchett J, Zuravleff JJ. *Staphylococcus aureus* nasal carriage and infection in patients on hemodialysis: efficacy of antibiotic prophylaxis. N Engl J Med. 1986;315:91–6.
3. Young BC, Golubchik T, Batty EM, Fung R, Larner-Svensson H, Votintseva AA, Miller RR, Godwin H, Knox K, Everitt RG, et al. Evolutionary dynamics of *Staphylococcus aureus* during progression from carriage to disease. Proc Natl Acad Sci USA. 2012;109:4550–5.
4. Munckhof WJ, Nimmo GR, Schooneveldt JM, Schlebusch S, Stephens AJ, Williams G, Huygens F, Giffard P. Nasal carriage of *Staphylococcus aureus*, including community-associated methicillin-resistant strains, in Queensland adults. Clin Microbiol Infect. 2009;15:149–55.
5. Salgado CD, Farr BM, Calfee DP. Community-acquired methicillin-resistant *Staphylococcus aureus*: a meta-analysis of prevalence and risk factors. Clin Infect Dis. 2003;36:131–9.
6. Herold BC, Immergluck LC, Maranan MC, Lauderdale DS, Gaskin RE, Boyle-Vavra S, Leitch CD, Daum RS. Community-acquired methicillin-resistant *Staphylococcus aureus* in children with no identified predisposing risk. JAMA. 1998;279:593–8.
7. Centers for Disease Control and Prevention. Four pediatric deaths from community-acquired methicillin-resistant *Staphylococcus aureus*—Minnesota and North Dakota, 1997–1999. MMWR Morb Mortal Wkly Rep. 1999;48:707–10.
8. Wertheim HF, Vos MC, Ott A, van Belkum A, Voss A, Kluytmans JA, van Keulen PH, Vandenbroucke-Grauls CM, Meester MH, Verbrugh HA. Risk and outcome of nosocomial *Staphylococcus aureus* bacteraemia in nasal carriers versus non-carriers. Lancet. 2004;364:703–5.
9. von Eiff C, Becker K, Machka K, Stammer H, Peters G. Nasal carriage as a source of *Staphylococcus aureus* bacteremia, Study Group. N Engl J Med. 2001;344:11–6.
10. Enright MC, Robinson DA, Randle G, Feil EJ, Grundmann H, Spratt BG. The evolutionary history of methicillin-resistant *Staphylococcus aureus* (MRSA). Proc Natl Acad Sci USA. 2002;99:7687–92.
11. Liu Y, Wang H, Du N, Shen E, Chen H, Niu J, Ye H, Chen M. Molecular evidence for spread of two major methicillin-resistant *Staphylococcus aureus* clones with a unique geographic distribution in Chinese hospitals. Antimicrob Agents Chemother. 2009;53:512–8.
12. Noble WC. Carriage of *Staphylococcus aureus* and beta haemolytic streptococci in relation to race. Acta Derm Venereol. 1974;54(5):403–5.
13. Kinsman OS, McKenna R, Noble WC. Association between histocompatability antigens (HLA) and nasal carriage of *Staphylococcus aureus*. J Med Microbiol. 1983;16:215–20.

14. Larsen AR, Stegger M, Sorum M. spa typing directly from a mecA, spa and pvl multiplex PCR assay-a cost-effective improvement for methicillin-resistant *Staphylococcus aureus* surveillance. Clin Microbiol Infect. 2008;14:611–4.
15. Fernandes P, Ferreira BS, Cabral JM. Solvent tolerance in bacteria: role of efflux pumps and cross-resistance with antibiotics. Int J Antimicrob Agents. 2003;22:211–6.
16. Zhang K, McClure JA, Elsayed S, Louie T, Conly JM. Novel multiplex PCR assay for characterization and concomitant subtyping of staphylococcal cassette chromosome mec types I to V in methicillin-resistant *Staphylococcus aureus*. J Clin Microbiol. 2005;43:5026–33.
17. Enright MC, Day NP, Davies CE, Peacock SJ, Spratt BG. Multilocus sequence typing for characterization of methicillin-resistant and methicillin-susceptible clones of *Staphylococcus aureus*. J Clin Microbiol. 2000;38:1008–15.
18. Ben Slama K, Gharsa H, Klibi N, Jouini A, Lozano C, Gomez-Sanz E, Zarazaga M, Boudabous A, Torres C. Nasal carriage of *Staphylococcus aureus* in healthy humans with different levels of contact with animals in Tunisia: genetic lineages, methicillin resistance, and virulence factors. Eur J Clin Microbiol Infect Dis. 2010;30:499–508.
19. Tenover FC, Arbeit RD, Goering RV, Mickelsen PA, Murray BE, Persing DH, Swaminathan B. Interpreting chromosomal DNA restriction patterns produced by pulsed-field gel electrophoresis: criteria for bacterial strain typing. J Clin Microbiol. 1995;33:2233–9.
20. Yan X, Song Y, Yu X, Tao X, Yan J, Luo F, Zhang H, Zhang J, Li Q, He L, et al. Factors associated with *Staphylococcus aureus* nasal carriage among healthy people in Northern China. Clin Microbiol Infect. 2015;21:157–62.
21. Wang JT, Liao CH, Fang CT, Chie WC, Lai MS, Lauderdale TL, Lee WS, Huang JH, Chang SC. Prevalence of and risk factors for colonization by methicillin-resistant *Staphylococcus aureus* among adults in community settings in Taiwan. J Clin Microbiol. 2009;47:2957–63.
22. Qu F, Cui E, Guo T, Li H, Chen S, Liu L, Han W, Bao C, Mao Y, Tang YW. Nasal colonization of and clonal transmission of methicillin-susceptible *Staphylococcus aureus* among Chinese military volunteers. J Clin Microbiol. 2009;48:64–9.
23. Cohen PR. The skin in the gym: a comprehensive review of the cutaneous manifestations of community-acquired methicillin-resistant *Staphylococcus aureus* infection in athletes. Clin Dermatol. 2008;26:16–26.
24. Chen CJ, Hsu KH, Lin TY, Hwang KP, Chen PY, Huang YC. Factors associated with nasal colonization of methicillin-resistant *Staphylococcus aureus* among healthy children in Taiwan. J Clin Microbiol. 2010;49:131–7.
25. Mainous AG 3rd, Hueston WJ, Everett CJ, Diaz VA. Nasal carriage of *Staphylococcus aureus* and methicillin-resistant S aureus in the United States, 2001–2002. Ann Fam Med. 2006;4:132–7.
26. Kitti T, Boonyonying K, Sitthisak S. Prevalence of methicillin-resistant *Staphylococcus aureus* among university students in Thailand. Southeast Asian J Trop Med Public Health. 2012;42:1498–504.
27. Walsh EE, Greene L, Kirshner R. Sustained reduction in methicillin-resistant *Staphylococcus aureus* wound infections after cardiothoracic surgery. Arch Intern Med. 2010;171:68–73.
28. Hamdan-Partida A, Sainz-Espunes T, Bustos-Martinez J. Characterization and persistence of *Staphylococcus aureus* strains isolated from the anterior nares and throats of healthy carriers in a Mexican community. J Clin Microbiol. 2010;48:1701–5.
29. Du J, Chen C, Ding B, Tu J, Qin Z, Parsons C, Salgado C, Cai Q, Song Y, Bao Q, et al. Molecular characterization and antimicrobial susceptibility of nasal *Staphylococcus aureus* isolates from a Chinese medical college campus. PLoS ONE. 2011;6:e27328.
30. Gushiken CY, Medeiros LB, Correia BP, Souza JM, Moris DV, Pereira VC, Giuffrida R, Rodrigues MV. Nasal carriage of resistant *Staphylococcus aureus* in a medical student community. An Acad Bras Cienc. 2016;88:1501–9.
31. Al-Rawahi GN, Schreader AG, Porter SD, Roscoe DL, Gustafson R, Bryce EA. Methicillin-resistant *Staphylococcus aureus* nasal carriage among injection drug users: six years later. J Clin Microbiol. 2008;46:477–9.
32. Graham PL 3rd, Lin SX, Larson EL. A U.S. population-based survey of *Staphylococcus aureus* colonization. Ann Intern Med. 2006;144:318–25.
33. Giarola LB, Dos Santos RR, Bedendo J, da Silva Junior WV, Borelli SD. HLA molecules and nasal carriage of *Staphylococcus aureus* isolated from dialysis and kidney transplant patients at a hospital in Southern Brazil. BMC Res Notes. 2012;5:90.
34. Chen B, Dai X, He B, Pan K, Li H, Liu X, Bao Y, Lao W, Wu X, Yao Y, et al. Differences in *Staphylococcus aureus* nasal carriage and molecular characteristics among community residents and healthcare workers at Sun Yat-Sen University, Guangzhou, Southern China. BMC Infect Dis. 2015;15:303.
35. Bogaert D, van Belkum A, Sluijter M, Luijendijk A, de Groot R, Rumke HC, Verbrugh HA, Hermans PW. Colonisation by Streptococcus pneumoniae and *Staphylococcus aureus* in healthy children. Lancet. 2004;363:1871–2.
36. Chen FJ, Huang IW, Wang CH, Chen PC, Wang HY, Lai JF, Shiau YR, Lauderdale TL. mecA-positive *Staphylococcus aureus* with low-level oxacillin MIC in Taiwan. J Clin Microbiol. 2012;50:1679–83.
37. Zhao C, Liu Y, Zhao M, Yu Y, Chen H, Sun Q, Jiang W, Han S, Xu Y, Chen M, et al. Characterization of community acquired *Staphylococcus aureus* associated with skin and soft tissue infection in Beijing: high prevalence of PVL + ST398. PLoS ONE. 2012;7:e38577.
38. Yu F, Li T, Huang X, Xie J, Xu Y, Tu J, Qin Z, Parsons C, Wang J, Hu L, et al. Virulence gene profiling and molecular characterization of hospital-acquired *Staphylococcus aureus* isolates associated with bloodstream infection. Diagn Microbiol Infect Dis. 2012;74:363–8.
39. Chen H, Liu Y, Jiang X, Chen M, Wang H. Rapid change of methicillin-resistant *Staphylococcus aureus* clones in a Chinese tertiary care hospital over a 15-year period. Antimicrob Agents Chemother. 2010;54:1842–7.
40. Murchan S, Kaufmann ME, Deplano A, de Ryck R, Struelens M, Zinn CE, Fussing V, Salmenlinna S, Vuopio-Varkila J, El Solh N, et al. Harmonization of pulsed-field gel electrophoresis protocols for epidemiological typing of strains of methicillin-resistant *Staphylococcus aureus*: a single approach developed by consensus in 10 European laboratories and its application for tracing the spread of related strains. J Clin Microbiol. 2003;41:1574–85.
41. Tristan A, Bes M, Meugnier H, Lina G, Bozdogan B, Courvalin P, Reverdy ME, Enright MC, Vandenesch F, Etienne J. Global distribution of Panton-Valentine leukocidin–positive methicillin-resistant *Staphylococcus aureus*, 2006. Emerg Infect Dis. 2007;13:594–600.
42. Spaan AN, Henry T, van Rooijen WJ, Perret M, Badiou C, Aerts PC, Kemmink J, de Haas CJ, van Kessel KP, Vandenesch F, et al. The staphylococcal toxin Panton-Valentine Leukocidin targets human C5a receptors. Cell Host Microbe. 2013;13:584–94.
43. Otto M. Community-associated MRSA: what makes them special? Int J Med Microbiol. 2013;303:324–30.
44. Sanchini A, Campanile F, Monaco M, Cafiso V, Rasigade JP, Laurent F, Etienne J, Stefani S, Pantosti A. DNA microarray-based characterisation of Panton-Valentine leukocidin-positive community-acquired methicillin-resistant *Staphylococcus aureus* from Italy. Eur J Clin Microbiol Infect Dis. 2011;30:1399–408.
45. Argudin MA, Mendoza MC, Rodicio MR. Food poisoning and *Staphylococcus aureus* enterotoxins. Toxins (Basel). 2010;2:1751–73.
46. He W, Chen H, Zhao C, Zhang F, Li H, Wang Q, Wang X, Wang H. Population structure and characterisation of *Staphylococcus aureus* from bacteraemia at multiple hospitals in China: association between antimicrobial resistance, toxin genes and genotypes. Int J Antimicrob Agents. 2013;42:211–9.
47. Wu D, Li X, Yang Y, Zheng Y, Wang C, Deng L, Liu L, Li C, Shang Y, Zhao C, et al. Superantigen gene profiles and presence of exfoliative toxin genes in community-acquired meticillin-resistant *Staphylococcus aureus* isolated from Chinese children. J Med Microbiol. 2010;60:35–45.
48. Xie X, Bao Y, Ouyang N, Dai X, Pan K, Chen B, Deng Y, Wu X, Xu F, Li H, et al. Molecular epidemiology and characteristic of virulence gene of community-acquired and hospital-acquired methicillin-resistant *Staphylococcus aureus* isolates in Sun Yat-sen Memorial hospital, Guangzhou, Southern China. BMC Infect Dis. 2016;16:339.
49. Mehndiratta PL, Gur R, Saini S, Bhalla P. *Staphylococcus aureus* phage types and their correlation to antibiotic resistance. Indian J Pathol Microbiol. 2010;53:738–41.
50. Treesirichod A, Hantagool S, Prommalikit O. Nasal carriage and antimicrobial susceptibility of *Staphylococcus aureus* among medical students at the HRH Princess Maha Chakri Sirindhorn Medical Center, Thailand: a cross sectional study. J Infect Public Health. 2013;6:196–201.

25

Antimicrobial susceptibility among Gram-positive and Gram-negative organisms collected from the Latin American region between 2004 and 2015 as part of the Tigecycline Evaluation and Surveillance Trial

Silvio Vega[1*] and Michael J. Dowzicky[2]

Abstract

Background: The in vitro activity of tigecycline and comparator agents was evaluated against Gram-positive and Gram-negative isolates collected in Latin American centers between 2004 and 2015 as part of the Tigecycline Evaluation and Surveillance Trial (T.E.S.T.) global surveillance study.

Methods: Minimum inhibitory concentrations (MICs) were determined using the broth microdilution methodology according to the Clinical and Laboratory Standards Institute (CLSI) guidelines. Antimicrobial susceptibility was determined using CLSI breakpoints, except for tigecycline for which the US Food and Drugs Administration breakpoints were used.

Results: A total of 48.3% (2202/4563) of *Staphylococcus aureus* isolates were methicillin-resistant *S. aureus* (MRSA). All MRSA isolates were susceptible to linezolid and vancomycin, and 99.9% (2199/2202) were susceptible to tigecycline. Among *Streptococcus pneumoniae* isolates, 13.8% (198/1436) were penicillin-resistant; all were susceptible to linezolid and vancomycin, and 98.0% (194/198) were susceptible to tigecycline. Susceptibility was >99.0% for linezolid and tigecycline against *Enterococcus faecium and Enterococcus faecalis* isolates. A total of 40.8% (235/576) *E. faecium* and 1.6% (33/2004) *E. faecalis* isolates were vancomycin-resistant. Among the Enterobacteriaceae, 36.3% (1465/4032) of *Klebsiella pneumoniae* isolates, 16.4% (67/409) of *Klebsiella oxytoca* isolates and 25.4% (1246/4912) of *Escherichia coli* isolates were extended-spectrum β-lactamase (ESBL) producers. Of the ESBL-producing *K. pneumoniae* and *E. coli* isolates, susceptibility was highest to tigecycline [93.4% (1369/1465) and 99.8% (1244/1246), respectively] and meropenem [86.9% (1103/1270) and 97.0% (1070/1103), respectively]. A total of 26.7% (966/3613) of *Pseudomonas aeruginosa* isolates were multidrug-resistant (MDR). Among all *P. aeruginosa* isolates, susceptibility was highest to amikacin [72.8% (2632/3613)]. A total of 70.3% (1654/2354) of *Acinetobacter baumannii* isolates were MDR, and susceptibility was highest to minocycline [88.3% (2079/2354) for all isolates, 86.2% (1426/1654) for MDR isolates]. Tigecycline had the lowest MIC_{90} (2 mg/L) among *A. baumannii* isolates, including MDR isolates.

Conclusions: This study of isolates from Latin America shows that linezolid, vancomycin and tigecycline continue to be active in vitro against important Gram-positive organisms such as MRSA, and that susceptibility rates to meropenem and tigecycline against members of the Enterobacteriaceae, including ESBL-producers, were high. However, we

*Correspondence: silviove@yahoo.com
[1] Complejo Hospitalario Metropolitano, Caja del Seguro Social, Panama City, Panama
Full list of author information is available at the end of the article

report that Latin America has high rates of MRSA, MDR *A. baumannii* and ESBL-producing Enterobacteriaceae which require continued monitoring.

Keywords: Gram-negative, Gram-positive, Latin America, Resistance, Surveillance, Susceptibility, Tigecycline

Background

Resistance among clinically important organisms to antimicrobial agents is severely threatening the repertoire of treatment options for common infections. The challenge is intensified by the fact that several of these organisms are resistant to multiple antimicrobials. Antimicrobial resistance is a global problem, with some regions noted to have higher rates of resistance than others. For example, Latin America is reported to have high rates of extended-spectrum β-lactamase (ESBL) producing Enterobacteriaceae, methicillin-resistant *Staphylococcus aureus* (MRSA), and multidrug-resistant (MDR) *Acinetobacter* spp. [1–4]. Also of concern are carbapenemase-producing *Klebsiella pneumoniae*. There have been many outbreaks in the Latin American region [5], particularly in Panama where there was an outbreak from 2011 to 2013 that was difficult to control [6]. Carbapenemases of the metallo-β-lactamases type, such as NDM-1 and VIM, have also emerged in the region [5, 7]. The lack of effective antibiotics against these multi-resistant strains has resulted in an increased use of colistin, and colistin-resistant strains of Enterobacteriaceae, *Pseudomonas* spp. and *Acinetobacter* spp. are beginning to appear [8].

The Tigecycline Evaluation and Surveillance Trial (T.E.S.T.) is an ongoing global surveillance study that has monitored the in vitro activity of tigecycline and comparator agents since 2004. Tigecycline is a broad-spectrum glycylcycline with activity against Gram-positive and Gram-negative organisms. In this report we examine the activity of tigecycline against Gram-positive and Gram-negative organisms collected from centers across Latin America between 2004 and 2015. Data from isolates collected in Latin America in the earlier years of the T.E.S.T. study have previously been presented. Rossi et al. [9] reported antimicrobial resistance between 2004 and 2007, Fernández-Canigia et al. [10] presented antimicrobial susceptibility between 2004 and 2010 (Gram-negative isolates only), and Garza-González et al. [11] presented susceptibility data for *S. aureus* isolates collected between 2004 and 2010.

Methods

The Latin American countries that participated in T.E.S.T. were Argentina, Brazil, Chile, Colombia, El Salvador, Guatemala, Honduras, Jamaica, Mexico, Nicaragua, Panama, Puerto Rico and Venezuela. Not all study centers submitted isolates during all study years. All body sites were acceptable sources for isolate collection and a maximum of 25% of isolates could be from urine. Isolates were collected from both inpatients and outpatients with documented hospital- or community-acquired infections, and one isolate was permitted per patient.

Detailed materials and methods for the T.E.S.T. study have been described in previous publications (e.g. [12]). Isolate identification and susceptibility testing were performed at the individual centers. Minimum inhibitory concentrations (MICs) were determined using the broth microdilution methodology according to the Clinical and Laboratory Standards Institute (CLSI) guidelines [13]. Antimicrobial susceptibility was determined using breakpoints approved by the CLSI [14], except for tigecycline for which the US Food and Drugs Administration (FDA) breakpoints were used [15]. When determining *Streptococcus pneumoniae* susceptibility to penicillin, oral penicillin V breakpoints were used. In 2006, four antimicrobials (azithromycin, clarithromycin, erythromycin and clindamycin) were added to the *S. pneumoniae* T.E.S.T. panel and, where available, isolates were tested retrospectively.

ESBL production among *Klebsiella* spp. and *Escherichia coli* were determined by IHMA according to CLSI guidelines using cefotaxime, cefotaxime–clavulanic acid, ceftazidime and ceftazidime–clavulanic acid disks. *Haemophilus influenzae* isolates were tested for β-lactamase production using center specific methodology.

In this study, MDR was defined as resistance to three or more classes of antimicrobial agents. The classes used to define MDR *Acinetobacter baumannii* were aminoglycosides (amikacin), β-lactams (cefepime, ceftazidime, ceftriaxone or piperacillin–tazobactam), carbapenems (imipenem or meropenem), fluoroquinolones (levofloxacin) and tetracyclines (minocycline). The classes used to define MDR *Pseudomonas aeruginosa* were aminoglycosides (amikacin), β-lactams (cefepime, ceftazidime or piperacillin–tazobactam), carbapenems (imipenem or meropenem) and fluoroquinolones (levofloxacin).

Results

Data are presented for a total of 31,933 isolates collected in Latin America between 2004 and 2015 (Table 1); 9918 were Gram-positive and 22,015 were Gram-negative. The majority of isolates came from three countries: Mexico (26.3%), Argentina (22.6%) and Colombia (14.7%). The numbers of centers that participated in each country were as follows: Mexico, 16; Colombia, 14; Argentina, 12;

Table 1 Number of isolates collected by year from T.E.S.T. Latin America centers, 2004–2015

Country	Number of isolates[a]													
	2004	2005	2006	2007	2008	2009	2010	2011	2012	2013	2014	2015	2011–2015	2004–2015
Central America														
Guatemala	4	0	172	213	187	531	562	1	0	0	0	159	160	1829
Honduras	0	0	93	97	0	244	1	0	0	0	0	0	0	435
Panama	0	1	182	90	205	185	182	0	189	196	195	195	775	1620
Rest of Latin America														
Argentina	450	1064	612	1142	1402	1113	900	199	0	0	0	332	531	7214
Brazil	83	291	161	236	482	583	20	0	0	0	8	344	352	2208
Chile	5	228	318	624	446	359	0	0	61	197	217	330	805	2785
Colombia	0	76	461	122	1176	1072	719	341	166	189	196	182	1074	4700
Mexico	0	105	1111	1010	1921	1586	1242	94	182	456	193	513	1438	8413
Venezuela	1	0	181	358	240	574	200	137	0	0	0	318	455	2009
All Latin America[b]	543	1765	3661	3899	6059	6434	3982	772	598	1038	809	2373	5590	31,933

[a] Not all countries in Latin America participated in T.E.S.T. every year

[b] Includes all countries in Latin America that participated in T.E.S.T. Individual data for El Salvador, Nicaragua, Jamaica and Puerto Rico not present as contributed isolates in ≤2 years

Chile, 6; Venezuela, 6; Brazil, 4; Guatemala, 4; Honduras, 2; Panama, 2. Four countries submitted isolates in ≤2 of the 12 years of study (El Salvador 2009, 2010; Nicaragua 2006, 2007; Jamaica 2006; Puerto Rico 2006) and so are not included in the country by country analysis. They are included the analysis of data for Latin America as a whole. The number of isolates of each organism, by year, are shown in Additional file 1: Table S1, S2.

Gram-positive organisms

Data on rates of Gram-positive resistant phenotypes of *S. aureus, S. pneumoniae, Enterococcus faecium* and *Enterococcus faecalis* are presented by country in Table 2 and by year in Fig. 1. Pooled (2004–2015) antimicrobial susceptibility data for these organisms, as well as *Streptococcus agalactiae*, are presented in Table 3, and year by year susceptibility data are presented in Additional file 1: Table S1.

A total of 4563 isolates of *S. aureus* were collected in Latin America between 2004 and 2015, and almost half (48.3%) were MRSA (Table 2). Rates of MRSA were highest in Guatemala and Chile (67.3 and 62.0%, respectively) and lowest in Panama and Colombia (39.7 and 40.0%, respectively). MRSA rates appeared stable,

Table 2 Rates of Gram-positive resistant phenotypes collected from Latin America by country, 2004–2015

Country	Methicillin-resistant *S. aureus*		Penicillin-resistant *S. pneumoniae*		Vancomycin-resistant *E. faecium*		Vancomycin-resistant *E. faecalis*	
	n/N	%	n/N	%	n/N	%	n/N	%
Central America								
Guatemala	226/336	67.3	0/15	0.0	6/29	20.7	0/116	0.0
Honduras	30/62	48.4	2/10	20.0	1/10	10.0	0/31	0.0
Panama	89/224	39.7	11/108	10.2	2/11	18.2	0/114	0.0
Rest of Latin America								
Argentina	454/947	47.9	35/412	8.5	60/115	52.2	2/408	0.5
Brazil	141/290	48.6	12/112	10.7	34/44	77.3	19/133	14.3
Chile	254/410	62.0	24/146	16.4	33/59	55.9	4/163	2.5
Colombia	261/653	40.0	25/187	13.4	33/86	38.4	5/314	1.6
Mexico	547/1243	44.0	73/350	20.9	55/175	31.4	2/565	0.4
Venezuela	136/265	51.3	14/81	17.3	9/38	23.7	1/121	0.8
All Latin America[a]	2202/4563	48.3	198/1436	13.8	235/576	40.8	33/2004	1.6

[a] Includes all countries in Latin America that participated in T.E.S.T. Individual data for El Salvador, Nicaragua, Jamaica and Puerto Rico not present as contributed isolates in ≤2 years

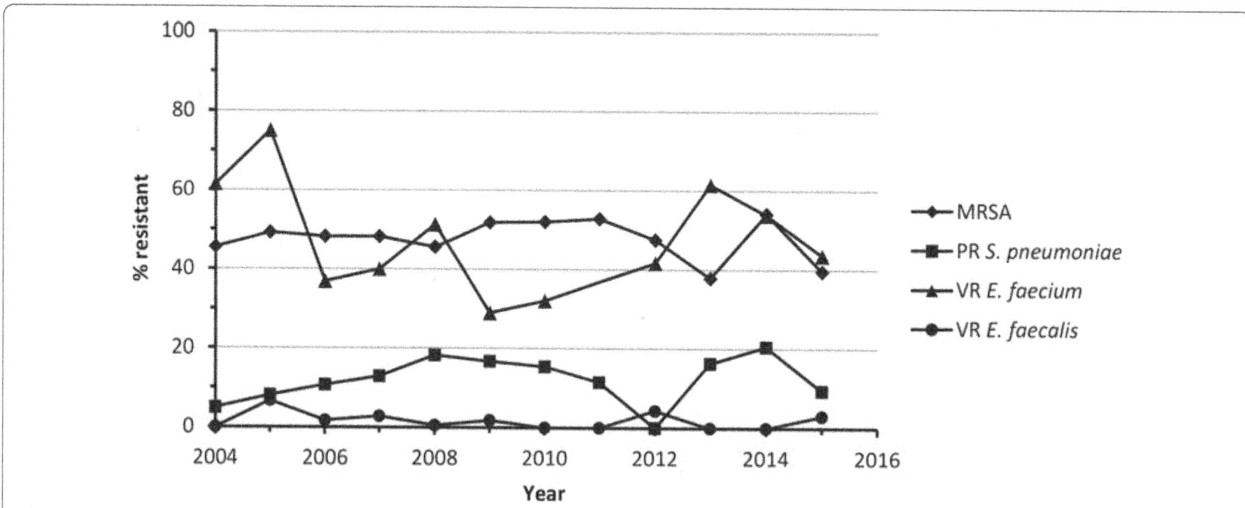

Fig. 1 Rates of Gram-positive resistant phenotypes collected from Latin America by year, 2004–2015. MRSA N values: 2004, 30/66; 2005, 131/266; 2006, 247/512; 2007, 258/535; 2008, 374/821; 2009, 479/924; 2010, 325/625; 2011, 57/108; 2012, 47/99; 2013, 55/145; 2014, 60/111; 2015, 139/351. PR *S. pneumoniae* N values: 2004, 2/41; 2005, 10/123; 2006, 19/178; 2007, 30/232; 2008, 49/269; 2009, 43/258; 2010, 14/91; 2011, 6/52; 2012, 0/14; 2013, 8/49; 2014, 9/44; 2015, 8/85. VR *E. faecium* N values: 2004, 8/13; 2005, 9/12; 2006, 24/65; 2007, 22/55; 2008, 60/117; 2009, 40/138; 2010, 25/78; 2012, 5/12; 2013, 16/26; 2014, 7/13; 2015, 17/39. Data point for VR *E. faecium* for 2011 omitted as N < 10. VR *E. faecalis* N values: 2004, 0/25; 2005, 7/104; 2006, 4/231; 2007, 6/216; 2008, 2/404; 2009, 7/389; 2010, 0/258; 2011, 0/40; 2012, 2/46; 2013, 0/71; 2014, 0/56; 2015, 5/164. *MRSA* methicillin-resistant *S. aureus*, *PR* penicillin-resistant, *VR* vancomycin-resistant

although some variability occurred in the more recent years [between 2004 and 2015 rates were lowest in 2013 (37.9%; 55/145) and highest in 2014 (54.1%; 60/111)] (Fig. 1). All *S. aureus* isolates, including MRSA isolates, were susceptible to linezolid and vancomycin (Table 3). Susceptibility rates among all *S. aureus* to tigecycline and minocycline were 99.9 and 97.6%, respectively (Table 3). Among MRSA isolates the rates of susceptibility to tigecycline and minocycline were 99.9 and 96.2%, respectively. Rates of susceptibility were stable over time against both *S. aureus* and MRSA (Additional file 1: Table S1). One exception was levofloxacin, susceptibility to which increased over the course of the study for all *S. aureus* isolates [56.1% (37/66) in 2004 and 74.9% (263/351) in 2015] and for MRSA isolates [3.3% (1/30) in 2004 and 46.8% (65/139) in 2015] (Additional file 1: Table S1).

Over the 2004–2015 time period, 1436 isolates of *S. pneumoniae* were submitted, of which 13.8% were penicillin-resistant (Table 2). Resistance to penicillin ranged from 0% (0/15) in Guatemala to 20.9% (73/350) in Mexico. Rates of penicillin resistance were ≤21.0% between 2004 and 2015, and ranged from 0% (0/14) in 2012 to 20.5% (9/44) in 2014 (Fig. 1). The number of penicillin-resistant isolates was ≤10 for seven years of the study (2004, 2005 and 2011–2015). All *S. pneumoniae* isolates were susceptible to linezolid and vancomycin (Table 3). Susceptibility rates for all *S. pneumoniae* isolates were ≥94.0% for levofloxacin, tigecycline, ceftriaxone and amoxicillin–clavulanic acid. Year by year data shows susceptibility rates were stable for levofloxacin (≥97.0% in all years) and ceftriaxone (≥89.0% in all years), however susceptibility rates were more variable for the other agents on the panel (Additional file 1: Table S1). All *S. pneumoniae* isolates were susceptible to tigecycline between 2010 and 2015, prior to that susceptibility increased from 78.0% (32/41) in 2004 to 99.2% (256/258) in 2009. Conversely, susceptibility to minocycline decreased between 2004 and 2009 [from 92.7% (38/41) to 32.2% (83/258)], and higher rates of susceptibility were reported in all subsequent years, with a rate in 2015 of 71.8% (61/85) (Additional file 1: Table S1). Susceptibility to levofloxacin and tigecycline among penicillin-resistant isolates was also high (98.0% for each for the 2004–2015 pooled time period); however, susceptibility to ceftriaxone and amoxicillin–clavulanic acid among penicillin-resistant isolates was reduced (69.2 and 63.6%, respectively) (Table 3).

A total of 1339 isolates of *S. agalactiae* were submitted to T.E.S.T. between 2004 and 2015 in Latin America (Table 3). Susceptibility to the majority of agents was unchanged over the course of the study (Additional file 1: Table S1) and all isolates were susceptible to ampicillin, linezolid, meropenem, penicillin and vancomycin (Table 3). More than 97.0% were susceptible to tigecycline, ceftriaxone and levofloxacin; however, susceptibility to minocycline was lower (27.6%) and variable over the course of the study (Table 3; Additional file 1: Table S1).

A total of 576 isolates of *E. faecium* were collected in Latin America between 2004 and 2015, and vancomycin

Table 3 Antimicrobial activity among Gram-positive organisms collected in Latin America, 2004–2015

Species (no. isolates) and antimicrobial agent	MIC (mg/L)			Susceptibility	
	MIC_{50}	MIC_{90}	MIC range	% S	% R
Staphylococcus aureus (4563)					
Amoxicillin–clavulanic acid	2	≥16	≤0.03 to ≥16	–	–
Ampicillin	16	≥32	≤0.06 to ≥32	–	–
Ceftriaxone	8	≥128	≤0.03 to ≥128	–	–
Levofloxacin	0.25	32	≤0.06 to ≥64	58.2	39.8
Linezolid	2	4	≤0.5 to 4	100	0.0
Meropenem (N = 3998)[a]	0.5	≥32	≤0.12 to ≥32	–	–
Minocycline	≤0.25	1	≤0.25 to ≥16	97.6	0.8
Penicillin	≥16	≥16	≤0.06 to ≥16	5.5	94.5
Piperacillin–tazobactam	2	≥32	≤0.25 to ≥32	–	–
Tigecycline	0.12	0.25	≤0.008 to 2	99.9	–
Vancomycin	1	1	≤0.12 to 2	100	0.0
Staphylococcus aureus, methicillin-resistant (2202/4563)					
Levofloxacin	8	32	≤0.06 to ≥64	20.3	77.4
Linezolid	2	2	≤0.5 to 4	100	0.0
Minocycline	≤0.25	1	≤0.25 to ≥16	96.2	1.3
Tigecycline	0.12	0.25	≤0.008 to 2	99.9	–
Vancomycin	1	1	≤0.12 to 2	100	0.0
Streptococcus pneumoniae (1436)					
Amoxicillin–clavulanic acid	≤0.03	2	≤0.03 to ≥16	94.6	2.0
Ampicillin (N = 1434)	≤0.06	2	≤0.06 to ≥32	–	–
Azithromycin (N = 1247)	0.12	64	≤0.03 to ≥128	72.6	26.9
Ceftriaxone	0.06	1	≤0.03 to ≥128	94.9	1.0
Clarithromycin (N = 1247)	0.03	64	≤0.015 to ≥128	72.7	26.8
Clindamycin (N = 1247)	0.06	64	≤0.015 to ≥128	88.0	11.9
Erythromycin (N = 1247)	0.06	64	≤0.015 to ≥128	71.7	27.3
Levofloxacin	1	1	≤0.06 to 32	98.9	0.3
Linezolid	1	1	≤0.5 to 2	100	–
Meropenem (N = 1256)[a]	≤0.12	0.5	≤0.12 to 16	79.6	7.7
Minocycline	1	8	≤0.25 to ≥16	59.8	28.8
Penicillin	≤0.06	2	≤0.06 to ≥16	54.7	13.8
Piperacillin–tazobactam	≤0.25	2	≤0.25 to ≥32	–	–
Tigecycline	0.015	0.06	≤0.008 to 0.5	95.5	–
Vancomycin	0.25	0.5	≤0.12 to 1	100	–
Streptococcus pneumoniae, penicillin-resistant (198/1436)					
Amoxicillin–clavulanic acid	2	8	≤0.03 to ≥16	63.6	13.1
Ampicillin (N = 197)	4	8	0.12 to ≥32	–	–
Azithromycin (N = 179)	16	≥128	≤0.03 to ≥128	41.3	58.1
Ceftriaxone	1	2	≤0.03 to ≥128	69.2	6.1
Clarithromycin (N = 179)	4	≥128	≤0.015 to ≥128	41.3	58.7
Clindamycin (N = 179)	0.12	≥128	≤0.015 to ≥128	62.0	38.0
Erythromycin (N = 179)	8	≥128	≤0.015 to ≥128	41.3	58.7
Levofloxacin	1	1	0.25 to 4	98.0	0.0
Linezolid	1	1	≤0.5 to 2	100	–
Meropenem (N = 184)[a]	0.5	1	≤0.12 to 16	7.6	43.5
Minocycline	4	≥16	≤0.25 to ≥16	32.8	55.6
Piperacillin–tazobactam	4	8	0.5 to ≥32	–	–
Tigecycline	0.015	0.03	≤0.008 to 0.5	98.0	–

Table 3 continued

Species (no. isolates) and antimicrobial agent	MIC (mg/L)			Susceptibility	
	MIC_{50}	MIC_{90}	MIC range	% S	% R
Vancomycin	0.5	0.5	≤0.12 to 1	100	–
Streptococcus agalactiae (1339)					
Amoxicillin–clavulanic acid	0.06	0.12	≤0.03 to ≥16	–	–
Ampicillin	≤0.06	0.12	≤0.06 to 0.25	100	–
Ceftriaxone	0.06	0.12	≤0.03 to 2	99.8	–
Levofloxacin	0.5	1	≤0.06 to ≥64	97.7	1.7
Linezolid	1	1	≤0.5 to 2	100	–
Meropenem (N = 1198)[a]	≤0.12	≤0.12	≤0.12 to 0.5	100	–
Minocycline	8	≥16	≤0.25 to ≥16	27.6	61.8
Penicillin	≤0.06	0.12	≤0.06 to 0.12	100	–
Piperacillin–tazobactam	≤0.25	0.5	≤0.25 to ≥32	–	–
Tigecycline	0.03	0.06	≤0.008 to 0.5	99.9	–
Vancomycin	0.5	0.5	≤0.12 to 1	100	–
Enterococcus faecium (576)					
Amoxicillin–clavulanic acid	≥16	≥16	≤0.03 to ≥16	–	–
Ampicillin	≥32	≥32	≤0.06 to ≥32	26.0	74.0
Ceftriaxone	≥128	≥128	≤0.03 to ≥128	–	–
Levofloxacin	≥64	≥64	≤0.06 to ≥64	21.7	71.0
Linezolid	2	2	≤0.5 to 4	99.8	0.0
Meropenem (N = 524)[a]	≥32	≥32	≤0.12 to ≥32	–	–
Minocycline	2	≥16	≤0.25 to ≥16	62.0	19.8
Penicillin	≥16	≥16	≤0.06 to ≥16	22.6	77.4
Piperacillin–tazobactam	≥32	≥32	≤0.25 to ≥32	–	–
Tigecycline	0.06	0.25	≤0.008 to 1	99.5	–
Vancomycin	2	≥64	≤0.12 to ≥64	56.8	40.8
Enterococcus faecium, vancomycin-resistant (235/576)					
Amoxicillin–clavulanic acid	≥16	≥16	1 to ≥16	–	–
Ampicillin	≥32	≥32	2 to ≥32	0.9	99.1
Ceftriaxone	≥128	≥128	4 to ≥128	–	–
Levofloxacin	≥64	≥64	2 to ≥64	0.9	97.0
Linezolid	2	2	≤0.5 to 2	100	0.0
Meropenem (N = 213)[a]	≥32	≥32	≤0.12 to ≥32	–	–
Minocycline	≤0.25	≥16	≤0.25 to ≥16	71.5	17.0
Penicillin	≥16	≥16	4 to ≥16	1.3	98.7
Piperacillin–tazobactam	≥32	≥32	2 to ≥32	–	–
Tigecycline	0.06	0.25	≤0.008 to 1	98.7	–
Enterococcus faecalis (2004)					
Amoxicillin–clavulanic acid	0.5	1	≤0.03 to ≥16	–	–
Ampicillin	1	2	≤0.06 to ≥32	99.0	1.0
Ceftriaxone	≥128	≥128	≤0.03 to ≥128	–	–
Levofloxacin	1	≥64	≤0.06 to ≥64	69.4	29.1
Linezolid	2	2	≤0.5 to 4	99.8	0.0
Meropenem (N = 1771)[a]	4	8	≤0.12 to ≥32	–	–
Minocycline	8	≥16	≤0.25 to ≥16	34.9	30.4
Penicillin	2	4	≤0.06 to ≥16	98.4	1.6
Piperacillin–tazobactam	4	8	≤0.25 to ≥32	–	–
Tigecycline	0.12	0.25	≤0.008 to 1	99.7	–
Vancomycin	1	2	≤0.12 to ≥64	98.1	1.6

Table 3 continued

Species (no. isolates) and antimicrobial agent	MIC (mg/L)			Susceptibility	
	MIC_{50}	MIC_{90}	MIC range	% S	% R
Enterococcus faecalis, vancomycin-resistant (33/2004)					
Amoxicillin–clavulanic acid	1	≥16	0.25 to ≥16	–	–
Ampicillin	2	≥32	0.5 to ≥32	78.8	21.2
Ceftriaxone	≥128	≥128	128 to ≥128	–	–
Levofloxacin	32	≥64	1 to ≥64	6.1	93.9
Linezolid	1	2	1 to 2	100	0.0
Meropenem (N = 27)[a]	16	≥32	2 to ≥32	–	–
Minocycline	4	≥16	≤0.25 to ≥16	51.5	18.2
Penicillin	8	≥16	2 to ≥16	75.8	24.2
Piperacillin–tazobactam	8	≥32	2 to ≥32	–	–
Tigecycline	0.12	0.25	0.015 to 0.25	100	–

–, no CLSI breakpoints available

MIC minimum inhibitory concentration, MIC_{50} MIC required to inhibit growth of 50% of isolates, MIC_{90} MIC required to inhibit growth of 90% of isolates, *S* susceptible, *R* resistant

[a] Susceptibility data for imipenem were collected from 2004 to 2006, after which time imipenem was replaced by meropenem

resistance was seen in 40.8% (Table 2). Rates of vancomycin resistance among *E. faecium* isolates were highest in Brazil (77.3%), Chile (55.9%) and Argentina (52.2%). Rates of vancomycin resistance among *E. faecium* isolates were lower in countries in Central America (Guatemala, Honduras and Panama) than in the rest of the Latin America. Vancomycin resistance rates were variable over the course of the study (Fig. 1). High percentages (>99.0%) of *E. faecium* isolates were susceptible to linezolid and tigecycline (Table 3) and rates were unchanged over the course of the study (Additional file 1: Table S1). A single *E. faecium* isolate was non-susceptible to linezolid. Among the vancomycin-resistant isolates, all were susceptible to linezolid and 98.7% were susceptible to tigecycline (Table 3).

Of the 2004 *E. faecalis* isolates submitted between 2004 and 2015, 1.6% were vancomycin-resistant (Table 2). Rates of vancomycin resistance were ≤2.5% in all countries except Brazil, which had a resistance rate of 14.3%. None of the *E. faecalis* isolates submitted by Central American countries were resistant to vancomycin. No vancomycin-resistant *E. faecalis* isolates were collected in 2004, 2010, 2011, 2013 or 2014, and less than 10 isolates were collected for any other year (Additional file 1: Table S1). Susceptibility rates for all *E. faecalis* isolates were >98.0% for linezolid, tigecycline, ampicillin, penicillin and vancomycin (Table 3) and were unchanged over time (Additional file 1: Table S1). This high level of susceptibility to linezolid and tigecycline was maintained among vancomycin-resistant isolates, whereas susceptibility to ampicillin and penicillin decreased to 78.8 and 75.8%, respectively (Table 3). Susceptibility among all *E. faecalis* isolates to minocycline decreased from 56.0% (14/25) in 2004 to 20.0% (8/40) in 2011; rates after 2011 were variable but did show a trend towards increasing susceptibility (Additional file 1: Table S1).

Gram-negative organisms

Data on rates of Gram-negative resistant phenotypes of *K. pneumoniae*, *Klebsiella oxytoca*, *E. coli*, *P. aeruginosa*, *A. baumannii* and *H. influenzae* are presented by country in Table 4, and by year in Fig. 2 (with the exception of *K. oxytoca* and *H. influenzae*). Antimicrobial susceptibility data for these organisms, as well as *Enterobacter* spp. and *Serratia marcescens*, are presented in Table 5, and year by year susceptibility data are presented in Additional file 1: Table S2.

Among the 4032 *K. pneumoniae* isolates submitted between 2004 and 2015, 36.3% were ESBL-producers (Table 4) and rates of ESBL production ranged from 18.3% in Venezuela to 73.7% in Honduras. Figure 2a shows *K. pneumoniae* ESBL production rate was relatively stable for the 2004–2015 time period. Among *K. pneumoniae* isolates, susceptibility was highest to tigecycline, meropenem and amikacin (95.7, 90.9 and 86.9%, respectively); susceptibility among ESBL-producers was also highest to these agents (93.4, 86.9 and 75.3%, respectively) (Table 5). Susceptibility rates to tigecycline and meropenem were stable across the years of the study, whereas rates to amikacin were more variable (Additional file 1: Table S2). Among both all *K. pneumoniae* and ESBL-producers susceptibility to minocycline decreased from 2004 [80.6% (54/67) and 69.6% (16/23), respectively] until 2010 [44.4% (233/525) and 25.7% (48/187),

Table 4 Rates of Gram-negative resistant phenotypes collected from Latin America by country, 2004–2015

Country	ESBL-producing *K. pneumoniae*		ESBL-producing *K. oxytoca*		ESBL-producing *E. coli*		βLPos *H. influenzae*		MDR *A. baumannii*		MDR *P. aeruginosa*	
	n/N	%	n/N	%	n/N	%	n/N	%	n/N	%	n/N	%
Central America												
Guatemala	153/253	60.5	3/8	37.5	163/414	39.4	2/16	12.5	150/189	79.4	103/235	43.8
Honduras	56/76	73.7	1/1	100	31/78	39.7	2/8	25.0	39/51	76.5	15/47	31.9
Panama	79/210	37.6	2/4	50.0	49/225	21.8	12/78	15.4	95/122	77.9	21/176	11.9
Rest of Latin America												
Argentina	367/869	42.2	14/83	16.9	133/949	14.0	109/468	23.3	465/573	81.2	192/749	25.6
Brazil	122/270	45.2	3/26	11.5	51/300	17.0	19/96	19.8	148/174	85.1	73/232	31.5
Chile	216/341	63.3	6/34	17.6	130/386	33.7	31/130	23.8	145/217	66.8	81/286	28.3
Colombia	138/593	23.3	9/80	11.3	92/708	13.0	9/168	5.4	180/319	56.4	82/535	15.3
Mexico	241/1025	23.5	23/152	15.1	510/1405	36.3	65/232	28.0	297/518	57.3	283/1035	27.3
Venezuela	50/273	18.3	4/17	23.5	54/296	18.2	18/89	20.2	101/137	73.7	77/236	32.6
All Latin America[a]	1465/4032	36.3	67/409	16.4	1246/4912	25.4	270/1300	20.8	1654/2354	70.3	966/3613	26.7

ESBL extended-spectrum β-lactamase, *βLPos* β-lactamase positive, *MDR* multidrug-resistant

[a] Includes all countries in Latin America that participated in T.E.S.T. Individual data for El Salvador, Nicaragua, Jamaica and Puerto Rico not present as contributed isolates in ≤2 years

respectively] and then increased, resulting in higher rates of susceptibility to minocycline in 2015 [81.9% (263/321) and 84.7% (83/98), respectively) (Additional file 1: Table S2). The susceptibility rate to levofloxacin among all *K. pneumoniae* isolates was 65.3%, and among ESBL-producing isolates was 39.4% (resistance rates 31.6 and 55.6%, respectively) (Table 5) and although there was some variability no trend was seen over time (Additional file 1: Table S2).

A total of 409 *K. oxytoca* isolates were collected, of which 16.4% were ESBL-producers (Table 4). Among all *K. oxytoca* isolates, susceptibility rates were highest to tigecycline, meropenem and amikacin (98.0, 97.6 and 95.6%, respectively) (Table 5) and little variability was seen over time (Additional file 1: Table S2). Numbers of ESBL-producing *K. oxytoca* were low in each year (≤14 isolates); in years with ≥10 isolates rates of susceptibility were highest to tigecycline, meropenem and amikacin (Additional file 1: Table S2).

Of the *E. coli* isolates collected, 25.4% were ESBL-producers and the percentage of isolates that produced ESBLs was highest in Honduras, Guatemala and Mexico (Table 4). Among all *E. coli* isolates, susceptibility was highest to tigecycline and meropenem (99.7 and 98.1%, respectively), and these rates were similar among the ESBL-producers (99.8 and 97.0%, respectively) (Table 5). Rates of susceptibility to tigecycline and meropenem were stable across the 2004–2015 time period (Additional file 1: Table S2). Susceptibility to minocycline decreased between 2004 and 2010/2011 and then increased, resulting in a similar rate of susceptibility in 2004 and 2015 [76.7% (56/73) and 81.7% (343/420), respectively] (Additional file 1: Table S2). For the other agents on the panel, susceptibility rates were lower among ESBL-producing *E. coli* compared with *E. coli* isolates overall. The rate of levofloxacin susceptibility among all *E. coli* isolates was 47.8%, and among ESBL-producing *E. coli* isolates was 11.8% (resistance rates were 48.8 and 84.4%, respectively). Susceptibility to meropenem was lower among *K. pneumoniae* isolates (90.9%) than *E. coli* isolates (98.1%).

Enterobacter spp. and *S. marcescens* were highly susceptible to tigecycline (95.7 and 94.8%, respectively), meropenem (95.1 and 95.0%, respectively), and amikacin (90.2 and 83.4%, respectively) (Table 5), and rates were stable across the 2004–2015 time period (Additional file 1: Table S2).

Of the 3613 *P. aeruginosa* isolates submitted by Latin American centers between 2004 and 2015, 26.7% were MDR (Table 4). The countries that submitted the highest percentages of MDR *P. aeruginosa* isolates were Guatemala, Venezuela, Honduras and Brazil (43.8, 32.6, 31.9 and 31.5%, respectively). The year on year rates of MDR were variable across the 2004–2015 time period, however <20% of *P aeruginosa* were MDR between 2012 and 2015 (Fig. 2b). Breakpoints were available for six of the agents on the panel. Of these, the agents with the highest rate of susceptibility against *P. aeruginosa* was amikacin (72.8%) (Table 5). Susceptibility to amikacin increased between 2011 [59.1% (39/66)] and 2014 [92.1% (82/89)] although there was a small decrease in 2015 [83.8% (228/272)] (Additional file 1: Table S2). Among all *P. aeruginosa* isolates, 56.8% were susceptible to ceftazidime. Among

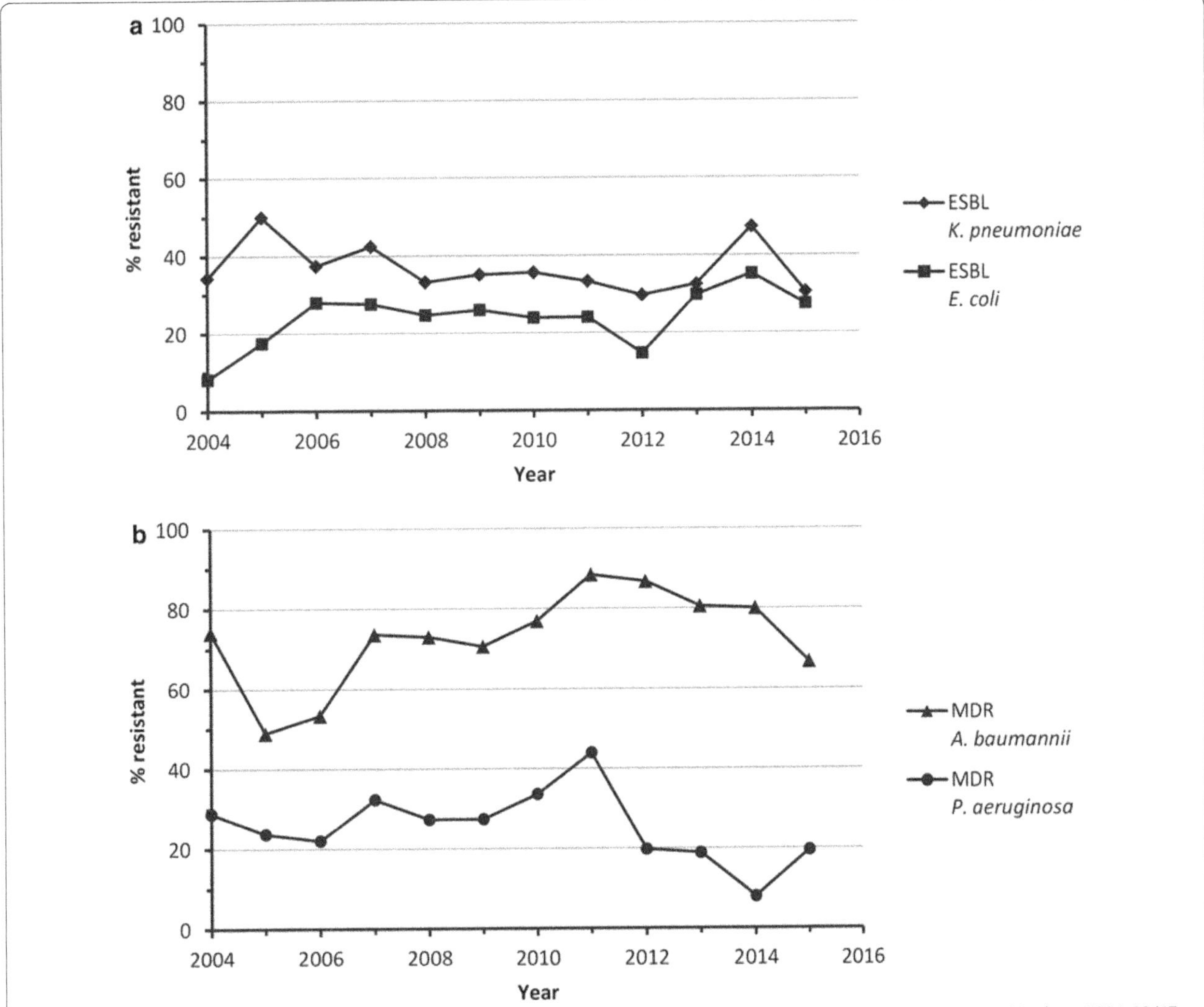

Fig. 2 Rates of Gram-negative resistant phenotypes collected from Latin America by year, 2004–2015. **a** ESBL *K. pneumoniae* N values: 2004, 23/67; 2005, 101/202; 2006, 166/444; 2007, 196/462; 2008, 263/791; 2009, 299/851; 2010, 187/525; 2011, 29/87; 2012, 22/74; 2013, 38/117; 2014, 43/91; 2015, 98/321. ESBL *E. coli* N values: 2004, 6/73; 2005, 37/211; 2006, 164/588; 2007, 147/534; 2008, 220/893; 2009, 272/1050; 2010, 158/660; 2011, 30/125; 2012, 15/102; 2013, 45/151; 2014, 37/105; 2015, 115/420. **b** MDR *A. baumannii* N values: 2004, 40/54; 2005, 66/135; 2006, 131/246; 2007, 209/284; 2008, 343/470; 2009, 344/487; 2010, 240/312; 2011, 38/43; 2012, 39/45; 2013, 62/77; 2014, 48/60; 2015, 94/141. MDR *P. aeruginosa* N values: 2004, 17/59; 2005, 40/169; 2006, 94/427; 2007, 124/384; 2008, 200/732; 2009, 206/753; 2010, 161/479; 2011, 29/66; 2012, 13/66; 2013, 22/117; 2014, 7/89; 2015, 53/272. ESBL-producing *K. oxytoca* and β-lactamase positive *H. influenzae* are not shown due to low number of isolates year on year. *ESBL* extended-spectrum β-lactamase, *MDR* multidrug-resistant

isolates that were MDR, susceptibility for all agents was <25.0%. The meropenem susceptibility rate among all *P. aeruginosa* isolates was 53.8% (resistance rate 36.9%).

Over the 2004–2015 time period, 2354 *A. baumannii* isolates were submitted, and 70.3% were MDR (Table 4). By country Brazil and Argentina had the highest levels of MDR (85.1 and 81.2%, respectively). Figure 2b shows variability in rates of MDR among *A. baumannii* across the 2004–2015 time period; however, between 2011 and 2015 MDR rates decreased each year from 88.4% (38/43) in 2011 to 66.7% (94/141) in 2015. The agents with the lowest MIC_{90} values among all *A. baumannii* isolates were tigecycline and minocycline (2 and 8 mg/L, respectively); these values were the same among MDR *A. baumannii* isolates (Table 5). Among all *A. baumannii* isolates, 30.8% were sensitive to amikacin. Year on year data from 2006 onwards shows a trend towards decreasing susceptibility of *A. baumannii* to meropenem [from 34.7% (43/124) in 2006 to 20.6% (29/141) in 2015] (Additional file 1: Table S2). Over the course of the study rates of susceptibility to minocycline decreased from 98.1% (53/54) in 2004 to 83.0% (117/141) in 2015; however,

Table 5 Antimicrobial activity among Gram-negative organisms collected in Latin America, 2004–2015

Species (no. isolates) and antimicrobial agent	MIC (mg/L)			Susceptibility	
	MIC_{50}	MIC_{90}	MIC range	% S	% R
Klebsiella pneumoniae (4032)					
Amikacin	2	32	≤0.5 to ≥128	86.9	8.9
Amoxicillin–clavulanic acid	16	≥64	≤0.12 to ≥64	47.3	35.3
Ampicillin (N = 4024)	≥64	≥64	1 to ≥64	1.3	92.8
Cefepime	1	≥64	≤0.5 to ≥64	55.8	33.9
Ceftriaxone	2	≥128	≤0.06 to ≥128	49.1	49.7
Levofloxacin	0.25	≥16	≤0.008 to ≥16	65.3	31.6
Meropenem (N = 3555)[a]	≤0.06	1	≤0.06 to ≥32	90.9	7.3
Minocycline	4	≥32	≤0.5 to ≥32	61.4	25.2
Piperacillin–tazobactam	4	≥256	≤0.06 to ≥256	64.0	25.4
Tigecycline	0.5	2	≤0.008 to ≥32	95.7	0.9
Klebsiella pneumoniae, ESBL (1465/4032)					
Amikacin	8	≥128	≤0.5 to ≥128	75.3	16.4
Amoxicillin–clavulanic acid	32	≥64	≤0.12 to ≥64	12.8	57.7
Ampicillin	≥64	≥64	4 to ≥64	0.1	99.6
Cefepime	32	≥64	≤0.5 to ≥64	11.2	71.3
Ceftriaxone	≥128	≥128	≤0.06 to ≥128	1.0	97.8
Levofloxacin	8	≥16	≤0.008 to ≥16	39.4	55.6
Meropenem (N = 1270)[a]	≤0.06	4	≤0.06 to ≥32	86.9	10.2
Minocycline	4	≥32	≤0.5 to ≥32	51.6	31.5
Piperacillin–tazobactam	64	≥256	0.12 to ≥256	35.5	45.1
Tigecycline	0.5	2	0.03 to 16	93.4	1.4
Klebsiella oxytoca (409)					
Amikacin	2	8	≤0.5 to ≥128	95.6	2.9
Amoxicillin–clavulanic acid	4	32	0.25 to ≥64	70.4	17.6
Ampicillin	≥64	≥64	≤0.5 to ≥64	1.7	90.6
Cefepime	≤0.5	16	≤0.5 to ≥64	79.5	13.0
Ceftriaxone	0.12	≥128	≤0.06 to ≥128	69.7	27.6
Levofloxacin	0.06	≥16	≤0.008 to ≥16	82.9	15.6
Meropenem (N = 333)[a]	≤0.06	0.12	≤0.06 to 16	97.6	1.5
Minocycline	2	16	≤0.5 to ≥32	79.0	11.2
Piperacillin–tazobactam	2	64	≤0.06 to ≥256	84.6	9.8
Tigecycline	0.25	1	0.06 to 4	98.0	0.0
Klebsiella oxytoca, ESBL (67/409)					
Amikacin	4	32	≤0.5 to ≥128	89.6	6.0
Amoxicillin–clavulanic acid	16	≥64	0.25 to ≥64	26.9	35.8
Ampicillin	≥64	≥64	32 to ≥64	0.0	100
Cefepime	8	≥64	≤0.5 to ≥64	26.9	49.3
Ceftriaxone	64	≥128	≤0.06 to ≥128	3.0	91.0
Levofloxacin	2	≥16	0.03 to ≥16	55.2	41.8
Meropenem (N = 48)[a]	≤0.06	0.25	≤0.06 to 16	95.8	4.2
Minocycline	8	≥32	≤0.5 to ≥32	49.3	22.4
Piperacillin–tazobactam	8	≥256	≤0.06 to ≥256	61.2	22.4
Tigecycline	0.5	2	0.06 to 4	94.0	0.0
Escherichia coli (4912)					
Amikacin	2	8	≤0.5 to ≥128	95.8	2.2
Amoxicillin–clavulanic acid	8	32	≤0.12 to ≥64	51.7	22.0
Ampicillin	≥64	≥64	≤0.5 to ≥64	21.2	77.7

Table 5 continued

Species (no. isolates) and antimicrobial agent	MIC (mg/L)			Susceptibility	
	MIC_{50}	MIC_{90}	MIC range	% S	% R
Cefepime	≤0.5	≥64	≤0.5 to ≥64	67.6	23.2
Ceftriaxone	0.12	≥128	≤0.06 to ≥128	60.2	37.9
Levofloxacin	4	≥16	≤0.008 to ≥16	47.8	48.8
Meropenem (N = 4284)[a]	≤0.06	0.12	≤0.06 to ≥32	98.1	1.3
Minocycline	4	≥32	≤0.5 to ≥32	61.9	24.0
Piperacillin–tazobactam	2	32	≤0.06 to ≥256	85.7	6.9
Tigecycline	0.25	0.5	≤0.008 to ≥32	99.7	<0.1
Escherichia coli, ESBL (1246/4912)					
Amikacin	4	16	≤0.5 to ≥128	90.6	4.5
Amoxicillin–clavulanic acid	16	32	0.25 to ≥64	23.4	34.1
Ampicillin	≥64	≥64	1 to ≥64	0.7	99.0
Cefepime	32	≥64	≤0.5 to ≥64	11.0	71.6
Ceftriaxone	≥128	≥128	≤0.06 to ≥128	1.3	97.0
Levofloxacin	≥16	≥16	0.015 to ≥16	11.8	84.4
Meropenem (N = 1103)[a]	≤0.06	0.12	≤0.06 to ≥32	97.0	2.2
Minocycline	4	≥32	≤0.5 to ≥32	55.4	30.2
Piperacillin–tazobactam	8	128	≤0.06 to ≥256	74.4	10.6
Tigecycline	0.25	0.5	≤0.008 to 4	99.8	0.0
Enterobacter spp. (3818)					
Amikacin	2	16	≤0.5 to ≥128	90.2	5.9
Amoxicillin–clavulanic acid	≥64	≥64	≤0.12 to ≥64	5.1	91.8
Ampicillin (N = 3810)	≥64	≥64	≤0.5 to ≥64	3.7	90.0
Cefepime	≤0.5	≥64	≤0.5 to ≥64	70.5	17.6
Ceftriaxone	0.5	≥128	≤0.06 to ≥128	53.5	43.8
Levofloxacin	0.12	≥16	≤0.008 to ≥16	78.4	18.6
Meropenem (N = 3320)[a]	≤0.06	0.5	≤0.06 to ≥32	95.1	3.3
Minocycline	4	≥32	≤0.5 to ≥32	63.4	19.6
Piperacillin–tazobactam	4	≥256	≤0.06 to ≥256	71.9	16.8
Tigecycline	0.5	2	≤0.008 to ≥32	95.7	0.6
Serratia marcescens (1577)					
Amikacin	2	32	≤0.5 to ≥128	83.4	9.1
Amoxicillin–clavulanic acid	≥64	≥64	≤0.12 to ≥64	4.9	91.8
Ampicillin (N = 1575)	≥64	≥64	≤0.5 to ≥64	2.8	90.2
Cefepime	≤0.5	32	≤0.5 to ≥64	76.0	16.5
Ceftriaxone	0.5	≥128	≤0.06 to ≥128	67.1	29.7
Levofloxacin	0.25	8	≤0.008 to ≥16	84.9	10.6
Meropenem (N = 1347)[a]	≤0.06	0.5	≤0.06 to ≥32	95.0	3.7
Minocycline	4	16	≤0.5 to ≥32	64.1	14.8
Piperacillin–tazobactam	2	128	≤0.06 to ≥256	83.4	10.1
Tigecycline	1	2	≤0.008 to 16	94.8	0.8
Pseudomonas aeruginosa (3613)					
Amikacin	4	≥128	≤0.5 to ≥128	72.8	20.1
Amoxicillin–clavulanic acid	≥64	≥64	0.5 to ≥64	–	–
Ampicillin	≥64	≥64	1 to ≥64	–	–
Cefepime	8	≥64	≤0.5 to ≥64	60.4	25.4
Ceftazidime	8	≥64	≤1 to ≥64	56.8	33.4
Ceftriaxone	64	≥128	≤0.06 to ≥128	–	–
Levofloxacin	2	≥16	0.015 to ≥16	53.5	40.0

Table 5 continued

Species (no. isolates) and antimicrobial agent	MIC (mg/L)			Susceptibility	
	MIC_{50}	MIC_{90}	MIC range	% S	% R
Meropenem (N = 3151)[a]	2	≥32	≤0.06 to ≥32	53.8	36.9
Minocycline	≥32	≥32	≤0.5 to ≥32	–	–
Piperacillin–tazobactam	16	≥256	≤0.06 to ≥256	58.5	24.4
Tigecycline	8	16	≤0.008 to ≥32	–	–
Pseudomonas aeruginosa, MDR (966/3613)					
Amikacin	64	≥128	≤0.5 to ≥128	24.5	66.7
Amoxicillin–clavulanic acid	≥64	≥64	4 to ≥64	–	–
Ampicillin	≥64	≥64	1 to ≥64	–	–
Cefepime	≥64	≥64	≤0.5 to ≥64	8.8	72.6
Ceftazidime	32	≥64	2 to ≥64	8.7	81.5
Ceftriaxone	≥128	≥128	4 to ≥128	–	–
Levofloxacin	≥16	≥16	0.25 to ≥16	2.2	95.4
Meropenem (N = 861)[a]	≥32	≥32	≤0.06 to ≥32	4.6	90.0
Minocycline	≥32	≥32	≤0.5 to ≥32	–	–
Piperacillin–tazobactam	128	≥256	0.5 to ≥256	11.2	62.7
Tigecycline	16	≥32	0.25 to ≥32	–	–
Acinetobacter baumannii (2354)					
Amikacin	64	≥128	≤0.5 to ≥128	30.8	55.9
Amoxicillin–clavulanic acid	≥64	≥64	0.25 to ≥64	–	–
Ampicillin	≥64	≥64	≤0.5 to ≥64	–	–
Cefepime	32	≥64	≤0.5 to ≥64	22.0	65.2
Ceftazidime	32	≥64	≤1 to ≥64	17.2	74.9
Ceftriaxone	≥128	≥128	≤0.06 to ≥128	9.1	79.4
Levofloxacin	8	≥16	≤0.008 to ≥16	19.3	69.4
Meropenem (N = 2046)[a]	≥32	≥32	≤0.06 to ≥32	25.7	69.9
Minocycline	≤0.5	8	≤0.5 to ≥32	88.3	6.7
Piperacillin–tazobactam	≥256	≥256	≤0.06 to ≥256	17.2	74.8
Tigecycline	0.5	2	≤0.008 to ≥32	–	–
Acinetobacter baumannii, MDR (1654/2354)					
Amikacin	≥128	≥128	≤0.5 to ≥128	11.5	77.1
Amoxicillin–clavulanic acid	≥64	≥64	8 to ≥64	–	–
Ampicillin	≥64	≥64	≤0.5 to ≥64	–	–
Cefepime	≥64	≥64	≤0.5 to ≥64	5.3	82.3
Ceftazidime	≥64	≥64	≤1 to ≥64	4.3	89.8
Ceftriaxone	≥128	≥128	0.25 to ≥128	0.4	95.1
Levofloxacin	≥16	≥16	0.03 to ≥16	1.6	90.7
Meropenem (N = 1493)[a]	≥32	≥32	≤0.06 to ≥32	6.8	89.8
Minocycline	1	8	≤0.5 to ≥32	86.2	8.4
Piperacillin–tazobactam	≥256	≥256	≤0.06 to ≥256	1.7	93.3
Tigecycline	0.5	2	0.03 to ≥32	–	–
Haemophilus influenzae (1300)					
Amikacin (N = 1299)	4	8	≤0.5 to ≥128	–	–
Amoxicillin–clavulanic acid	0.5	2	≤0.12 to ≥64	99.4	0.6
Ampicillin	≤0.5	32	≤0.5 to ≥64	77.8	19.5
Cefepime	≤0.5	≤0.5	≤0.5 to 16	99.3	–
Ceftriaxone	≤0.06	≤0.06	≤0.06 to 32	99.7	–
Levofloxacin	0.015	0.03	≤0.008 to 2	100	–
Meropenem (N = 1075)[a]	≤0.06	0.12	≤0.06 to 0.5	100	–

Table 5 continued

Species (no. isolates) and antimicrobial agent	MIC (mg/L)			Susceptibility	
	MIC_{50}	MIC_{90}	MIC range	% S	% R
Minocycline (N = 1299)	≤0.5	1	≤0.5 to 16	98.8	0.5
Piperacillin–tazobactam	≤0.06	≤0.06	≤0.06 to 16	99.3	0.7
Tigecycline	0.12	0.25	≤0.008 to 2	97.8	–
Haemophilus influenzae, βLPos (270/1300)					
Amikacin	4	8	≤0.5 to 16	–	–
Amoxicillin–clavulanic acid	1	2	≤0.12 to ≥64	98.5	1.5
Ampicillin	16	≥64	≤0.5 to ≥64	0.7	92.6
Cefepime	≤0.5	≤0.5	≤0.5 to 16	98.9	–
Ceftriaxone	≤0.06	≤0.06	≤0.06 to 16	99.6	–
Levofloxacin	0.015	0.03	≤0.008 to 0.5	100	–
Meropenem (N = 236)[a]	≤0.06	0.12	≤0.06 to 0.5	100	–
Minocycline	≤0.5	1	≤0.5 to 16	98.1	0.7
Piperacillin–tazobactam	≤0.06	≤0.06	≤0.06 to 16	99.6	0.4
Tigecycline	0.12	0.25	≤0.008 to 0.5	98.5	–

–, no CLSI breakpoints available

MIC minimum inhibitory concentration, *MIC_{50}* MIC required to inhibit growth of 50% of isolates, *MIC_{90}* MIC required to inhibit growth of 90% of isolates, *S* susceptible, *R* resistant, *ESBL* extended-spectrum β-lactamase, *βLPos* β-lactamase positive, *MDR* multidrug-resistant

[a] Susceptibility data for imipenem were collected from 2004 to 2006, after which time imipenem was replaced by meropenem

susceptibility to amikacin increased reaching 50.4% (71/141) in 2015 (Additional file 1: Table S2). A similar pattern was seen among MDR *A. baumannii* (Additional file 1: Table S2).

Of the 1300 *H. influenzae* isolates submitted between 2004 and 2015, 20.8% were β-lactamase positive (Table 4). The country with the highest rate of β-lactamase positive isolates was Mexico (28.0%), whilst the lowest rate was in Colombia (5.4%). All *H. influenzae* isolates were susceptible to levofloxacin and meropenem (Table 5) and rates of susceptibility were consistent across the years of the study (Additional file 1: Table S2). Among all *H. influenzae* isolates and among β-lactamase positive isolates, susceptibility was ≥97.0% to ceftriaxone, amoxicillin–clavulanic acid, cefepime, piperacillin–tazobactam, minocycline and tigecycline.

Discussion

This study reports on the rates of resistant phenotypes and in vitro antimicrobial susceptibility among important Gram-positive and Gram-negative isolates collected in Latin America between 2004 and 2015. It provides an update to previous publications which reported T.E.S.T. data from Latin America [9–11]. Tigecycline maintained its in vitro activity against the isolates collected in this study (susceptibility >93.0%, MIC_{90} 2 mg/L for *A. baumannii*). As previously reported, tigecycline was not active against *P. aeruginosa* [16].

Historically, the prevalence of MRSA has been reported to be increasing in the Latin American region. For example, the SENTRY study reported a significant increase in MRSA rates in Latin America between 1997 and 2006 (from 33.8 to 40.2%; $p = 0.007$) [17]. Previous T.E.S.T. reports have suggested a stabilization of rates [11] and this T.E.S.T. study of data for isolates collected between 2004 and 2015 continues to suggest that rates are stable in the region, although with country variations. The overall rate of MRSA in this study was 48.3%, which is similar to a SENTRY report from Latin America for the 2011–2014 time period (44.7%) [18]. Recent studies from Europe (between 2012 and 2015) and the USA (between 2005 and 2011) have reported decreasing rates of MRSA [19, 20]. Such reports suggest that global efforts regarding infection control and antimicrobial stewardships are having an impact.

Linezolid and vancomycin are key tools in the treatment of MRSA as infections are often caused by organisms resistant to other antimicrobials. As reported by other studies in Latin America [1, 3, 18, 21], all *S. aureus* isolates (including MRSA) collected as part of T.E.S.T between 2004 and 2015 were susceptible to linezolid and vancomycin. Small numbers of tigecycline non-susceptible isolates were collected in the early years of the T.E.S.T. program, as previously reported by Garza-González et al. [11]. However, from 2010 onwards all *S. aureus* isolates (including MRSA) were susceptible to tigecycline. This was also the case in the Latin American SENTRY study in which all *S. aureus* isolates (including MRSA) collected over a similar time (2011–2014) were susceptible to tigecycline [18].

Linezolid-resistant *Enterococcus* spp. have previously been reported in Latin America [18]. However, none of the *Enterococcus* spp. isolates submitted to T.E.S.T. between 2004 and 2015 were linezolid-resistant. There were five intermediate (MIC 4 mg/L) isolates: 1 *E. faecium* collected in Argentina in 2009 and 4 *E. faecalis*, 3 collected in Mexico in 2009 and 1 in El Salvador in 2010. The rate of vancomycin-resistant *E. faecium* was 40.8%, which was lower than reported by Sader et al. [18] for the 2011–2014 time period (50.3%). Year on year rates of vancomycin resistance in this study were variable, although this is likely to be in part due to the low number of isolates collected in some years. Interestingly, the rates of vancomycin-resistant *E. faecium* were lower in the Central American countries included in this study (Guatemala, Honduras and Panama) compared with the rest of Latin America, although it should be noted that a relatively low number of *E. faecium* isolates were collected in Central America. Sader et al. [18] also reported variable *E. faecium* vancomycin resistance rates (26.3% in Argentina to 71.7% in Brazil between 2011 and 2014), although they did not report on the Central American region. The rate of vancomycin-resistant *E. faecalis* was low (1.6%), and this was consistent year by year. This rate was similar to that reported by Sader et al. (2.3%) [18], and similar the global rate for the 2004–2013 T.E.S.T. study period (2.2%) [4]. There was a striking regional pattern among *E. faecalis* isolates: none of the *E. faecalis* isolates collected in Central America as part of this study were vancomycin-resistant. Importantly, the high rates of susceptibility of these *Enterococcus* spp. to linezolid and tigecycline were maintained among vancomycin-resistant isolates. Indeed, Sader et al. [18] reported 100% susceptibility of *Enterococcus* spp. to tigecycline. Three *E. faecium* isolates collected in this T.E.S.T. study were non-susceptible to tigecycline, all of which were vancomycin-resistant (two collected in 2008 and one in 2012). All vancomycin-resistant *E. faecalis* isolates were susceptible to tigecycline.

High frequencies of ESBL-producing Enterobacteriaceae have been reported in Latin America by previous surveillance studies, particularly *K. pneumoniae* and *E. coli* [2]. In this update we have shown the rate of these organisms to be 36.3% and 25.4%. Sader et al. [18] reported higher rates of ESBL-producing *K. pneumoniae* and *E. coli* (57.3 and 37.7%, respectively) from the SENTRY study of Latin American centers (2011–2014). Differences could be in part due to the different countries included in each study, and variable rates of ESBL production across Latin America have previously been reported [2]. Furthermore, the rates of ESBL production in this T.E.S.T. study have been shown to vary widely by country. Year on year the rates of ESBL production were relatively stable which supports the findings of Kazmierczak et al. [22] for *K. pneumoniae* collected from intra-abdominal infections in Latin America between 2008 and 2012. We found a high percentage of resistance to fluoroquinolones (levofloxacin) among *E. coli* isolates (48.8%), reflecting the wide use of this antimicrobial in the treatment of urinary tract infections in Latin America. The resistance rate among ESBL-producing isolates of *E. coli* was higher (84.4%).

Carbapenem-resistant Enterobacteriaceae are of particular concern as they are increasingly reported globally and few treatment options are available for these types of infections [23, 24]. In this study, 3.8% (482/12,839) of Enterobacteriaceae were meropenem-resistant. This rate is the same as the Latin American rate of meropenem resistance reported by Sader et al. [18] for isolates collected between 2011 and 2014 (3.8%). The majority of meropenem-resistant Enterobacteriaceae in this T.E.S.T. study were *K. pneumoniae* isolates [54.1% (261/482)]. Carbapenem-resistant *K. pneumoniae* are often co-resistant with fluoroquinolones, tetracycline derivatives and aminoglycosides, and in this study approximately 50% of such isolates were non-susceptible to amikacin and/or minocycline and 90% were resistant to levofloxacin (data not shown). The World Health Organization performed a review of published studies (1946–2013) and reported that for patients with carbapenem-resistant *K. pneumoniae* infections there was a significant increase in all-cause mortality and 30-day mortality [25]. The agent most active against the carbapenem-resistant *K. pneumoniae* isolates in this study was tigecycline (87.3%, 233/267), followed by amikacin and minocycline [50.9% (136/267) and 48.3% (129/267) respectively].

Acinetobacter baumannii and *P. aeruginosa* are clinically important pathogens and major causes of health-care-associated infections [26, 27]. These pathogens are difficult to treat because, in addition to their intrinsic resistance to many antimicrobials, they have the ability to acquire resistance by a range of mechanisms [26]. In this study, 70.3% of the *A. baumannii* isolates and 26.7% of the *P. aeruginosa* isolates submitted between 2004 and 2015 were MDR. A study of T.E.S.T. data for 2004–2014 reported a global rate of MDR *A. baumannii* of 44.3% and Latin America had one of highest regional rates (Latin America, 70.5%; Middle East, 69.5%; Africa, 61.2%) [28]. Global rates of MDR *A. baumannii* isolates increased over the 2004–2014 time period, however the results of this study show rates of MDR in Latin American were variable between 2004 and 2015. Indeed, *A. baumannii* MDR rates decreased each year from 2011 to 2015. Among *A. baumannii* isolates, tigecycline had the lowest MIC_{90} (2 mg/L) of the antimicrobials on the T.E.S.T. panel. This MIC_{90} was comparable with the SENTRY study which reported an MIC_{90} of 2 mg/L for *Acinetobacter* spp.

collected in Latin America between 2011 and 2014 [18], and lower than the MIC_{90} reported by Jones et al. [1] for *Acinetobacter* spp. collected in Latin America in 2011 (MIC_{90} 4 mg/L). The antimicrobial with the highest rate of susceptibility against *A. baumannii* collected in this study was minocycline (88.3%). Susceptibility to meropenem was 25.7%, which is lower than the Latin American rate reported from the T.E.S.T. study for the 2004–2010 time period (33.9%) [10], and lower than the global rate for the 2004–2013 T.E.S.T. study period (54.8%) [4]. The year on year data from this study between 2006 and 2015 shows a trend of decreasing *A. baumannii* susceptibility to meropenem. *Acinetobacter* spp. strains resistant to carbapenems have increased in prevalence and present a serious treatment challenge to clinicians [27]. As a result older agents, such as colistin, have seen a resurgence in use; however, colistin-resistant and pan-drug-resistant strains have been reported [8, 27, 29] highlighting the importance of judicious antimicrobial use and stewardship.

It is notable, particularly in the case of the Enterobacteriaceae, that from the start of this study until 2009/2010 susceptibility to minocycline decreased and then from 2010/2011 onwards began to increase again so that rates in 2015 are similar to rates from 2004. This has also been reported in both a global analysis of the T.E.S.T. data and also among isolates from skin and soft tissue infections [4, 30]. The reasons for this are unclear although there was variability in center involvement throughout the study and the total number of isolates submitted peaked in 2009 with lower numbers of isolates submitted in subsequent years. To our knowledge this has not be reported by other surveillance studies and warrants further analysis.

Surveillance studies such as T.E.S.T are an invaluable tool for monitoring the rate of resistant pathogen phenotypes and antimicrobial susceptibility among clinical pathogens. However, there are a number of limitations to this study. For example, there was a yearly variation in the number of participating centers with a larger number of centers participating in the earlier years of the study than the latter. The center count was at its highest in 2008 (44 centers) and at its lowest in 2012 (4 centers). Furthermore, the number of isolates submitted varied widely from country to country, with almost half of isolates (48.9%) being submitted by Mexico and Argentina combined.

Conclusions

Antimicrobial resistance continues to be a problem in Latin America with high rates of MRSA, ESBL-producing Enterobacteriaceae and MDR *A. baumannii.* There are limited treatment choices for infections caused by such organisms; however, this study shows that linezolid, vancomycin and tigecycline continue to be active in vitro against Gram-positive organisms such as MRSA. Against resistant Gram-negative organisms, both in Latin America and globally, the rise in antimicrobial resistance is more troubling especially in the context of carbapenem resistance. In vitro, this study reported high percentages of susceptibility to meropenem and tigecycline among Gram-negative organisms (with the exception of *P. aeruginosa*). However, resistant isolates were identified and warrant continued monitoring.

Abbreviations

CLSI: Clinical and Laboratory Standards Institute; ESBL: extended-spectrum β-lactamase; FDA: US Food and Drugs Administration; MIC: minimum inhibitory concentration; MRSA: methicillin-resistant *staphylococcus aureus*; MDR: multidrug-resistant; T.E.S.T.: Tigecycline Evaluation and Surveillance Trial.

Authors' contributions

SV participated in data collection and interpretation as well as drafting and review of the manuscript. MJD was involved in the study design and data interpretation, and drafting and review of the manuscript. Both authors read and approved the final manuscript.

Author details

[1] Complejo Hospitalario Metropolitano, Caja del Seguro Social, Panama City, Panama. [2] Pfizer Inc, Collegeville, PA 19426, USA.

Acknowledgements

The authors would like to thank all T.E.S.T. Latin America investigators and laboratories for their participation in the study and would also like to thank the staff at IHMA for their coordination of T.E.S.T. Pfizer were involved in the study design and the decision to submit this article for publication.

Competing interests

SV has been speaker for Pfizer and MSD. MJD is an employee of Pfizer.

Funding

This study is sponsored by Pfizer. Medical writing support was provided by Wendy Hartley PhD and Helen Linley PhD at Micron Research Ltd., Ely, UK, and was funded by Pfizer. Micron Research Ltd. also provided data management services which were funded by Pfizer.

References

1. Jones RN, Guzman-Blanco M, Gales AC, et al. Susceptibility rates in Latin American nations: report from a regional resistance surveillance program (2011). Braz J Infect Dis. 2013;17:672–81.
2. Guzmán-Blanco M, Labarca JA, Villegas MV, Gotuzzo E, Latin America Working Group on Bacterial Resistance. Extended spectrum β-lactamase producers among nosocomial Enterobacteriaceae in Latin America. Braz J Infect Dis. 2014;18:421–33.
3. Biedenbach DJ, Hoban DJ, Reiszner E, et al. In vitro activity of ceftaroline against *Staphylococcus aureus* isolates collected in 2012 from Latin American countries as part of the AWARE surveillance program. Antimicrob Agents Chemother. 2015;59:7873–7.

4. Hoban DJ, Reinert RR, Bouchillon SK, Dowzicky MJ. Global in vitro activity of tigecycline and comparator agents: Tigecycline Evaluation and Surveillance Trial 2004–2013. Ann Clin Microbiol Antimicrob. 2015;14:27.
5. Nordmann P, Naas T, Poirel L. Global spread of carbapenemase-producing Enterobacteriaceae. Emerg Infect Dis. 2011;17:1791–8.
6. Zúñiga J, Cruz G, Pérez C, LCRSP Microbiology Group, Tarajia M. The combined-disk boronic acid test as an accurate strategy for the detection of KPC carbapenemase in Central America. J Infect Dev Ctries. 2016;10:298–303.
7. Pasteran F, Albornoz E, Faccone D, et al. Emergence of NDM-1-producing *Klebsiella pneumoniae* in Guatemala. J Antimicrob Chemother. 2012;67:1795–7.
8. Rossi F, Girardello R, Cury AP, Gioia TS, Almeida JN Jr, Duarte AJ. Emergence of colistin resistance in the largest university hospital complex of São Paulo, Brazil, over 5 years. Braz J Infect Dis. 2017;21:98–101.
9. Rossi F, García P, Ronzon B, Curcio D, Dowzicky MJ. Rates of antimicrobial resistance in Latin America (2004–2007) and in vitro activity of the glycylcycline tigecycline and of other antibiotics. Braz J Infect Dis. 2008;12:405–15.
10. Fernández-Canigia L, Dowzicky MJ. Susceptibility of important Gram-negative pathogens to tigecycline and other antibiotics in Latin America between 2004 and 2010. Ann Clin Microbiol Antimicrob. 2012;11:29.
11. Garza-González E, Dowzicky MJ. Changes in *Staphylococcus aureus* susceptibility across Latin America between 2004 and 2010. Braz J Infect Dis. 2013;17:13–9.
12. Morfin-Otero R, Noriega ER, Dowzicky MJ. Antimicrobial susceptibility trends among Gram-positive and -negative clinical isolates collected between 2005 and 2012 in Mexico: results from the Tigecycline Evaluation and Surveillance Trial. Ann Clin Microbiol Antimicrob. 2015;14:53.
13. Clinical Laboratory Standards Institute (CLSI). Methods for dilution antimicrobial susceptibility tests for bacteria that grow aerobically; approved standards—10th Edn. CLSI document M07-A10. 10th ed. Wayne: Clinical Laboratory Standards Institute (CLSI); 2015.
14. Clinical and Laboratory Standards Institute (CLSI). Performance standards for antimicrobial susceptibility testing—Twenty-Sixth Informational Supplement. CLSI document M100S. Wayne: Clinical Laboratory Standards Institute (CLSI); 2016.
15. Pfizer Inc. Tygacil®. Tigecycline FDA prescribing information. Collegeville: Pfizer Inc.; 2016.
16. Jones RN. Disk diffusion susceptibility test development for the new glycylcycline, GAR-936. Diagn Microbiol Infect Dis. 1999;35:249–52.
17. Picao R, Sader H, Jones R, Andrade S, Gales A. Analysis of resistance and vancomycin "reverse creep" in Latin American *Staphylococcus aureus*: 10-year report of the SENTRY Antimicrobial Surveillance Program (1997–2006). Clin Microbiol Infect. 2008;14:S173.
18. Sader HS, Castanheira M, Farrell DJ, Flamm RK, Mendes RE, Jones RN. Tigecycline antimicrobial activity tested against clinical bacteria from Latin American medical centres: results from SENTRY Antimicrobial Surveillance Program (2011–2014). Int J Antimicrob Agents. 2016;48:144–50.
19. Malani PN. National burden of invasive methicillin-resistant *Staphylococcus aureus* infection. JAMA. 2014;311:1438–9.
20. Antimicrobial resistance surveillance in Europe. Annual report of the European Antimicrobial Resistance Surveillance Network (EARS-Net) 2014.
21. Hoban D, Biedenbach D, Sahm D, Reiszner E, Iaconis J. Activity of ceftaroline and comparators against pathogens isolated from skin and soft tissue infections in Latin America—results of AWARE surveillance 2012. Braz J Infect Dis. 2015;19:596–603.
22. Kazmierczak KM, Lob SH, Hoban DJ, Hackel MA, Badal RE, Bouchillon SK. Characterization of extended-spectrum beta-lactamases and antimicrobial resistance of *Klebsiella pneumoniae* in intra-abdominal infection isolates in Latin America, 2008–2012. Results of the study for monitoring antimicrobial resistance trends. Diagn Microbiol Infect Dis. 2015;82:209–14.
23. Nordmann P. Carbapenemase-producing Enterobacteriaceae: overview of a major public health challenge. Med Mal Infect. 2014;44:51–6.
24. Tzouvelekis LS, Markogiannakis A, Piperaki E, Souli M, Daikos GL. Treating infections caused by carbapenemase-producing Enterobacteriaceae. Clin Microbiol Infect. 2014;20:862–72.
25. World Health Organization (WHO). Antimicrobial resistance: global report on surveillance. Geneva: WHO; 2014.
26. Zavascki AP, Carvalhaes CG, Picão RC, Gales AC. Multidrug-resistant *Pseudomonas aeruginosa* and *Acinetobacter baumannii*: resistance mechanisms and implications for therapy. Expert Rev Anti Infect Ther. 2010;8:71–93.
27. Gonzalez-Villoria AM, Valverde-Garduno V. Antibiotic-resistant *Acinetobacter baumannii* increasing success remains a challenge as a nosocomial pathogen. J Pathog. 2016;2016:7318075.
28. Giammanco A, Calà C, Fasciana T, Dowzicky MJ. Global assessment of the activity of tigecycline against multidrug-resistant Gram-negative pathogens between 2004 and 2014 as part of the Tigecycline Evaluation and Surveillance Trial. mSphere. 2017;2:e00310–6.
29. Manchanda V, Sanchaita S, Singh N. Multidrug resistant acinetobacter. J Glob Infect Dis. 2010;2:291–304.
30. Tärnberg M, Nilsson LE, Dowzicky MJ. Antimicrobial activity against a global collection of skin and skin structure pathogens: results from the Tigecycline Evaluation and Surveillance Trial (T.E.S.T.), 2010–2014. Int J Infect Dis. 2016;49:141–8.

List of Contributors

Akosua Adom Agyeman and Richard Ofori-Asenso
Research Unit, Health Policy Consult, Weija, Accra, Ghana

Birson Ingti1, Deepjyoti Paul, Anand Prakash Maurya and Amitabha Bhattacharjee
Department of Microbiology, Assam University, Silchar 788011, India

Debadatta Dhar Chanda and Atanu Chakravarty
Department of Microbiology, Silchar Medical College and Hospital, Silchar 788014, India

Debajyoti Bora
Department of Statistics, Dibrugarh University, Dibrugarh, India

Alexandra Brunner, Marta Marschalko and Sarolta Karpati
Department of Dermatology, Venerology and Dermatooncology, Semmelweis University, 41 Mária Street, Budapest, Hungary

Eva Nemes-Nikodem
Department of Laboratory Medicine, Semmelweis University, 41 Mária Street, Budapest, Hungary

Csaba Jeney, Dora Szabo and Eszter Ostorhazi
Institute of Medical Microbiology, Semmelweis University, 4 Nagyvárad Square, Budapest, Hungary.

P. T. Fowoyo
Biosciences Department, Salem University, P.M.B. 1060 Lokoja, Kogi State, Nigeria

S. T. Ogunbanwo
Microbiology Department, University of Ibadan, Ibadan, Oyo State,Nigeria

Rodrigo Trolezi, Juliana Maziero Azanha, Jéssica Luana Chechi, Ramon Kaneno, Ary Fernandes Junior and Sandra de Moraes Gimenes Bosco
Department of Microbiology and Immunology, Institute of Biosciences of Botucatu, UNESP Univ Estadual Paulista, Botucatu, SP 18618-970, Brazil

Natália Rodrigues Paschoal
School of Veterinary Medicine and Animal Science, UNESP Univ Estadual Paulista, Botucatu, SP, Brazil

Marcelo José Dias Silva and Wagner Vilegas
Institute of Chemistry, UNESP Univ Estadual Paulista, Araraquara, SP, Brazil

Viciany Eric Fabris
Department of Pathology, Botucatu School of Medicine, UNESP Univ Estadual Paulista, Botucatu, SP, Brazil

Mustafa Kolukirik
ENGY Environmental and Energy Technologies Biotechnology Research and Development Limited Company, Istanbul, Turkey

Mesut Yılmaz
Infectious Diseases and Clinical Microbiology, Istanbul Medipol University, Istanbul, Turkey

Orhan Ince and Canan Ketre
Istanbul Technical University, Istanbul, Turkey

Ayşe Istanbullu Tosun
Microbiology, Istanbul Medipol University, Istanbul, Turkey

Bahar K. Ince
Bogazici University, Istanbul, Turkey

Liangfei Xu, Xiaoxi Sun and Xiaoling Ma
Department of Laboratory Medicine, Anhui Provincial Hospital, Anhui Medical University, Hefei 230001, Anhui, China

Shiva Mirkalantari, Gholam Reza Irajian and Nour Amirmozafari
Microbiology Department, Faculty of Medicine, Iran University of Medical Sciences, Tehran, Iran

Amir-Hassan Zarnani
Dept. of Immunology, School of Public Health, Tehran University of Medical Sciences, Tehran, Iran

Immunology Research Center, Iran University of Medical Sciences, Tehran, Iran.

Mahboobeh Nazari
Monoclonal Antibody Reaserch Center, Avicenna Research Institute, ACECR, Tehran, Iran

Clotilde Silvia Cabassi, Andrea Sala, Davide Santospirito and Simone Taddei
Department of Veterinary Science, University of Parma, Via del Taglio 10, 43126 Parma, Italy

Giovanni Loris Alborali
Istituto Zooprofilattico Sperimentale della Lombardia e dell'Emilia Romagna, Via Bianchi 7/9, 25124 Brescia, Italy

Edoardo Carretto
Arcispedale S. Maria Nuova, Viale Risorgimento 80, 42123 Reggio Emilia, Italy

Giovanni Ghibaudo
Clinica Veterinaria Malpensa, Via Marconi 27, 21017 Samarate, VA, Italy

Geoffrey Omuse and Gunturu Revathi
Department of Pathology, Aga Khan University Hospital Nairobi, Nairobi, Kenya

Kristien Nel Van Zyl, Kim Hoek and Andrew Whitelaw
Division of Medical Microbiology, Department of Pathology, Stellenbosch University, Western Cape, South Africa

Shima Abdulgader
Division of Medical Microbiology, Department of Pathology, Faculty of Health Sciences, University of Cape Town, South Africa, Cape Town, South Africa

Samuel Kariuki
Center of Microbiology Research, Kenya Medical Research Institute, Nairobi, Kenya

Dietmar Enko, Gabriele Halwachs-Baumann, Robert Stolba and Gernot Kriegshäuser
Institute of Clinical Chemistry and Laboratory Medicine, General Hospital Steyr, Sierningerstraße 170, 4400 Steyr, Austria

Ortrun Rössler
Institute of Pathology, General Hospital Steyr, Sierningerstraße 170, 4400 Steyr, Austria

Ankit Belbase, Krishus Nepal, Bibhusan Neupane and Rikesh Baidhya
Department of Microbiology, GoldenGate International College, Battisputali, Kathmandu, Nepal

Narayan Dutt Pant
Department of Microbiology, Grande International Hospital, Dhapasi, Kathmandu, Nepal

Reena Baidya
Department of Pathology, B&B Hospital, Gwarko, Lalitpur, Nepal

Binod Lekhak
Central Department of Microbiology, Tribhuvan University, Kirtipur, Nepal

Tamer Akel
Department of Internal Medicine, Staten Island University Hospital, 475 Seaview Avenue, Staten Island, NY 10305, USA

Neville Mobarakai
Department of Infectious Diseases, Staten Island University Hospital, 475 Seaview Avenue, Staten Island, NY 10305, USA

Fatma Elzahraa Akram, Khaled Abou-Aisha and Mohamed El-Azizi
Department of Microbiology, Immunology, and Biotechnology, German University in Cairo, GUC, New Cairo City, Cairo, Egypt

Tarek El-Tayeb
National Institute for Laser Enhanced Sciences, Cairo University, Cairo, Egypt

Kimberley Lau
McMaster University, Hamilton, ON, Canada

Robert Slinger, Michael Slinger, Ioana Moldovan and Francis Chan
Department of Laboratory Medicine and Pathology, Children's Hospital of Eastern Ontario, University of Ottawa, 401 Smyth Rd, Ottawa, ON K1H 8L1, Canada

Tsedale Semunigus
Amhara Regional Health Bureau, North Shewa Zonal Health Bureau, Debre Birhan, Ethiopia

Belay Tessema, Setegn Eshetie and Feleke Moges
School of Biomedical and Laboratory Sciences, Department of Medical Microbiology, University of Gondar, Gonder, Ethiopia

A. Różańska, J. Wójkowska-Mach and M. Bulanda
Chair of Microbiology, Jagiellonian University Medical College, 18 Czysta Street, 31-121 Krakow, Poland
Institute of Nature Conservation Polish Academy of Sciences, Krakow, Poland

M. Borszewska-Kornacka
Clinic of Neonatology and Intensive Neonatal Care, Warsaw Medical University, Warsaw, Poland

E. Gulczyńska and M. Nowiczewski
Clinic of Neonatology, Polish Mother's Memorial Hospital-Research Institute, Lodz, Poland

E. Helwich
Clinic of Neonatology and Intensive Neonatal Care, Institute of Mother and Child, Warsaw, Poland

A. Kordek
Department of Neonatal Diseases, Pomeranian Medical University, Szczecin, Poland.

D. Pawlik
Clinic of Neonatology, Jagiellonian University Medical College, Krakow, Poland

Kaisheng Lai, Yanning Ma, Ling Guo, Jingna An, Liyan Ye and Jiyong Yang
Kaisheng Lai and Yanning Ma contributed equally to this work Department of Microbiology, Chinese PLA General Hospital, 301 Hospital, 28# Fuxing Road, Beijing 100853, China

Jian Wang, Yaping Pan, Jilu Shen and Yuanhong Xu
Department of Clinical Laboratory, The First Affiliated Hospital of Anhui Medical University, Anhui Medical University, Hefei 230022, Anhui, China

Makoto Saito, Hideki Hashimoto, Takumitsu Suzuki, Daisuke Jubishi1, and Hiroshi Yotsuyanagi
Department of Infectious Diseases, University of Tokyo Hospital, 7-3-1 Hongo, Bunkyo-ku, Tokyo 113-8655, Japan

Shuji Hatakeyama
Department of Infectious Diseases, University of Tokyo Hospital, 7-3-1 Hongo, Bunkyo-ku, Tokyo 113-8655, Japan
Division of General Internal Medicine, Division of Infectious Diseases, Jichi Medical University Hospital, 3311-1 Yakushiji, Shimotsuke-shi, Tochigi 329-0498, Japan

Makoto Kaneko and Yukio Kume
Department of Clinical Laboratory, University of Tokyo Hospital, 7-3-1 Hongo, Bunkyo-ku, Tokyo 113-8655, Japan

Takehito Yamamoto and Hiroshi Suzuki
Department of Pharmacy, University of Tokyo Hospital, 7-3-1 Hongo, Bunkyo-ku, Tokyo 113-8655, Japan

Doaa Mohammad Ghaith and Mai Mahmoud Zafer
Department of Clinical and Chemical Pathology, Faculty of Medicine, Cairo University, Cairo, Egypt.
Department of Microbiology and Immunology, Faculty of Pharmacy, Ahram Canadian University, Giza, Egypt.

Mohamed Hamed Al-Agamy
Department of Pharmaceutics, College of Pharmacy, King Saud University, Saudi Arabia
Department of Microbiology and Immunology, Faculty of Pharmacy, Al-Azhar University, Cairo, Egypt

Essam J. Alyamani and Rayan Y. Booq
National Center for Biotechnology, King Abdulaziz City for Science and Technology, Riyadh, Saudi Arabia.

Omar Almoazzamy
Department of Microbiology, Faculty of Science, Zagazig University, Zagazig, Egypt

Ekaterina A. Kletsova and Bettina C. Fries
Department of Medicine, Division of Infectious Diseases, Stony Brook University, Stony Brook, USA

Luis A. Marcos
Department of Medicine, Division of Infectious Diseases, Stony Brook University, Stony Brook, USA.

Global Health Institute, Stony Brook University, Stony Brook, NY, USA

Eric D. Spitzer
Department of Pathology, Stony Brook University, Stony Brook, NY, USA

Ling Qing, Hai-Yan Li and Hai-Hong Jiang
Departments of Reproductive Medicine, Urology, and Nursing, The First Affiliated Hospital of Wenzhou Medical University, #2-4P07 Nan Bai Xiang, Ouhai, Wenzhou 325000, Zhejiang, China

Qi-Xiang Song
Department of Urology, Changhai Hospital, Shanghai 200433, China

Jian-Li Feng
Department of Urology, The 324 Hospital of PLA, Chongqing 400020, China

Guiming Liu
Department of Surgery/Urology, Metro Health Medical Center, Case Western Reserve University, Cleveland, OH 44109, USA

B. J. Chen, X. Y. Xie, L. J. Ni, X. L. Dai, X. Q. Wu, H. Y. Li and S. Y. Huang
Department of Laboratory, Guangdong Provincial Key Laboratory of Malignant Tumor Epigenetics and Gene Regulation, Sun Yat-Sen Memorial Hospital, Sun Yat-Sen University, Guangzhou 510120, China

Y. Lu
Cross Infection Control Office, Sun Yat-Sen Memorial Hospital, Sun Yat-Sen University, Guangzhou 510120, Guangdong, China

Y. D. Yao
Breast Tumor Center, Sun Yat-Sen Memorial Hospital, Sun Yat-Sen University, Guangzhou 510120, Guangdong, China

Silvio Vega
Complejo Hospitalario Metropolitano, Caja del Seguro Social, Panama City,Panama

Michael J. Dowzicky
Pfizer Inc, Collegeville, PA 19426, USA

Index

A

Acute Pharyngitis, 46, 50-51

Agnps, 105-115

Amoxicillin, 32-35, 37, 99, 105-110, 113, 115, 117, 165, 199-202, 205-208

Anti-tb Treatment, 128

Antibiotic Resistance, 25, 30-33, 35, 37-38, 46, 70-71, 93, 110, 116-117, 139, 171, 195

Antimicrobial Peptide, 70-71, 75, 78

Antimicrobial Susceptibility, 18-19, 25, 27, 30-32, 38, 77, 80, 86-87, 93, 95-97, 116, 141-143, 145, 165-166, 170, 186, 195-197, 202, 208, 210-211

Atovaquone, 100, 103, 172-178

Azithromycin-resistance, 26, 30

B

B. Microti, 98-100, 173

Babesia, 98-104, 172, 177

Bacteraemia, 61-63, 146-147, 154, 158, 194-195

Biofilm, 93-97, 113, 116

Blaoxa-23-like, 165-166

Bloodstream Infections, 59, 61-63, 132-134, 136, 139, 146-147, 154-155

Bmi, 124-126, 128-130

Brucella, 64-69

Brucellosis, 64, 66-69

C

Campylobacter, 48, 92, 120-121

Cephalosporins, 18, 20-21, 23-24, 27, 30, 71-72, 165

Checkerboard Assay, 106-107, 111-113, 115

Chlamydia Trachomatis, 26, 179, 184-185

Clarithromycin, 16, 105-110, 112-115, 134, 197, 200

Coagulase-negative Staphylococci, 32-34, 37-38, 113

Cons, 32-35, 37, 150, 154-155

Crkp, 52-60, 62

Cskp, 52-60

Cystic Fibrosis, 70-72, 74, 77-78

D

Daptomycin, 156-163

Defined Daily Dose, 133-136, 139

Dha, 18-25

Dic, 98, 100-101, 103, 175

Dna, 18, 25, 32-34, 37, 46, 48-51, 73, 80-81, 86, 120, 123, 143-144, 166, 179-180, 183-185, 188, 193, 195

Dot, 3-4, 7, 12, 15, 132-139

E

E. Coli, 18-24, 65-66, 68, 75, 77-78, 118-119, 121, 123, 142, 196, 202-204, 209

Efa1/lifa, 118-123

Ehec, 118-123

Elisa, 57, 64-69

Enterobacteriaceae, 19, 24-25, 53, 61, 134, 141-142, 144-145, 155, 170, 196-197, 209-211

Epec, 118-123

G

Gas, 46-50

Gram-negative, 25, 60, 71, 78, 115, 134, 138, 141, 145, 153, 196-197, 202-205, 208, 210-211

Gram-positive, 71, 115, 134-135, 138, 153, 156-157, 163, 187, 196-200, 208, 210-211

H

H. Pylori, 88-91

Hiv, 2-3, 5-6, 15, 100, 103, 124-131, 172, 174

Homeless Individuals, 124-130

Human Babesiosis, 98, 100, 102-104, 177-178

I

Immunoassay, 51, 66, 88-91

Imp, 19-20, 22, 53, 141-145

Inducible Clindamycin Resistance, 85, 93-97, 187

L

Lc-bsi, 133-135, 137-138

Linezolid, 1-17, 82, 85, 93-96, 105-110, 113-116, 148, 155, 196, 199-202, 208-210

Lot, 106, 133, 139, 193

M

Mbc, 73, 75, 77, 107-108, 115

Mdr/xdr-tb, 2, 13

Meca Gene, 32-33, 37-38, 79, 96, 187-188, 190

Methicillin Resistance, 32, 34-35, 37-38, 79, 86, 93-94, 96, 116, 195

Mhb, 107-108, 115

Mlst, 79-84, 86, 106-107, 115, 141, 143, 164-166, 170, 188, 190, 192-193
Monotherapy, 30, 146-147, 151, 153-155
Mrsa, 38, 79-80, 82-87, 93, 95-97, 105-117, 148, 150, 154, 186-188, 190-199, 208, 210
Mssa, 79-80, 82-86, 93, 95-96, 116, 187, 193
Mycoplasma Genitalium, 26, 179, 185
Myelosuppression, 1, 3, 7-9, 11, 13-15

N
Nasal Carriage, 186-187, 189-195
Neisseria Gonorrhoeae, 26-27, 30-31, 179, 184
Nicus, 132, 135, 137-138

O
Oomycete, 39, 45

P
Polymyxins, 60, 72, 151, 153, 155, 164
Prothrombin Time, 156-160, 162-163
Pseudomonas Aeruginosa, 25, 49, 70-72, 75, 77-78, 116-117, 120, 141, 144-145, 165, 196-197, 206-207, 211
Pulmonary Tb, 3, 124-125
Pythiosis, 39-45
Pythium Insidiosum, 39, 41-42, 44-45

Q
Qpcr, 46-50, 118-123

R
Rna, 20, 23, 179-181, 183

S
S. Aureus, 33, 79-82, 84, 86-87, 93-97, 106, 110, 112, 114, 186-194, 196-199, 208
Sat, 179-180, 183-184
Scanning Electron Microscopy, 40, 42, 70, 73, 75
Sperm Dna, 179-180, 183-185
Staphylococcus Aureus, 34, 38, 49, 51, 79, 83, 86-87, 93, 97, 105-106, 115-117, 120, 140, 150, 154-155, 157, 165, 186-187, 191, 193-196, 200, 210-211

T
Tigecycline, 19, 21, 60, 63, 82, 85, 146-155, 166, 196-197, 199-211
Tuberculosis, 1-3, 15-17, 124-125, 128-131, 184

V
Vancomycin, 82, 85, 93-97, 105-110, 113-115, 134, 140, 148-150, 154-155, 157, 186-187, 196, 198-202, 208-209, 211
Virb12, 64-69

W
Warfarin, 156-163

X
Xdr, 1-3, 5-6, 10-13, 15-17, 71-72, 75, 77, 147-148, 150, 154, 164, 166

www.ingramcontent.com/pod-product-compliance
Lightning Source LLC
Chambersburg PA
CBHW082044190326
41458CB00010B/3457
9781632427021